Cerebrospinal Fluid in Neurology and Psychiatry

Cerebrospinal Fluid in Neurology and Psychiatry

Edited by

H. McConnell MD, FRCPC
Departments of Physiology and Psychological Medicine
University of Otago Medical School
Dunedin, New Zealand.

Currently at
Allegheny Neuropsychiatric Institute
Medical College of Pennsylvania
Departments of Neurology and Psychiatry
Allegheny Campus, Oakdale
Pennsylvania, USA.

and

J. Bianchine MD, PhD
Department of Pharmacology
Ohio State University
College of Medicine and Adria Laboratories
Columbus, Ohio, USA.

SPRINGER-SCIENCE+BUSINESS MEDIA, B.V.

First edition 1994

© 1994 Springer Science+Business Media Dordrecht
Originally published by Chapman & Hall in 1994
Softcover reprint of the hardcover 1st edition 1994

Typeset in 10/11.5pt Times by Farrand Press, London, UK

ISBN 978-0-412-53570-3   ISBN 978-1-4899-3372-0 (eBook)
DOI 10.1007/978-1-4899-3372-0

A catalogue record for this book is available from the British Library

∞ Printed on permanent acid-free text paper, manufactured in accordance with ANSI/NISO Z 39.48-1992 and ANSI/NISO Z39.48-1984 (Permanence of Paper).

This book is dedicated to my father,
Dr Ross S. McConnell,
and to my late brother, Tommy.

Contents

The authorship of any section within a chapter is that of the writer(s) given immediately below the chapter title, except where different authors' names are noted below any one section.

Contributors

J. Bianchine, MD, PhD, Adria Laboratories, P.O. Box 16529, Columbus, Ohio 43216-6529, USA.

J. Brillman, MD, Chairman, Department of Neurology, Medical College of Pennsylvania, Allegheny Campus, Allegheny General Hospital, 320, North Avenue, Pittsburg, Pennsylvania 15212, USA.

H. McConnell, MD, FRCPC, Present Address: Allegheny Neuropsychiatric Institute, Medical College of Pennsylvania, Allegheny Campus, 7777 Steubenville Pike, Oakdale, Pennsylvania 15071, USA.

H. Nukada, MBChB, MD, Neurology Department, University of Otago, Dunedin, New Zealand.

D. Rillstone, MBChB, University of Otago Medical School, Dunedin, New Zealand. Present address: Department of Medicine, Kew Hospital, Private Bag, Invercargill, New Zealand.

U. Roelcke, MD, Department of Neurology, University of Heidelberg, Heidelberg, Germany. Present address: Paul Scherrer Institute, Med, PET, CH-5232, Villigen, Switzerland.

T. Scott, MD, Department of Neurology, Medical College of Pennsylvania, Allegheny Campus, Allegheny General Hospital, 320 E. North Avenue, Pittsburgh, Pennsylvania 15212, USA.

A. Wilder-Smith, MBChB, Department of Paediatrics, University of Berne, Berne, Switzerland. Present address: Roggernweg 8, 3646 Einigen, Switzerland.

E. Wilder-Smith, MD, Neurology Department, University of Berne, Berne, Switzerland. Present address: Roggernweg 8, 3646 Einigen, Switzerland.

Preface

Scientists have speculated as to the nature of cerebrospinal fluid (CSF) – "the third circulation" or "vital spirit" for centuries. Just what is this mysterious bathing solution of the central nervous system? Is it a vehicle of transport for an "animal spirit" directing all our activities, as thought by Galen (Singer, 1956) or but a "modified tap water" (Halliburton, 1917)? With the advent of lumbar puncture, cerebrospinal fluid has become a readily available and important means of studying disease affecting the nervous system. In recent years, many sophisticated tools including computer guided gas chromatography/mass spectrometry and high performance liquid chromatography have made it possible to identify and quantify many constituents of this fluid.

The CSF has an enormous, though largely "untapped", potential in aiding diagnosis and evaluating treatment of many neurological, psychiatric and systemic disorders. As the ependyma is only a diffusional barrier between the CSF and extracellular fluid of the brain for many compounds, changes in the concentration of these compounds in the CSF may reflect disease processes in the brain.

It is 100 years since Quincke first introduced lumbar puncture as a diagnostic tool, measuring the CSF for pressure, glucose, protein and cell count. A century later, many clinicians stop at measuring just these same parameters. Why, after a century of lumbar puncture, has the analysis of CSF lagged so far behind that of other body fluids, particularly blood and urine? Are there other parameters that can be looked at, and what do they tell us?

In recent years there have been several excellent reviews of the experimental, physiologic and neurologic aspects of CSF, including those of Wood (1980, 1983), Davson, Welch and Segal (1987), Herndon and Brumback (1989), Rosenberg (1990), and, of course, Fishman's (1992) recently revised classic. In the ensuing chapters we will take a somewhat different perspective on the physiology and neurology of CSF, focusing on some of the neurochemical aspects of the fluid as well as some of the new potential diagnostic markers. Within the last few years there have been promising markers proposed for paraneoplastic syndromes, Alzheimer's disease, Creutzfeldt-Jacob disease, the lysosomal storage diseases, cerebral amyloid angiopathy, HIV dementia, among others. We will also explore some of the exciting advances in the neurochemistry of psychiatric illness where CSF is a promising tool. Although the only clear indication to date for lumbar puncture in psychiatry is to exclude neurological illness, CSF studies have shed some light on the neurochemistry of schizophrenia, affective illness, anorexia nervosa and other psychiatric illnesses. With the introduction of new technologies in the neurosciences, the overlap between neurology and psychiatry is becoming more important and the general psychiatrist and neuropsychiatrist must be aware of the neurochemical advances in both fields. An extensive bibliography is provided to guide the reader to the most pertinent original studies, review articles, and references of historical note in the field, covering both the neurological and psychiatric aspects.

This book is not intended to be an exhaustive review of the ever-growing literature of CSF studies, but rather a guide to some of the practical and theoretical aspects of CSF for the clinician and clinically-oriented neuro-scientist and a look at the exciting recent developments of the diagnostic and therapeutic potential of CSF.

H. McConnell, MD
J. Bianchine, MD, PhD

Acknowledgements

We gratefully thank, first of all, Drs H. Nukada, E. Wilder-Smith, A. Wilder-Smith, J. Brillman, T. Scott, U. Roelcke and D. Rillstone for their valuable contributions. We would also like to thank the many people who have reviewed various sections of the book and provided valuable suggestions, in particularly Professors J. Hubbard, A. McKnight, S. Romans, T. Silverstone, M. Pollock and J. Brillman and Drs R. Nada Raja, B. Spittle, S. Ng, R. Miller, E. Teghavi and I. Jajour.

We would also like to acknowledge the support of Val Dempster, M. McConnell, C.Z., L.M., A. O'Brien, of Drs T. Heads, H. Campbell, P. Taylor and P. Cheung, the technical assistance of M. Bevin, and particularly of Susan Wolkow, and the support of the Dawn Short Trust of the New Zealand Branch of the Royal Australia/New Zealand College of Psychiatrists. We thank Christine Cooper, Prescilla North and Judy Swaine for their expert secretarial assistance in preparing this book and the wonderful staffs of the Otago, Allegheny General, and Ohio State University Medical Libraries. We must also thank the staff of Farrand Press, who have prepared manuscript for Chapman & Hall, for their patience and expert editorial assistance.

Glossary

AAN	American Academy of Neurology	HPA	hypothalamic-pituitary-adrenal axis
ACE	Angiotensin converting enzyme		
ACP	American College of Physicans	HSV	herpes simplex virus
ACTH	adrenocorticotrophin	5-HIAA	5-hydroxyindoleacetic acid
ACh	Acetylcholine	5-HT	5-hydroxytryptamine (serotonin)
AChE	acetylcholinesterase	5-HTP	5-hydroxytryptophan
ADD	attention deficit disorder	HVA	homovanillic acid
ADH	antidiuretic hormone	ICP	intracranial pressure
AIDS	acquired immunodeficiency syndrome	ISF	interstitial fluid
		LCSF	lumbar cerebrospinal fluid
ALS	amyotrophic lateral sclerosis	LCM	lymphocytic choriomeningitis
ARD	AIDS-related dementia	LDH	lactate dehydrogenase
AVP	arginine vasopressin	LP	lumbar puncture
B.b.	*Borrelia burgdorferi*	MAOI	monoamine oxidase inhibitor
B.B.B.	blood brain barrier	MBP	myelin basic protein
cAMP	adenosine-3,5-cyclic monophosphate	MHPG	methoxy hydroxy phenyl glycol
		MRI	magnetic resonance imaging
CCK	cholecystokinin	MSH	melanocyte stimulating hormone
CEA	carcinoembryonic antigen	NE	norepinephrine
cGMP	guanosine-3,5-cyclic monophosphate	NMDA	N-methyl-D-aspartate
		NNA	neuronal nuclear antibodies
CIDP	chronic inflammatory polyradiculoneuropathy	NPH	normal pressure hydrocephalus
		NPY	neuropeptide Y
CIE	counter immunoelectrophoresis	NT	neurotensin
CJD	Creutzfeld-Jacob disease	OSAI	organism-specific antibody index
CMV	cytomegalovirus	PCA	Purkinje cell antibody
CPK	creatinine phosphokinase	PCR	polymerase chain reaction
CRH	corticotrophin releasing hormone	PET	positron emission tomography
CSF	cerebrospinal fluid	PG	prostaglandins
CT	computerised tomography	PLPH	post-lumbar puncture headache
DA	dopamine	PMN	polymorphonuclear leucocyte
DBH	dopamine-β-hydroxylase	PTC	pseudotumour cerebri
DBI	diazepam-binding inhibitor	REM	rapid eye movement
DOPA	dihydroxyphenylalanine	SAH	subarachnoid haemorrhage
DOPAC	3,4-dihydroxyphenylacetic acid	SIE	stroke in evolution
ECF	extracellular fluid	SLE	systemic lupus erythematosus
ECM	erythema chronicum migrans	SLI	somatostatin-like immunoreactivity
EEG	electroencephalogram	SSPE	subacute sclerosing panencephalitis
ELI	enkephalin-like immunoreactivity	TCA	tricyclic antidepressant
FTA-ABS	fluorescent treponal antibody absorption test	TD	tardive dyskinesia
		TIA	transient ischaemic attack
GABA	gamma-aminobutyric acid	TRH	thyrotrophin releasing hormone
GFAP	glial fibrillary acidic protein	VCSF	ventricular cerebrospinal fluid
GH	growth hormone	VDRL	Venereal Disease Research Laboratory
GTS	Gilles de la Tourette syndrome		
HCG	human chorionic gonadotrophin	VIP	vasoactive inhibitory polypeptide
HIV	human immunodeficiency virus	VMA	vanillylmandelic acid

1. Historical Perspective

The roots of our current knowledge of CSF date back to the times of the Ancients. The existence of the meninges has been known for over 5000 years and that of the ventricular system for over 3000 years (Woollam, 1957). For all these years, with the exception of the last century, these two structures have been implicated as centres of human activity and thought (Woollam, 1957).

It was the Edwin Smith Surgical Papyrus that provided the first description of a fluid contained within the brain (Breasted, 1930). This document was written around 1700 BC, but its contents probably date to the pyramid age 3000-2500 BC. It describes several cases of head injuries which refer to the cerebral convolutions, the meninges, and to the cerebrospinal fluid. It is in this document that the word "brain" appears for the first time implying "marrow of the skull" (Clarke and O'Malley, 1968; Breasted, 1930).

Hippocrates, in the 4th century BC, described a fluid drawn from the body and collecting in the brain in his early studies of hydrocephalus. However, he considered this fluid only to be pathological in origin and did not recognise it as a normal constituent of the brain. Hippocrates spoke of the brain as a gland attracting water from the body (Woollam, 1957). He considered that "abnormal moistness" of the brain caused it to move and that "madness comes from its moistness".

Aristotle spoke of two meningeal membranes, pia mater and dura mater, and also of the ventricles (Clarke and O'Malley, 1968). Contrary to the teachings of Hippocrates and Plato, he gave supremacy to the heart as the centre of thought and intelligence claiming the role of the brain to be that of tempering the heat of the heart. It was Herophilus in the 3rd century BC who first described the choroid plexus and the fourth ventricle and also restored the brain as being the seat of thought and intelligence, speaking of the ventricles as being the seat of the soul. Although he carried out over 600 human dissections, it is not known whether he was aware of the presence of CSF, as his writings have unfortunately not survived (Clarke and O'Malley, 1968; Millen and Woollam, 1962; Levinson, 1923).

In the 2nd century AD Galen presented the "pneumatic" theory of the ventricles and CSF which persisted for well over 1000 years (Torack, 1982). He believed that the "pneumas" (spirits) transported by this fluid provided energy and motion for the entire body. Passage of these "pneumas" into the ventricular system was achieved by air coming through the cribriform plate and rete mirabile – a structure present in oxen and analogous to the circle of Willis in humans. The "pneuma zotican" (vital spirit) derived from the heart where it was formed from the external pneuma mixing with the "pneuma physicon" (natural spirit). In the ventricles it was transformed into the "pneuma psychicon" (animal spirit) which traversed the nerves "as sunshine passes through air or water" and thus, moved the muscles (Woollam, 1957). This was accomplished "by boiling" and "sieving" in the rete mirabile and further refined in the anterior ventricles. The ventricles were also seen as serving an excretory function for these "pneumas".

Galen believed the CSF was formed by the choroid plexus in the lateral ventricles and then flowed into the third and fourth ventricles. These liquid excretions were thought to pass from the fourth ventricle through either the cribriform plate, being discharged as nasal secretions, or through tubes originating near the infundibulum leading to the palate (Torack, 1982). Galen also described an opening of the fourth ventricle that appears to describe the foramen of Magendie some 1600 years before Magendie (Torack, 1982). Galen's "pneumatic" theory was probably based on Herophilus' original description of the ventricles and a similar theory of Erasistratus (Millen and Woollam, 1962). The strong theological influence of the time and the rise of the Christian Church may account for the wide acceptance of Galen's ideas, which remained largely unchallenged until the 16th century. His postulated three "pneumas" may be seen as analogous to the concept of the Trinity in Christianity. His pneumatic theory may be viewed as being monotheistic and consistent with the idea of the body as an instrument of the soul and thus acceptable to Christians, Jews and Arabs (Woollam, 1957).

In medieval manuscripts Galen's ideas were rather amplified to give specific mental functions to the ventricles – ascribing to the anterior (lateral) ventricles the powers of the imagination, cognition being assigned to the middle (third) ventricle and memory to the posterior (fourth) ventricle (Woollam, 1957).

In the 16th century the anatomy of the ventricular system became better elucidated, first with Leonardo Da Vinci producing a wax cast of the human ventricular system in 1504 (although his findings were not well known until the 19th century) and then with Vesalius giving the first accurate and detailed account of the ventricular system, showing that the rete mirabile did not exist in humans (Clarke and O'Malley, 1968). Varolius (1543-1575), who had described the pons, insisted that it was fluid and not pneumas that filled the ventricles (Levinson, 1923).

The 17th century was marked by the works of Thomas Willis, who showed that CSF was not secreted into the palate, and of Richard Lower who demonstrated nasal secretions to be a consequence of respiratory and not of CNS function (Torack, 1982). The anatomy and physiology of the ventricular system were further elucidated in the early 18th century by von

Haller, a Swiss anatomist and botanist, who first defined the CSF pathways and described the lateral foramina 50 years before Luschka. This work paved the way for the first truly descriptive treatise on CSF, attributed to Cotugno, in 1764. Cotugno pointed out that earlier anatomists had not appreciated the presence of this fluid because it was lost in the process of decapitation prior to dissection, pointing out that CSF was a normal body fluid rather than a pathological phenomenon. The importance of his work was not realised until much later, being embedded within a longer treatise on sciatica (Peltier, 1988).

Chemical and physiological studies of CSF were thus not begun until Magendie in 1825. It was Magendie who first termed this fluid "liquid cephalo-spinal" (cerebrospinal fluid) and first described the buoyancy and protective function of CSF (Millen and Woollam, 1962). Magendie was an extremely controversial figure in his day and his debates with Sir Charles Bell over the function of the spinal cord roots are well known (Flourens, 1858). It was actually during one of Magendie's dissections of nerve roots that he noted a clear fluid around the roots and thus described CSF to be a physiological fluid. His initial papers on cerebrospinal fluid in 1825 and 1827 met with a scathing editorial in the *Lancet* (*Lancet*, IX pp. 71-2, 1828) directed very personally towards him, speaking of his "carelessness" and "ill founded self confidence".

Even today Magendie remains a controversial figure in the history of physiology. Torack (1982) points out that Magendie's concept of CSF circulation was indeed far less accurate than that of either Cotugno or von Haller and that he perpetuated many misconceptions. Magendie claimed that the CSF was formed at the surface of the brain, secreted by the arachnoid and flowed into the ventricles via the foramen of Magendie, the complete reversal of the more correct description of CSF circulation previously described by von Haller. While he gave full credit to Cotugno for his original description of CSF, he was particularly disdainful of his colleagues who subscribed to vitalism and dissected cadavers without doing animal experiments. He was critical of both the eminent von Haller and of Bichat (Torack, 1982). The ideas of the anatomist Bichat were held in high esteem at the end of the 19th century; his concept of the spinal cord being surrounded by an enclosed sac analogous to the pericardial sac was well accepted (Bichat and Traite, 1802) and probably contributed to the difficulty that Magendie faced in having his "rediscovery" of the cerebrospinal fluid accepted in the 19th century.

These problems are discussed further by van den Doel (1987), who noted that in various stories by Balzac, as well as in several medical text books published well into the second half of the 19th century, there was general acceptance of the diagnosis of "serous apoplexy". This was felt to be a diagnosis in most cases based on the finding of quantities of cerebrospinal fluid at autopsies, considered to be a symptom of disease.

It was thus not until the latter part of the 19th century that CSF became generally accepted as a normal physiological fluid. The first generally accepted anatomical and physiological treatise on cerebrospinal fluid, which validated Magendie's views and restored some of the previous accurate observations of von Haller and of Cotugno, was that of Key and Retzius in 1876.

In 1885, Corning injected cocaine between the spinous processes of T11-12 in a man with spinal weakness, making his legs "sleepy" and thus set the stage for spinal anaesthesia, and in 1889, Wynter treated a case of tuberculous meningitis with lumbar CSF drainage (Levinson, 1923).

In 1891, Quinke first introduced lumbar puncture as a diagnostic tool, analysing the fluid for protein, sugar, pressure and cell count. He paved the way for the use of lumbar puncture for intrathecal therapy which was first employed in 1899 by Kocher for a case of tetanus (Fishman, 1980).

The early part of this century was marked by Goldmann's (1913) introduction of the concept of the blood-brain barrier and by Cushing's and Weed's works on the role of the choroid plexus and CSF circulation (Walker, 1971). Walter Dandy introduced pneumoencephalography in 1919. In 1942, Kabat first used electrophoresis to show that the CSF had a different protein make-up than serum, isolating prealbumin (protein "X") and subsequently performing quantitative immunochemical precipitation of albumin and IgG. This heralded the beginning of routine CSF protein analysis (Thompson, 1988).

The last 30 years have seen the development of many important tools in the study of CSF, including isovolumetric pressure transducers, electron microscopy, radioisotope tagging, ventriculo-cisternal perfusion methods, microsurgical methods, improved analytical methods such as gas chromatography, high performance liquid chromatography, mass spectrometry, and the imaging procedures myelography, computerised tomography, and magnetic resonance imaging. These advances have led to a better understanding of CSF absorption, secretion, and membrane transport principles and have further elucidated the chemical composition and ultrastructural relationships of the CSF.

Clarke and O'Malley (1968), Millen and Woollam (1962), Fishman (1992), Woollam (1957), Torack (1982), Herndon (1989a), and Sakula (1991) have all provided excellent reviews of the history of CSF and Thompson (1988) has reviewed historical aspects of the CSF proteins.

2. Cerebrospinal Fluid Dynamics

Functions of CSF

A large variety of functions have been attributed to the cerebrospinal fluid in the past. However, there are currently only four principal roles attributed to the CSF:
1   mechanical protection and support,
2   intracerebral transport,
3   provision of an internal milieu, and
4   a lymphatic role.

Mechanical protection and support

The CSF provides mechanical protection from trauma for the delicate brain, nerve roots, and blood vessels by supplying buoyancy. The buoyancy effect is due to the difference in the specific gravities of the CSF (1.007) and brain (1.040). A brain weighing 1500 g in air will weigh only 50 g when immersed in CSF because of this buoyancy effect (Carpenter, 1978). The relative weight of the spinal cord is similarly decreased by as much as 96.38% (Szukiewicz and Jaskolska, 1982). In this way the buoyancy of the CSF acts as an important protective device against stretching and compressive forces.

Intracerebral transport

Another major function of CSF is to provide intracerebral transport and homeostasis for the extracellular fluid (ECF) compartment of the brain. As the CSF oscillates and flows over the ventricular and pial surfaces, it sweeps up compounds originating in adjacent brain tissues and carries them along its path. This exposes distant parts of the CNS to these compounds.

Evidence for a physiological role of neurotransmitter substances in the CSF comes from studies of the predictable effects of intraventricular administration of biogenic amines and endorphins, and from the prompt and dramatic increase in CSF beta-endorphin levels after thalamic and periaqueductal gray stimulation in humans (Milhorat and Hammock, 1983; Hosobuchi and Bloom, 1983)

Hormone transfer is one example of the transport function of the CSF. Cells within the hypothalamus produce many of the releasing-hormones for pituitary control. These hypothalamic peptides are released into the CSF and may not only affect pituitary function, but may also be involved in many other specific roles such as regulation of pain, sleep, and various behaviours (Milhorat and Hammock, 1983; Rapoport, 1976). This is possible because they are transported to many other regions of the CNS. CSF transport of biogenic amines may also have important effects on pituitary and CNS activity (Milhorat, 1975; Milhorat and Hammock, 1983). Peptide and other hormone transport in the CSF are discussed further in Chapter 6.

Provision of an internal milieu

Since CSF serves as a bathing solution for the central nervous system, it is not surprising that it provides an important function in maintaining the chemical environment of the CNS. It has only to diffuse a maximum distance of 2 cm to be able to reach any part of the central nervous system (Davson, 1967). The CSF is separated from the ECF of the brain and spinal cord only by a thin layer of ependyma-glial and pia-glial cells. It may well also be in more direct contact with the ECF by way of the Virchow-Robin perivascular spaces. These spaces extend from the subarachnoid space to a variable depth and may allow free diffusion of some solute. The chemical makeup of the ECF and the CSF is a function of this "brain-CSF barrier" as well as of the "blood-brain" and "blood-CSF" barriers. These serve to guard the relative constancy of the brain interspaces from wide variations in plasma composition and from many potentially toxic large or polar molecules (Milhorat, 1975). These "barriers" will be discussed in more detail in a later section.

The composition of the CSF is quite different from plasma. It does not merely represent an ultrafiltrate of plasma, but rather an energy requiring secretion. The CSF is the product of metabolic activity by the brain and choroid plexus, providing a proper environment for CNS function.

While the study of the extracellular fluid (ECF) of the brain poses technical difficulties, preliminary evidence indicates that ECF has concentrations of bicarbonate, potassium, and chloride similar to CSF (Cserr, 1975). The concentrations of K^+, Mg^{++}, and Ca^{++} in mammalian CSF are remarkably resistant to changes in plasma concentrations of these ions. However, the function of the CNS is quite sensitive to changes in CSF ionic composition. Alterations in CSF K^+, Ca^{++}, and Mg^{++} produce marked changes in blood pressure, heart rate, the rate and depth of breathing, gastric motility, emotional state, and neuronal electrical activity (Rapoport, 1976; Bradbury and Sarna, 1977; Hochwald, 1983). Cerebral blood flow, CNS metabolism, and the brainstem respiratory center are all profoundly affected by even small changes in the acid-base status of the CSF (Milhorat, 1975; Hochwald, 1983). Receptors in the third ventricle which monitor the drive for thirst and ADH release are very sensitive to changes in the concentrations of Na^+ in the CSF.

In addition to inorganic compound homeostasis, the organic constituents of CSF are carefully regulated as well. The CSF is thought to have a limited role in the chemical regulation of nutrients entering the CNS. Some nutritive substances, e.g. glucose, amino acids, and fatty acids, enter the CNS principally through carrier-mediated systems within the brain capillaries, passing directly through the blood-brain barrier (BBB) into the extracellular fluid (ECF) of the brain (Spector and Ellis, 1984). However, other substances, e.g. certain vitamins including folate, ascorbic acid, and pyrimidine deoxynucleosides will enter the brain ECF primarily via the CSF, passing through the blood-CSF barrier. These substances utilise specific transport systems in the choroid plexus (Spector and Ellis, 1984). This nutritive function of the CSF for the CNS is believed to play only a small role in adult mammals, being of much more significance in embryos and in lower vertebrates (Cserr, 1975).

Lymphatic role

The brain lacks the conventional lymphatic mechanism for removal of the products of metabolism. The blood-brain interface poses a barrier for water soluble substances unless there exists a specific transport system capable of removing that specific compound. Evidence for a major excretory role for cerebral capillaries is lacking. Parenchymal capillaries are impermeable to high molecular weight, water soluble materials. The hydrostatic pressure in cerebral capillaries is greater than that in the ECF, and the number of transport systems known to exist in the capillary endothelium are too few to explain the removal of the cerebral metabolic end products (Milhorat, 1976; Oldendorf, 1977). Thus cerebral wastes are believed to be transferred to the CSF by both diffusion and bulk flow of the ISF of the brain (Cserr, 1974), after which they are removed primarily via the arachnoid villi to the dural sinus. In various other mammalian species, substances move through the subarachnoid space across the cribriform plate and into the nasal mucosa (Rosenberg, 1990). Whether or not a similar process occurs in humans is unknown.

An excretory role of the CSF and ISF is well accepted. The choroid plexus possesses many transport systems capable of removing metabolites and drugs from the CSF to the blood. Absorption of the CSF via the arachnoid villi may also provide a "sink" or drain for substances which have accumulated in the brain and passed on to the CSF. These metabolic end products are thought to gain access to the CSF by bulk flow of ECF and net diffusion (Davson, 1967). Their removal then from CSF via active transport and bulk absorption provides an essential function for brain tissue which, otherwise, lacks any type of lymphatic apparatus. This lymphatic role of the CSF is also important in the removal of substances foreign to the central nervous system. The "third circulation", as a dynamic circular drain for neural tissue, is capable of removing proteins, drugs, toxins, and cellular elements in pathological states (Milhorat, 1975).

Anatomical Aspects

In about the fourth week of gestation the neural groove undergoes closure dorsally and, after segmentation, forms the cerebral ventricles. The caudal aspect forms the spinal cord while the cephalic segment dilates to become the brain and ventricular system (Rosenberg, 1990). The prosencephalon (forebrain), mesencephalon (midbrain) and rhombencephalon (hind brain) form from three rostral bulges in the initially straight tube. The ventricular system and central canal of the spinal cord form from the fluid-filled central cavity of the neural tube (Brumback, 1989a). Sac-like invaginations of the roof plate form at about 6-8 weeks and develop into the choroid plexuses of the fourth, lateral, and third ventricles in that order. At four months gestation, the foramina of Luschka and Magendie develop from weak spots in the roof plate of the rhombencephalon, allowing free communication within the ventricular system (Langman, 1978).

The ventricular system contains about 23 ml of the 140 ml total volume of the CSF. The remaining volume is contained within the subarachnoid space, about 30 ml of which is within the spinal subarachnoid space (Davson, 1967). A single layer of ependymal cells lines the ventricles. Vascular invaginations of the pia matar – the "tela choroidea" – serve to suspend the choroid plexuses within the ventricles. There are small plexuses located in the roofs of the third and fourth ventricles in addition to the two large ones found in the floor of the lateral ventricles. The plexuses play a key role in the constant renewal of CSF by the secretion and absorption of some 0.35 ml/min or 400-500 ml per day. This represents enough fluid to replace the entire volume three times daily.

The lateral ventricles are about 9.2 cm in length and consist of the frontal, occipital, and temporal horns, the body, and the collateral trigone (atrium). They communicate with the third ventricle via the two interventricular foramina of Monro (see Figs. 2-1 and 2-2). The third ventricle is about 20-30 mm in height and, in about 75% of brains, there is a mass of tissue connecting the thalamus of each side, called the massa intermedia, located in the middle of the third ventricle. The tela choroidea, a thin layer of ependyma and pia mater from which the choroid plexus originates, forms the roof of the third ventricle. The diencephalon makes up the lateral walls, and the floor of the third ventricle becomes continuous with the ventral wall of the cerebral aqueduct posteriorly. The aqueduct is approximately 11 mm long and connects the third ventricle to the fourth ventricle. The floor of the fourth ventricle extends from the cerebral aqueduct overlying the pons and medulla to the central canal of the spinal cord and is bounded by the superior and inferior cerebellar peduncles. The lateral recesses of the fourth ventricle form channels that curve around the inferior cerebellar peduncle to open into the lateral foramina of Luschka. The pontine segment of the roof is formed by the superior medullary velum and the medullary portion formed by the inferior medullary velum and tela choroidea. The foramen of Magendie is located in the midline at the caudal aspect of the roof. An opening for the central spinal canal is found on the caudal aspect of the fourth ventricle, but usually there is little if any communication with the fourth ventricle, the lumen being occluded at multiple sites (Brumback, 1989a).

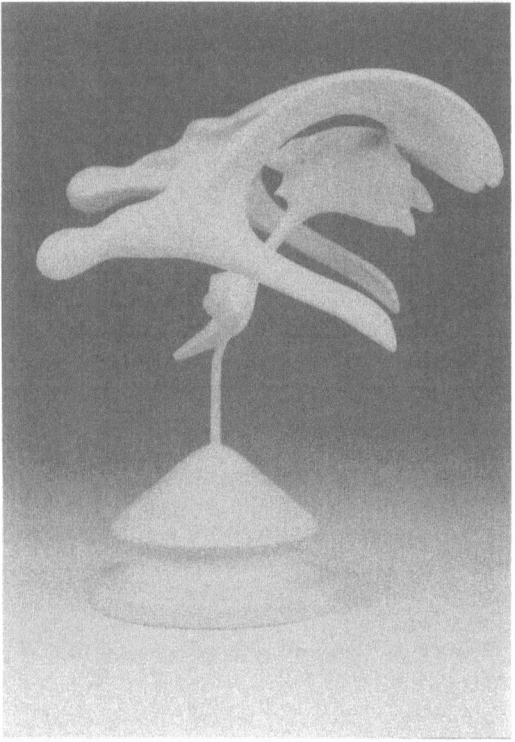

FIG. 2.1. Lateral view of cast of the human ventricular system.

The internal cerebrospinal fluid of the ventricles and central canal of the spinal cord connects with the fluid of the subarachnoid space via the two lateral foramina of Luschka and the medial foramen of Magendie (Fig. 2.2). The external CSF flows within the cerebral and spinal subarachnoid spaces.

Several small pockets of fluid, called cisterns, are found at different locations in the subarachnoid space, the largest being the cisterna magna.

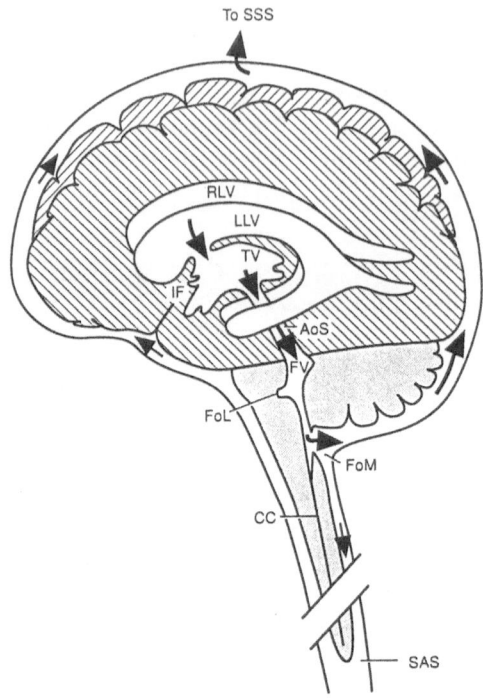

FIG. 2.2. Schematic diagram of the CSF circulation.
RLV right lateral ventricle; LLV left lateral ventricle; IF interventricular foramina; TV third ventricle; AoS aqueduct of Sylvius; FV fourth ventricle; FoL foramina of Luschka; FoM foramen of Magendie; CC Central Canal; SAS subarachnoid space; SSS superior sagittal sinus.

The CSF has a net flow from its primary source, the choroid plexus in the ventricles, through the foramina of Luschka and Magendie, into the subarachnoid space of the brain and spinal cord. From there it flows both cranially toward the arachnoid villi, where a large part of the CSF is absorbed, and caudally to the spinal subarachnoid space (Millen and Woollam, 1962). The fluid travels from the fourth ventricle through the cisterna magna and circulates through the subarachnoid space of the cerebellar hemispheres to the cisterna ambiens and the basilar cistern. Currents in the posterior cisterna magna direct some of the CSF to flow down the spinal subarachnoid space. The CSF then travels from the basilar and ambient cisterns to the interpeduncular and prechiasmatic cisterns and on to the lateral and frontal hemispheric subarachnoid space, to the posterior cerebral hemispheric subarachnoid space and cephalad to the arachnoid villi associated with the superior sagittal sinus. Within the spinal subarachnoid space, the CSF flows predominantly caudally in the posterior portion and cephalad in the anterior portion. There is a potential circulation into the spinal central canal to the "terminal" or "fifth" ventricle above the filum terminale but this central canal is closed by the age of 12 in humans. The fluid movement is predominantly laminar in the subarachnoid space and undirectional in the ventricles (Tourtellotte and Shorr, 1982; Brumback, 1989a).

Barriers in the CNS

In 1885 Paul Ehrlich discovered that injection of an acidic dye, coerulein-S, would cause staining of all the organs except the brain. He postulated that the brain had a lower affinity for the dye. In 1913 Edwin Goldmann, a former student of Ehrlich, injected the dye trypan blue intravenously in animals, finding again that the brain was spared of staining, with the exception of the choroid plexuses. He then went on to inject the dye directly into the CSF of dogs and rabbits, finding the brain to stain a deep blue. The dye did not exit into the bloodstream and stain the other internal organs. He thus first clearly demonstrated the presence of the blood-brain-barrier (Bakay, 1956; Goldstein and Betz, 1986).

The barriers in the CNS serve to protect the brain from endogenous and exogenous toxins in the blood, to hinder the escape of neurotransmitters and other active compounds from interstitial fluid into blood and to provide a separate internal environment to be maintained for the CNS by regulating the homeostasis of H^+, HCO_3^-, Ca^{++}, Mg^{++}, nutrients and other substances (Bradbury, 1979). Cerebral blood flow and ventilation are regulated by the relative impermeability of the barriers to H^+ and HCO_3^- and the high permeability of the barriers to CO_2 regulates the pH of the cerebral interstitial fluid. The only other such blood-interstitital fluid barriers functioning in mammals besides the blood-retinal and blood-nerve barriers, are those of the placenta and the testis (Bradbury, 1979).

Homeostasis of the fluid environment of the CNS is controlled by selective transport processes found in cerebral capillaries, the choroid plexus, and other cellular linings of the CSF-containing compartment. Some authors (Rapoport, 1976) use the term blood-brain barrier (BBB) to include both the capillary-glial barrier and the choroid plexus. The choroid plexus does ultimately separate the blood and the brain if the substance passes through the CSF-brain interface. However, as this discussion is concerned with CSF reflecting cerebral metabolic processes, the more limited use of the term BBB for only the capillary-glial barrier is used.

There are three principal barriers or interfaces in the CNS involved in the regulation of the composition of CSF: blood-brain, blood-CSF, and CSF-brain (Fig. 2-3).

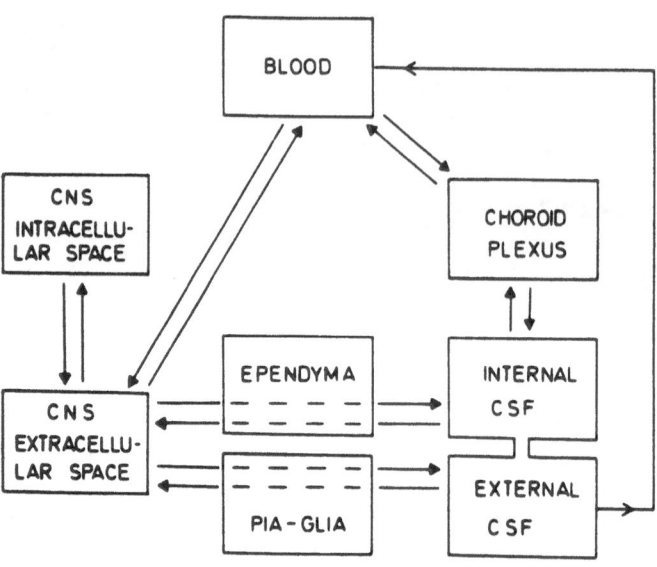

FIG. 2.3. Schematic diagram of the exchange of substances between blood, CNS and CSF (from Bulat and Zivkovic, 1978).

Blood-brain interface

As explained above, this consists primarily of the capillary-glial barrier, for the purposes of this discussion. The unique physiological aspects of the BBB as compared to other capillary-tissue interfaces in the body can be attributed, in part, to the following ultrastructural features: (a) the presence of tight junctions between the capillary endothelial cells, (b) glial foot processes surrounding the capillaries, (c) fewer pinocytotic vesicles in the endothelium, (d) increased number of mitochondria in the endothelium and (e) the relative paucity of pericapillary connective tissue (Levin, 1977; Fishman, 1980). These characteristics are depicted in Fig. 2-4. The BBB may be viewed as a sheet of cells connected by tight junctions on a basement membrane with low permeability to hydrophilic non-electrolytes and very low ionic permeability. Passive solute permeability occurs predominantly at the intercellular junctions and there is also facilitated transport of organic solutes (Crone, 1986).

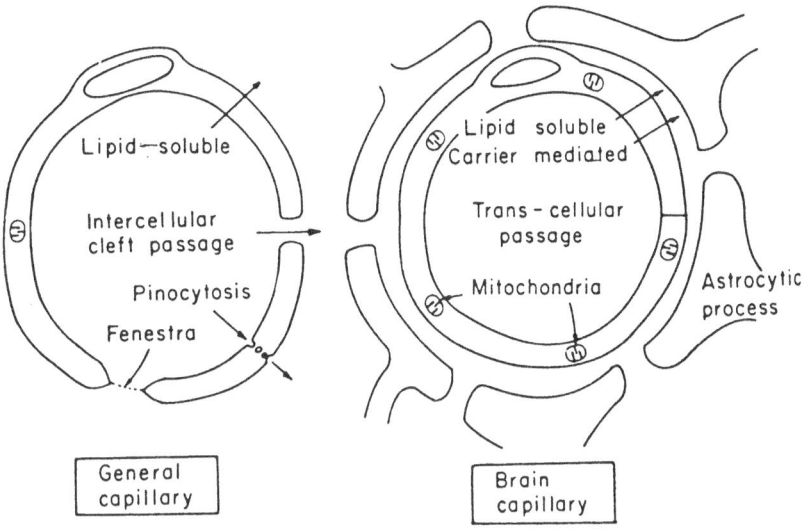

FIG. 2.4. Schema of structural differences between general and brain capillaries (see text for description) from Oldendorf (1977), with permission.

These factors serve to restrict the entry of macromolecules and polar (non-lipid soluble) substances. There is also evidence that specific active transport systems and enzymes within the capillary endothelium play an important role in homeostasis (Levin, 1977) and delivery of nutrients to the CNS (Spector and Ellis, 1984; Bradbury, 1984). These will be discussed further in a later section. Examples of important substances entering the CNS primarily via the blood-brain interface include amino acids, fatty acids, and glucose (Spector and Ellis, 1984; Bradbury, 1984).

CSF-brain interface

The CSF-brain interface consists of the ependyma-glial and pia-glial cells. The epithelial cells of the ependyma lining the ventricular surface have cilia in direct contact with the CSF in many areas, similar to those seen in the trachea. These do not function to move particles as they do in the trachea, but rather appear to mix molecules on the surface and increase transport (Rosenberg, 1990). The walls of the ventricles and spinal canal are lined with only a single layer of ependymal cells.

In general, exchange between the CSF and brain ECF occurs between adjacent ependymal cells by diffusion and by pinocytosis, while the cilia of the ependymal cells aid the mixing of the ECF and CSF at the interface

(Cserr, 1974: Rapoport, 1976; Davson *et al.*, 1987). As these cells are not connected by tight junctions, they pose neither a diffusional barrier to small solutes nor a barrier to macromolecular exchange except for a few unique areas where the underlying blood-brain barrier is absent. In these areas, the ventricle is covered with a specialised epithelium which possesses tight junctions between adjacent cells and is capable of halting intercellular movement of colloidal markers (Milhorat, 1976).

One example of this is the ependyma of the median eminence. Specialised cells called tanycytes connect the nuclei of the hypothalamus with the ventricular surface on the floor of the third ventricle. They are connected by tight junctions and the ventricular surface of these cells possess microvilli instead of cilia. The tanycytes serve an important barrier function protecting the structures of the median eminence from molecules entering from the CSF and have also been suggested as possibly serving as a mechanism by which hormones may be transported between the CSF and the hypothalamus (Rosenberg, 1990).

The pia-glial interface is considered to have permeability properties quite similar to the ependyma-glial interface, and often is not considered separately. However, the pia possesses a vascular supply, and its role in transport of compounds between CSF and brain or blood also needs to be investigated. Experiments by Wright *et al.*, (1971) and Levin *et al.*, (1974) support a role for the pial vessels in transporting selective substances from the CSF to the blood. Water and phenylalanine were transferred, and, in the case of the amino acid, the process was saturable. Na^+, for example, did not pass into the pial vasculature. Levin *et al.* proposed that the endothelial cells of pial vessels may have similar transport properties and regulatory functions as the cerebral capillaries.

Blood-CSF interface

The blood-CSF barrier or interface is composed of the pial blood vessels already discussed, the dura-arachnoid membrane, choroid plexus, arachnoid villi and peripheral nerves. The choroid plexus and arachnoid villi are to be discussed in further detail in the next section. The epineurium of the peripheral nerves and the dura are derived from mesoderm whereas the arachnoid, pia and their peripheral nerve counterparts, perineurium and endoneurium, are neural crest derivatives (Rapoport, 1976). Maturation of this interface occurs maximally during the third month of life after which it decreases rapidly (Statz and Felgenhauer, 1983).

The dura-arachnoid complex is composed of three layers. The outer layer or dura is a thick mat of collagen which stains with an intravenous injection of trypan blue. The next two layers make up the avascular arachnoid. The middle layer consists of several layers of flat arachnoid cells that are connected with rings of tight junctions. It is this middle layer that prevents tracers in either the blood or CSF from reaching the opposite compartment. The inner arachnoid layer consists of loosely associated arachnoid cells (Davson, 1967; Rapoport, 1976), and arachnoid trabeculae extend from the arachnoid to the pia.

The choroid plexus is a complex regulator of the blood-CSF interface. Not only is the choroid plexus the major site of CSF formation, but it possesses many selective transport mechanisms capable of moving substances in a direction opposite to the main secretory flow. Some of the experimental techniques that have been of value in elucidating choroidal function and CSF formation are ventriculo-cisternal perfusion, isolated perfused choroid plexus, in vivo exposed choroid plexus, open drainage, micropuncture of the principal vein of the choroid plexus, and kinetic studies.

The choroid plexus appears in the ventricles as a velvety vascular membrane that oscillates with the pulsations of the CSF. It possesses a vascular core with large fenestrated capillaries, an incomplete lining membrane of pial origin, and a fibrillar stroma. Lining this stroma is the lamina epithelialis – a low columnar to high cuboidal epithelium with basal infoldings and an apical brush border with occasional cilia. These epithelial cells are connected by apical tight junctions and are separated from the stroma by a basement membrane (Milhorat, 1976; Conly and Ronald, 1983).The stroma of the choroid plexus is accessible to substances in the blood, but the apical tight junctions of the epithelial cells prevent these substances from entering the CSF (Rosenberg, 1990). The choroidal cilia become increasingly less frequent in man after infancy (Milhorat, 1976).

The choroid plexus receives its arterial supply from the anterior choroidal artery (from the internal carotid) as well as from the posterior cerebral artery. The superior cervical ganglion and the nervous network around the internal carotid artery innervate the plexus. Vagal stimulation will result in dilation of the choroidal artery plexus, while sympathetic stimulation results in its constriction (DeJong, 1979). Edvinsson et al. (1983) have reviewed the autonomic nervous system regulation of the choroid plexus.

The choroid plexus has a key role in maintaining the composition of the CSF and, thus, the composition of cerebral interstitial fluid. The choroid plexus has been shown to transport bidirectionally a number of biologically important substances and has been compared to a miniature kidney, that, along with the BBB, closely regulates the neuronal environmental (Pollay, 1974).

Exchanges of substances between the blood and the CSF have been studied using ventriculocisternal perfusion. When a substance disappears from the CSF between the lateral ventricle and the cisterna magna, it may either have been lost to the brain by diffusion or been absorbed by the choroid plexus. Evidence supporting this role of the choroid plexus has come from perfusion studies localising the site of absorption to near the choroid plexus. However, the site of solute transport cannot be proven by this method. To test whether the substance may be transported out of the CSF by the choroid plexus, the isolated perfused choroid plexus has been used to demonstrate the plexus' ability to accumulate the substances *in vitro*. Substances that have been found to be accumulated by the isolated choroid plexus are listed in Table 2-1 (Cserr, 1971; Rapoport, 1976, and Lorenzo and Spector, 1976).

TABLE 2-1. *Substances accumulated in isolated choroid plexus by carrier-mediated energy dependent transport process.*

Monovalent anions	Primary amines	Amino acids
iodide	5-HT	*neutral*
thiocyanate	NE	L-proline
		DL-hydroxyproline
Divalent anions	*Tertiary amines*	glycine
sulfate	dihydromorphine	L-valine
thiosulfate	dextrophan	L-alanine
	morphine	L-methionine
Organic Compounds	nalorphine	D-cysteine
diodrast	codeine	DL--aminobutyric
iodipamide	levorphan	acid
o-iodohippurate	methorphan	L-tyrosine
p-aminohippurate	atropine	L-phenylalanine
phenosulfonphthalein	lysergic acid diethylamide	
iodopyracet	methadone	*Basic*
methotrexate		L-histidine
penicillin	*Quaternary amines*	L-lysine
salicylic acid	hexamethonium	L-arginine
5-HIAA	decamethonium	
ascorbic acid	N-methylnicotinamide	*Acidic*
PGE	nicotinamide	L-asparatate
p-aminosalicylic acid	methylatropine	
	acetylcholine	*Monosaccharidos*
	choline	
Purines		glucose
xanthine		galactose
Aminoglycosides		
gentamicin		

Modified from Cserr, 1971; Lorenzo and Spector, 1976; Rapoport, 1976.

These accumulatory processes show the usual characteristics of carrier-mediated, energy dependent transport systems (Cserr, 1975). Each class of compounds is believed to be transported by its own carrier system in the choroid plexus as judged by competition of compounds for uptake (Cserr, 1971). Even though the substance is transported *in vivo* as demonstrated by ventriculocisternal perfusion, and is accumulated by the isolated perfused choroid plexus, one cannot rule out tissue binding or intracellular accumulation by the choroid plexus (Cserr, 1975). Gradients across the choroid plexus have been found for several colored organic acids, and an organic acid transport system in the choroid plexus is fairly well accepted. Although the evidence for other transport systems is not as rigorous, they too probably function in the choroid plexus.

Rapid exchanges between the CSF and blood are also possible by bidirectional carrier-mediated diffusion through the capillary endothelial cells. An example of this is the rapid equilibration in the CSF glucose levels following changes in blood glucose levels (Fishman, 1980).

Other studies using radioisotopes have helped to delineate the kinetics and membrane-permeability characteristics of the blood-CSF barrier (see review of Davson *et al.*, 1987) and the CSF/serum ratios of albumin, IgG, alpha2-macroglobulin and other proteins have been useful in distinguishing various different components of the blood-CSF barrier for proteins (Keir and Thompson, 1986).

The cranial and spinal nerves present other routes where the CSF and blood can meet. The olfactory, optic, and acoustic cranial nerves have connective tissue sheaths which are continuous with the subarachnoid space (Davson *et al.*, 1987). Injection of coloured dyes into the subarachnoid space results in colouring of the optic tracts and nerves as far as the epichoroidal and episcleral tissues within minutes (Davson *et al.*, 1987). The cytoplasmic processes of the olfactory receptor cells provide an important route of entry into the CNS of some viruses, and the area where the optic nerve enters the globe of the eye may also present a route of entry of blood-borne substances into the CSF (Rapoport, 1976).

Sensory ganglia of both spinal and cranial nerves are not protected by a barrier system and are thus more accessible to intravascular substances. In contrast to the above mentioned cranial nerves, the arachnoid of the spinal nerves fuses with the pia in the region of the emerging root, and spinal arachnoid villi located at this site may provide a route of drainage for substances from the CSF into the lymph nodes and blood (Davson, 1967). Whether or not CSF is normally absorbed at these spinal sites is not known, but it is possible that spinal (and transventricular) absorption processes could be compensatory mechanisms of absorption in communicating hydrocephalus (Cutler and Spertell, 1982).

Physiological aspects of the barriers

The three anatomical interfaces just discussed act as an integrated whole in the homeostasis of the brain fluids. The blood-brain and blood-CSF barriers serve to exclude large molecules like proteins and to regulate the entry of small ones by requiring them to cross the lipid-bilayer of the plasma membranes. Water-soluble molecules cross the barriers poorly whereas lipid soluble molecules cross readily, e.g. nicotine, ethanol and heroin. The readiness with which these substances cross the barriers may in part account for their high abuse potential.

Active transport systems are also present on the luminal and antiluminal endothelial cell membranes. These may be "symmetric", i.e. bidirectional, for example glucose and large neutral amino acids, or "asymmetric", i.e. unidirectional, usually directing molecules such as K^+ and small neutral amino acids like glycine out of the CNS (Goldstein and Betz, 1986; Shapiro, 1988).

The main physiological and biochemical characteristics which contribute to the overall barrier-effect may be summarized as follows (Levin, 1977; Fishman, 1980): (a) the capillary endothelial permeability, (b) the "sink action" of the CSF, (c) active transport mechanisms of the choroid plexuses and capillary endothelium, (d) metabolite exchange mechanisms, (e) enzyme activity within the endothelium and (f) electrical potential difference. The first two of these factors have already been discussed and the active transport mechanisms will be looked at further in the next section. Here we will look at the roles of metabolite exchange, enzymes, and electrical potential differences in the regulation of CSF composition.

The anti-luminal surface of the endothelial membrane of the blood-brain barrier has a coupled Na^+ - K^+ pump which is important for transepithelial transport. The surface of the cell membrane facing the CSF of the epithelial cells of the choroid plexus also has a Na^+ - K^+ -stimulated ATPase. Both systems in the endothelial cells and the choroid plexus epithelial cells are thus able to pump potassium away from the brain or CSF and probably pump sodium in the opposite direction (Crone, 1986). There is thus a net secretion of sodium from blood to interstitial fluid and to CSF whereas potassium tends to be removed from the ISF and CSF. There are also specific transport mechanisms for glucose, amino acids, and precursors of neurotransmitters. Neurotransmitters themselves tend not to be transported across the blood-brain-CSF barriers.

There is evidence that various metabolites may cross the different interfaces without changing their concentration in their respective fluid compartments (Cohen and Lajtha, 1972; Levin, 1977). The process may be very rapid and occur without any net change in metabolite concentration (Levin, 1977). The significance of this exchange is not yet clear.

Enzyme systems may play an important role in transforming various substances in the endothelium of the brain capillaries. The enzyme DOPA-decarboxylase, for example, has been found in rat endothelial cells.

This enzyme converts L-DOPA, which is capable of crossing the BBB, to dopamine which is not capable of crossing the BBB (Levin, 1977). Some enzyme systems may thus act as a chemical barrier for some substances.

Different investigators have found electrical potentials between CSF and blood ranging from 0 to +15 mV (Fishman, 1992). This has been shown to vary with pH. The genesis of this potential and its significance as a BBB diffusion potential gradient are not known. It is, however, thought to be of importance by some in the distribution of ions and in acid-base balance (Welch, 1975a,b).

These physiologic mechanisms act together to maintain the relative constancy of the CSF and brain ECF. Osmotic differences will vary directly with changes in plasma but are sustained only briefly. Toxins, metabolic waste products, and cellular debris are removed. The permeability characteristics favour passage of small molecular weight and lipid-soluble molecules. The passage of ions, organic acids and bases depend primarily on bidirectional active transport by the choroid plexus and endothelium.

Both the blood-brain and blood-CSF interfaces regulate the fluid environment of the CSF. Factors which are known to affect the entry, distribution, and final concentration of a compound in the CSF include: plasma concentration, physical and chemical properties of the compound, degree of binding to plasma proteins, cerebral blood flow, regional vascularity, permeability of cerebral blood vessels, rate of diffusion through interstitial spaces and CSF, uptake and metabolism by cells, rate of bulk flow of CSF, and rate of diffusion and transport between the brain, CSF, and blood vessels (Lorenzo and Spector, 1976).

The regulation of the organic composition of the CSF is an important issue. The blood-CSF and blood-brain barrier transport processes are responsible for protecting the CNS from accumulating potentially harmful substances such as exogenous drugs and endogenous metabolites that are produced by or enter into the CNS. The relative role of the blood-brain and blood-CSF interfaces in this regulation is controversial. The choroid plexus and pia-arachnoid membranes are probably the primary sites of these regulatory transport processes.

The ability of the choroid plexus to accumulate organic anions is poorly developed in the newborn dog (Miller and Ross, 1976). This ability is developed during the early weeks of life, and it is speculated that this may be partly the reason why newborns are particularly vulnerable to the entry of drugs into the CNS. In addition, experiments with newborn rats (Bass and Lundborg, 1976) provide evidence that postnatal development of the barrier function of brain capillaries parallels the maturation of transport mechanisms for the removal of organic acids.

The barriers of the CNS prevent many therapeutic agents from entering the CNS. For example, penicillin, a water soluble cyclic peptide, often fails to reach effective concentrations within the CNS. Not only do these barriers inhibit entry, but also the penicillin that does reach the CSF is cleared by an active transport system which hastens its removal. This clearance mechanism from CSF to blood can work against a concentration gradient and is believed to be carrier mediated. The choroid plexus *in vitro* can concentrate penicillin, and is thought to be the site for this efflux transport mechanism. Although an efflux system at the blood-brain interface is possible, it is believed that if present, it would not be as effective as that of the choroid plexus (Lorenzo and Spector, 1976). Penicillin is cleared from the CSF to the blood much faster than it can enter by that route. This is fairly general for many drugs except for example salicylic acid and possibly morphine (Lorenzo, 1977). Although levels of salicylic acid in the CSF are lower than theoretically predicted on the basis of physicochemical properties, the weak organic acid transport system has a low affinity for the compound and is not thought to significantly alter the CSF levels.

Drug delivery to the brain can be enhanced by administering them into the carotid or vertebral systems after first using osmotic agents, e.g. mannitol to "open" the BBB. The tight junctions can be reversibly separated by osmotic agents allowing drugs which ordinarily penetrate the BBB poorly to enter (Neuwelt and Rapoport, 1984; Goldstein, 1988; Rapoport *et al.*, 1972). Fishman (1992, pp. 55-62) has reviewed some of the newer strategies to enhance drug delivery to the CNS.

The evidence for an organic cation transport system out of the CSF is less convincing than that for the organic acids. The best evidence for this system comes from the competitive disappearance of hexamethonium, N-methylnicotinamide (NMN) and other organic cations following injection of these compounds into the lateral ventricle of rabbits and sampling of cisternal CSF (Miller and Ross, 1976). Neither this technique nor ventriculo-cisternal perfusion reveals the site of this transport, but perfusion techniques can give some idea of the capacity of the system.

A number of organic cations are accumulated *in vitro* by the choroid plexus (Table 2.1). Dibenamide, a specific blocker for organic cation transport in the kidney, is effective in blocking the choroid plexus cation uptake (Miller and Ross, 1976). The sites of this choroid plexus uptake are not known. In fact, several drugs, for example gentamicin, morphine, and atropine, which are accumulated actively by the choroid plexus, are not significantly removed from the CSF by this method (Lorenzo, 1977; Lorenzo and Spector, 1976). They are cleared primarily by the bulk flow of the CSF and diffusion. Uptake of these compounds by the choroid plexus *in vitro* could be associated with low affinity but not transport or intracellular accumulation of the drug. In experiments with rabbits, NMN, a quaternary ammonium compound, is not bound to homogenates of choroid plexus and appears to be transported out of the CSF by the choroid plexus, although at a low rate (Miller and Ross, 1976). There is evidence that, in the frog, the arachnoid removes quaternary ammonium compounds from the CSF (Wright, 1977).

The interested reader is referred to the extensive reviews of the blood-brain-CSF barriers of Rapoport (1976), Bradbury (1979), Suckling *et al.* (1986), Davson *et al.* (1987, pp.35-452), and Neuwett (1989).

Physiological Considerations

Production of CSF

Both diffusion and secretory mechanisms are believed to play an important role in CSF production (DeJong, 1979). The choroid plexus is the principal source of CSF. The blood-CSF barrier in the choroid plexus consists of (1) apical tight junctions between epithelial cells prohibiting intercellular movement of large molecules, (2) a bidirectional active transport system of epithelial cell enzymes; and (3) intracellular pinocytotic vesicles and lysosomal enzymes (Milhorat and Hammock, 1983).

The epithelial cells of the choroid plexus are ideally suited for transporting and secreting fluids and solutes. The CSF produced by the choroid plexus is believed to be formed by two major processes in series – filtration and secretion. First, the blood plasma is filtered across the choroidal capillaries to the interstitial spaces of the plexus. It passes to the fibrillar stroma beneath the epithelium by hydrostatic pressure (McComb, 1983). Then that protein-rich fluid is acted upon by the lamina epithelium to produce the CSF (Welch, 1975a). The protein in the plasma filtrate is believed to be taken up by the epithelium in small pinocytotic vesicles, transported to the Golgi region of the cell, and digested by the lysosomal enzymes contained in the vesicles which fuse with the protein-containing vesicles (Milhorat, 1976).

The basic mechanism of CSF secretion by the choroid plexus is believed to be osmotically obligated water flow across the lamina epithelialis secondary to an electrically silent Na^+ transport (Davson, 1967; Pollay, 1974; Pollay, 1975). Minor ions may be able to pass through the apical tight junctions via hydrostatic pressure or a separate transport mechanism. Factors playing an important role in the secretion mechanism include a metabolic energy supply, active Na^+ transport with passive water transfer, possibly a Cl^- pump, bicarbonate movement, and Na^+-K^+ ATPase (Segal and Pollay, 1977; McComb, 1983). These factors have been elucidated largely by observing the effects of metabolic and transport inhibitors such as ouabain, acetazolamide, furosemide, DNP and cyanide on CSF production. Ouabain, a Na^+-K^+ ATPase inhibitor, will nearly abolish choroidal CSF secretion experimentally, and acetazolamide, a carbonic anhydrase inhibitor, will diminish CSF production by about 50%. Na^+ - K^+ ATPase is located on the apical surface of the epithelial cells and carbonic anhydrase is contained within the cell (Rosenberg, 1990). These observations suggest that Na^+-K^+ ATPase and carbonic anhydrase both play a key role in choroidal CSF production (Brumback, 1989a).

Cholera toxin administered intravenously results in a large increase in the production of CSF. Because cholera toxin stimulates adenylate cyclase, Epstein et al. (1977) suggest that cAMP plays a role in CSF production. The basal surface of the epithelial cells has areas that stain for cyclic nucleotide, further supporting a role for cAMP (Rosenberg, 1990). This effect of cholera toxin is blocked by indomethacin which is an antagonist of prostaglandins, suggesting a possible role for prostaglandins in CSF formation as well (McComb, 1983).

Steardo and Nathanson (1987) have also demonstrated recently that the peptide atrial natriuretic factor (ANF) will decrease CSF formation when infused into the CSF. ANF is released by the cardiac atria in response to fluid overload and is thought to act on cyclic GMP.

In addition, sympathetic nerves in the choroid plexus have an inhibitory effect on CSF production which is believed to be exerted primarily on the plexus epithelium rather than on the choroidal vasculature and blood flow (Lindval et al., 1978). The epithelium and vascular smooth muscle cells of the choroid plexuses receive both adrenergic and cholinergic innervation which also regulate CSF production. Sympathetic stimulation will cause a 30% reduction in CSF production, while sympathectomy will increase production by about 30% and cholinomimetic agents will also reduce CSF formation, suggesting that the choroid plexus contains muscarinic receptors (Edvinsson et al., 1983).

Decreased metabolism due to hypothermia and hyperosmolarity are other factors which may reduce CSF formation (Rosenberg, 1990).

The choroid plexus is not the only source of CSF. The failure of plexectomy to cure hydrocephalus as well as experiments involving isolated aqueduct of Sylvius perfusion and inhibitors of choroidal secretion have provided evidence for the extrachoroidal secretion of CSF. Assessing the quantity of the rates of choroidal versus extrachoroidal CSF secretion is technically difficult. Estimates have ranged from 30% to 70% of the total CSF being produced by the choroid plexus (Segal and Pollay, 1977; Milhorat, 1976; Welch, 1975b; Krieg, 1979). As the secretion of CSF continues after plexectomy and has a normal composition, this extrachoroidal secretion also appears to be regulated and to play a role in the homeostasis of the fluid environment of the CNS.

The ECF of the brain is believed to be the primary source of extrachoroidal CSF with the cerebral capillaries providing the regulation. Evidence supporting the concept that bulk movement of fluid from the brain interstitium to the CSF does occur has come from studies using blue dextran 2000 injected into the caudate nucleus of rat brains that were edematous (Cserr, 1974,1975; Cserr and Tang, 1975). By following the intracranial distribution of the dextran, these experiments demonstrated the movement of bulk fluid through the interstitial spaces of the brain and along the course of cerebral blood vessels. This technique is not sensitive enough to be done in a non-oedematous brain (Lorenzo, 1975). Additional evidence for the bulk flow of ECF to the CSF come from Na^+ exchange kinetic studies (Milhorat, 1976; Welch, 1975a), and from studies following the intracerebral distribution of extracellular markers introduced into the parenchyma (Cserr et al., 1977; McComb, 1983).

Absorption of the CSF

The arachnoid villi serve as the main site of absorption of the CSF into the dural sinuses. The arachnoid cells are joined by tight junctions (Rosenberg, 1990). CSF is formed at a hydrostatic pressure head of about 15 cm H_2O (Rapoport, 1976) and it is the hydrostatic pressure difference between the CSF and the sagital sinus that drives the CSF across the arachnoid villi. The rectified channels seem to act like pores that are wide enough to permit molecules the size of serum globulins (about 100 Angstroms) to pass. The channels may be even wider, as labelled erythrocytes in the CSF appear fairly rapidly in the blood (Ekstedt, 1975; Davson et al., 1987).

There is controversy over the nature of these channels and over the physiological mechanisms of transport across them. "Open" channels (solely pressure-dependent), "closed" channels (covered by a continuous tight-junctioned endothelial membrane) and transendothelial vacuolisation (temporarily creating open channels through the villus) have all been proposed (McComb, 1983; Fishman, 1980). Transport mechanisms across the villi which have been implicated include bulk absorption, diffusion, active transport, phagocytosis, degradation, and pinocytosis (Hochwald, 1983; McComb, 1983). Tripathi and Tripathi (1974) have described vacuoles transporting CSF through the arachnoid cells to the venous system. These vacuoles may be large enough to encompass intact red blood cells.

Though the bulk of CSF is absorbed by the arachnoid villi to the dural sinus, other subsidiary sites of absorption probably play a role as well. The leptomeninges, ventricular ependyma and the lymphatics of the spinal and cranial nerves have all been implicated as sites of bulk absorption (Milhorat, 1975; Milhorat et al., 1983), but whether these function in the physiological absorption of the fluid is not known.

The absorption of CSF will start at a pressure of 7 cm H_2O and increases linearly at a rate of 7.6 µl/min up to a pressure of about 25 cm H_2O (Cutler and Spertell, 1982; Brumback, 1989a). At 25 cm H_2O pressure the absorption rate is 90 ml/h, 4 1/2 times the constant CSF formation rate. An equilibrium between the formation and absorption rates occurs at about 11 cm H_2O (Brumback, 1989a).

The brain parenchyma is not believed to be a significant site of CSF absorption (Welch, 1975a) but probably does act as a conduit for CSF to go from the ventricles into the prelymphatic channels of blood vessels or into the subarachnoid space (McComb, 1983). Some components of the CSF may disappear by simple diffusion into the brain parenchyma. Examples of this include CO_2, H^+, lactate, and ammonia ions. Lipid soluble drugs such as procaine are thought to diffuse rapidly through the CNS. Bidirectional carrier mediated diffusion through the capillary endothelial cells also allows for rapid exchanges between the CSF and blood (Fishman, 1992). Active transport occurs primarily through the choroid plexus, although ependymal and endothelial sites of transport have also been implicated (Fishman, 1992). The bidirectional transport of the choroid plexus was discussed earlier. The choroid plexus may also be able to absorb by pinocytosis, at rates of up to 1/10 that of CSF secretion. This mechanism may be important at high pressures and low secretion rates (Welch, 1975a).

In summary, CSF reabsorption occurs primarily via the arachnoid villi into the dural sinus, though other subsidiary sites have been proposed. The rate of absorption is directly dependent on the CSF hydrostatic pressure and, normally, is the same as the rate of secretion. Bulk flow, active transport, vacuolar transport, and both passive and facilitated diffusion are all important mechanisms of absorption (McComb, 1983).

CSF circulation

The anatomy of CSF circulation was dealt with in an earlier section (see Fig. 2.2). The force behind this circulation is primarily the hydrostatic pressure at which it is formed (about 15 cm H_2O). The choroid plexus also generates a pulse pressure which adds some additional force (Wood, 1980a). Cilia on the ependymal cells aid in its propulsion. A CSF-venous gradient of 5-6 cm H_2O adds some momentum to this flow (Wood, 1980a). The CSF flow in the subarachnoid space is laminar while flow through the ventricles is unidirectional. Radionucleotide cisternography studies of CSF currents have shown very variable intracranial distribution and rates of cephalad movement of CSF (Brumback, 1989a).

Pressure dynamics

The effects of increased intracranial pressure (ICP) have been known since the times of the ancient Egyptians, being first written of in the Smith Papyrus (Bruce, 1980). The pressure of the CSF was not actually measured though until 1891 when Quinke first introduced lumbar puncture as a diagnostic tool (Fishman, 1992).

Increased CSF pressure (as measured by lumbar puncture) is seen in congestive heart failure, acute obstruction of the superior vena cava, obstruction of venous sinuses, inflammation of the meninges, acute hypo-osmolarity (as in haemodialysis), impaired CSF resorption (as with elevated CSF protein and subarachnoid haemorrhage), cerebral oedema of any cause, or impaired CSF circulation due to mass lesions, adhesions, narrowing of the foramina of Monro, Luschka, or Magendie or acqueductal stenosis (Krieg, 1979; De Jong, 1979).

The lumbar(LCSF) pressure may decrease in shock, severe dehydration, fainting, degenerative diseases of the brain, cachexia, barbituate intoxication, acute hyperosmolarity, leakage of CSF, complete spinal subarachnoid block, decreased CSF formation (following trauma, spinal puncture, or intracranial surgery), depression, and in states of decreased arterial and venous pressures (De Jong, 1979; Krieg, 1979; Tourtellotte and Shorr, 1982).

The ICP is a dynamic pressure, depending primarily on the pressure-volume relationships of the intracranial contents, being the brain, blood, CSF, and ECF. These in turn are affected by alterations in the rate of CSF production and absorption, osmotic pressure, hydrostatic pressures, rates of diffusion and secretion, the subarachnoid reservoir size, the dural elasticity, osmotic equilibrium with the blood, venous and arterial pressures, blockage of the CSF circulation, and the effects of disease states and drug administration (De Jong, 1979). Sympathetic adrenergic activity may also influence ICP by its effects on CSF formation and on cerebral blood volume (Edvinsson *et al.,* 1983).

The brain is thought to occupy 80% of the intracranial space, while the CSF and blood (primarily in the venous sinuses and pial veins) each account for about 10% (Bruce, 1980). The thick, essentially non-distensible bone of the skull serves to protect and support the brain parenchyma. In doing so, it also forms a physical boundary for the effectively non-compressible contents which fill the intracranial space.

In contrast to the Monroe-Kellie Doctrine of the early 19th century, however, the brain and spinal cord are not now thought of as being contained within a totally non expandable fixed-volume container. Though the skull is not able to expand its volume, volume changes in the epidural venous plexus will allow the spinal dural sac to partially expand in order to accommodate very small volumetric changes of the brain and spinal cord (Bruce, 1980). In addition, the extracranial vascular system may serve as a vent for the blood and CSF compartments of the intracranial space (Langfitt, 1972) The stability of the normal ICP is thus a function of the relationships of the brain, blood, CSF, and ECF volumes, the sum of which must be a constant given complete expansion of the dural sac.

Anything causing a rise in the ICP must be compensated for by a shift in the relative volumes of the different intracranial compartments. An expansion of parenchyma is accommodated, for example, by displacement of the fluid compartments. The ICP begins to rise when the volume added becomes greater than the volume displaced. Once the finite volume of displaceable fluid has been reached, even very small increases in volume will result in great increases in ICP. The rate of volume change is also important. A rapid rate of volume increase will also result in a greater rise in ICP than will a slowly expanding mass (Langfitt, 1972; Davson, 1967). Acute mass lesions do not increase ICP until they reach about 90 ml in volume, or larger volumes if they are chronic (Tourtellotte and Shorr, 1982).

These same relations also hold true if it is the fluid compartments increasing in volume and causing displacement of brain tissue (e.g. via herniation or pressure-atrophy as in hydrocephalus). The CSF acts as a major buffering component for the pressure. Its displacement into the spinal sac and increased absorption in the presence of increased ICP are major mechanisms of compensation. CSF production, however, is unaffected by changes in ICP unless it is high enough to impede blood flow of the choroid plexus (Bruce, 1980).

Under normal conditions the ICP will, following Pascal's law, be transmitted equally along the CSF pathways as well as between intracranial compartments (Langfitt, 1972). The CSF pressure is then equal at all points in a horizontal plane. The difference in pressure between two horizontal planes is equal to the weight of the corresponding vertical column of CSF (Magnaes, 1983). Pathological obstruction of the fluid compartments or displacement of brain parenchyma as with mass lesions will, however, result in pressure gradients between compartments (Jennett, 1972; Langfitt, 1972).

The CSF pressure, in the absence of significant pressure gradients, reflects the ICP. The normal CSF pressure is usually measured by lumbar puncture with the patient's craniovertebral axis horizontal and using the pressure level of the right atrium as the zero reference. The normal limits vary from study to study but are approximately 5-15 mmHg (which corresponds to 65-195 mm CSF or mm H_2O) (Davson, 1967; Fishman, 1992). The normal range of CSF pressure in the newborn is 15-80 mm CSF, increasing to the values for young adults by the age of 6-8 years onward. There is a slight tendency toward lower pressure with increasing age in the elderly (Tourtellotte and Shorr, 1982). The average LCSF pressure in the sitting position is about 490 mm H_2O with the level of zero CSF pressure around C3 (Magnaes, 1983). The level of zero pressure in the sitting position moves cranially when the filling pressure of CSF is increased and caudally when the filling pressure is decreased (e.g. with CSF shunts).

Small pulsations in the CSF pressure are usually seen. In normal subjects pulsations may be observed synchronous with respiration (ranging 2-5 mm) and with systole (ranging 1-2 mm).

Because the brain and CSF are enclosed in a rigid cranium, the CSF oscillates with the arterial pulse as the volume of the brain expands with each heart beat. CSF is displaced from the ventricles and cerebral subarachnoid space into the spinal subarachnoid space (Bering, 1974). The process is reversed in diastole as the blood drains away and decreases the volume of the intracerebral contents. With each cycle there is a small net displacement of CSF from the ventricles equal to the ventricular CSF secretion. It has been estimated that approximately 13.75 ml of CSF moves out of the head and into the spinal cord and back again with each heart beat (Bering, 1974).

Three different types of abnormal pressure pulses have been identified: (1) rhythmic variations related to Cheyne-Stokes respirations; (2) "B-waves" related to the Traube-Hering-Breuer waves of systemic blood pressure; and (3) "plateau waves" related to intracranial hypertension (Fishman, 1992; Langfitt, 1972). These plateau waves (or "A waves") are most frequently observed in posterior fossa tumours but may also be seen in other tumour states, trauma, hydrocephalus, in other causes of intracranial hypertension, and in rapid eye movement (REM) sleep in patients with normal pressure hydrocephalus. They may gradually increase in amplitude and duration in a series of waves and be followed by a "terminal wave". This is thought to represent the point at which ICP rises to the level of systemic arterial pressure (SAP) resulting in the cessation of cerebral blood flow (CBF) (Langfitt, 1972; Nornes et al., 1975). Figure 2-5 shows these plateau waves as measured with an intracranial pressure transducer. Plateau waves can produce large elevations of CSF pressure of 130 cm or more and may last 20 min or longer (Brumback, 1989a).

The ICP has been shown to be affected by many physiologic factors including the arterial and venous blood pressures, posture, blood gases, temperature, and thoracic influences. Though chronic increases in SAP do not influence CSF pressure, acute, rapid changes will produce transitory parallel changes, which are dampened to some degree. This may be seen clinically in patients with increased ICP secondary to phaeochromocytoma or hypertensive encephalopathy. If the CSF pressure is increased to a degree approaching that of the diastolic pressure, arterial hypertension may occur with elevated ICP (De Jong, 1979; Davson, 1967; Fishman, 1980).

Increased intracranial venous pressure has a more profound effect on ICP. This is seen in patients with congestive heart failure and in mediastinal tumours causing superior vena caval obstruction. Another example is the Queckenstedt Test, in which changes in the CSF pressure are seen to parallel the jugular venous pressure upon jugular compression and release.

The increased intracranial venous pressure is one major factor underlying the increased lumbar CSF pressure seen in a shift from the horizontal to vertical posture and in changes associated with the Valsalva manoeuvre. In the former instance, the pressure influences of the hydrostatic column, the elasticity of the subarachnoid space, and other factors play important roles as well. Actions resulting in a Valsalva manoeuvre (e.g. coughing, sneezing) elevate the intrathoracic pressure causing a transient rise in central venous pressure. The CSF pressure, elevated by the resultant increased intracranial venous pressure, returns to normal when the straining is stopped. This may be followed by a "secondary overshoot" rise caused by a transient increase in arterial pressure (Davson, 1967; Fishman, 1992).

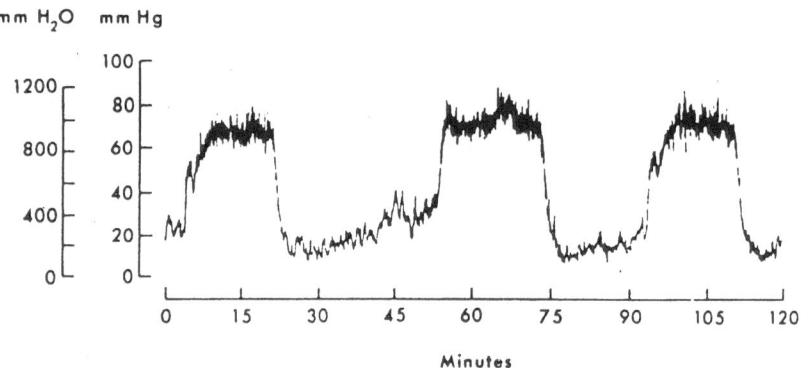

FIG. 2.5. Plateau waves visualised with an intracranial pressure transducer (from Fishman, 1980), with permission.

Both hypoxia and hypercarbia will induce cerebral vasodilation and increase cerebral blood flow (CBF) causing a secondary rise in ICP. Conversely, a respiratory alkalotic state will decrease CBF and cause vasoconstriction, secondarily lowering the ICP. This is thought to be due largely to the hydrogen ion concentration directly affecting arteriolar tone (Fishman, 1980). The effect of hypothermia in decreasing ICP is also attributed to vasoconstriction and a lowering of CBF (Davson, 1967).

The CBF is a function of vascular resistance and of the inflow and outflow pressures. In the presence of increased ICP this translates into the formula:

$$CBF = (SAP - ICP) / CVR$$

where CVR is cerebrovascular resistance, and SAP-ICP represents the cerebral perfusion pressure (CPP) (Langfitt, 1972). The cerebral perfusion pressure is normally considered the pressure of the internal carotid artery minus that of the jugular vein. Cerebral venous pressure increases as the ICP increases and the two pressures are roughly the same with increased ICP until the veins collapse (Langfitt, 1972). The CBF will autoregulate to both decreases in SAP and increases in ICP in the same way.

With intact autoregulation, it will remain fairly constant until the CPP is reduced to 40-50 mm Hg. Increased ICP will not produce any deleterious effects in cerebral metabolism until the CPP is lowered such that CBF falls to 40-45% of normal or until cerebral herniation occurs. The effects of herniation are believed to be due to both cerebral distortion and secondary regional ischaemia (Bruce, 1980). In injured and diseased brains, these relationships between ICP and CBF become much more difficult to predict. Oedema, for example, may compress the microcirculation and markedly decrease CBF while ICP may be only minimally elevated. Cerebrovascular dilatation may cause both CBF and ICP to rise by increasing cerebral blood volume (Langfitt, 1972).

Marmarou *et al.* (1978) have found that under normal conditions, the major determinants of CSF pressure are the dural sinus pressure, the CSF formation rate, the absorption resistance of CSF, and CSF compliance. They isolated the cerebral and spinal compartments by inflating a balloon positioned epidurally at C-6 in anaesthetised cats and evaluated the compliance (change in CSF volume per unit change in pressure) and absorption rates. They calculated that 68% of total compliance and 84% of total CSF absorption were contributed by the cerebral compartment. The compliance is not constant, but rather decreases as pressure increases and the volume-pressure curve of the CSF is exponential in form. They found that the compliance affected only the transient behaviour and not the equilibrium level of CSF pressure, so that, under normal conditions the CSF pressure (P) may be determined by the dural sinus pressure (Pd) and the product of formation rate (If) and absorption resistance (R):

$$P = Pd + IfR$$

The dural sinus pressure accounts for approximately 90% of the CSF pressure while IfR contributes about 10% and any influence of systemic blood pressure on ICP is normally dampened by the effects of autoregulation of cerebral blood flow (Hochwald, 1983).

The interested reader is referred to the extensive review of Davson *et al.* (1987, pp 731-82).

Hydrocephalus

Hydrocephalus is a result of disturbances in the cerebrospinal fluid dynamics and is characterised by increased CSF volume resulting in dilation of cerebral ventricles. Depending on the underlying pathogenesis, hydrocephalus is divided clinically into four types: obstructive, communicating, normal pressure, and *"ex vacuo"* hydrocephalus. Obstructive hydrocephalus occurs with impairment of the CSF circulation in either intraventricular or extraventricular pathways. In communicating hydrocephalus, no obstruction of the CSF pathways can be demonstrated and there is either overproduction or defective absorption of CSF or venous drainage insufficiency. Normal pressure hydrocephalus may follow trauma, meningitis, subarachnoid haemorrhage or be associated with an occult mass lesion and is characterized by normal CSF pressure at lumbar puncture and the absence of papilloedema. Its pathophysiology is not as clear, but may be related to insufficiency of the transcortical subarachnoid space, with or without impaired absorption, and decreased conductance to CSF outflow (Prockop and Shah, 1989).NPH may be associated with episodic increased ICP during REM sleep with plateau waves and this finding may serve as a guide for the selection of patients for surgical shunting (Fishman, 1992). *Ex vacuo* hydrocephalus is due to loss of cerebral tissue as in Alzheimer's disease.

The three forms of CSF disturbance which most often lead to hydrocephalus will be considered separately:
1   impaired CSF circulation,
2   underabsorption of CSF,
3   oversecretion of CSF.

Impaired CSF circulation

This is the most common form of hydrocephalus, causing dilatation of CSF pathways proximal to the site of obstruction and is generally referred to as obstructive hydrocephalus. From a clinical point of view, it is useful to divide this into two types: (1) lesions restricting the ventricular system and (2) lesions restricting the subarachnoid space.

A wide spectrum of congenital and acquired disease, ranging from neural tube defects to post-inflammatory fibrosis and mass lesions, may lead to the development of obstructive hydrocephalus. Dilatation of ventricles mostly follows the laws of a simple pressure/volume relationship. However, larger volume areas such as the lateral ventricles will dilate faster under the same pressure than areas with a smaller surface area such as the aqueduct of Sylvius or the third ventricle (Adams and Victor, 1985).

Underabsorption of CSF

A less common cause of hydrocephalus is impaired absorption of CSF either due to defective arachnoid villi or less commonly to raised intracranial venous pressure or impaired cerebral venous drainage. Blockage of arachnoid villi absorption may be achieved by red blood cells (as in subarachnoid haemorrhage), protein content exceeding 500 mg/dl (as in tumour, infection or rarely neuropathy), malignant cells, or fibrosis (as sequillae of meningeal inflammation of any cause) (Prockop and Shah, 1989). The resulting picture is that of communicating hydrocephalus where no obstruction to flow in the ventricular system can be demonstrated and all ventricles, including the aqueduct of Sylvius are enlarged. Raised intracranial venous pressure (via a dynamic block to the resorption of CSF) may occasionally, especially in children, lead to the same picture (Rosman, and Shands, 1978).

Whereas secretion of CSF is virtually independent of CSF pressure, its absorption is linearly related to CSF pressure. Hence any decrease in absorption leads to a rise in CSF pressure and dilation of cerebral ventricles. There is, however, a problem in explaining how blockage at the level of the arachnoid villi causes gross dilation of the cerebral ventricles, since there will be increased CSF pressure both on the surface of the brain in the subarachnoid space and within the ventricles. Pressure from the subarachnoid space is directed inwards, counteracting any expansion in size of the ventricles. Well-documented examples of hydrocephalus due to blockage of the arachnoid villi are uncommon (Adams and Victor, 1985). Blockage of the basilar subarachnoid space could on its own result in and explain ventricular dilation.

Changes in the "viscoelasticity" of the brain and of pulse pressure from the choroid plexus are thought to play an important part in the development of early ventricular dilation (Mori, 1990). Mori (1990) suggests that more attention should be paid to the intraparenchymal CSF compartment, alterations of which cause changes in brain compliance. With increased compliance, choroid plexus pulse waves could result in ventricular enlargement in the face of normal intraventricular pressure.

Oversecretion of CSF

Choroid plexus papilloma is the only known cause of oversecretion hydrocephalus (Milhorat, 1985). Caution needs to be exercised in attributing this association casually, since considerable doubt exists as to which feature of choroid plexus papilloma contributes most to the development of hydrocephalus (Leech, 1989). Other pathophysiological features of choroid plexus papilloma include obstruction of intraventricular CSF flow and blockage of CSF absorption due to raised protein levels and haemorrhage.

The interested reader is referred to the reviews of Milhorat (1985), Davson et al. (1987) and Leech (1989).

Spontaneous Hypoliquorrhoea Syndrome

The association of headaches with low spinal fluid pressure was first postulated by August Bier in 1898 as resulting from continuous leakage of cerebrospinal fluid (CSF) through the dural rent, following his own lumbar puncture-induced headache (see Chapter 4). Schaltenbrand was the first to describe a rare identical syndrome occurring spontaneously with no discernible precipitating cause and referred to it as "spontaneous aliquorrhoea" (Schaltenbrand, 1938). The syndrome has also been termed "spontaneous or primary intracranial hypotension", "spontaneous hypoliquorrhoea syndrome", or "spontaneous low CSF pressure headache". Fewer than 30 cases have been reported in the literature to date (Schaltenbrand, 1938; Hesser, 1946; Lindqvist and Moberg, 1949; Nosik, 1955; Bell et al., 1960; Lasater, 1970; Diamond and Baltes, 1973; Labadie et al., 1976; Lipman, 1977; Murros and Fogelholm, 1983; Baker, 1983; Gaukroger and Brownridge, 1987; Gibson et al., 1988; Rando and Fishman, 1992).

The clinical picture consists of a dull or throbbing fronto-occipital headache aggravated by the erect position and relieved by the supine position which may be accompanied by nausea, vomiting, backache, blurred vision, diplopia, photophobia, tinnitus, vertigo, and mental confusion (Fernandez, 1990). Characteristically jugular compression alleviates the symptoms (Mumenthaler, 1990). Neck stiffness can also be present, referred to as pseudomeningitis (Lindquist and Moberg, 1949; Bell et al., 1960). Neurological exam and ophthalmoscopic examination of the fundi are normal, although abducens paralysis has been reported in a few cases (Gibson et al., 1988; Bell et al., 1960).

Lumbar puncture is a necessity for the diagnosis. Pressure determination in the lateral recumbent position is usually below 40 mmHg (Bell et al., 1960) and can even be zero. Jugular compression as well as placing the patient in a sitting position may result in a small rise. If the spinal fluid pressure is lower than or the same as atmospheric pressure, no fluid may be obtained (Bell et al., 1960). CSF findings can be normal (Fernandez, 1990), however, a mild to moderate elevation of protein (usually less than 100 mg/dl), an increased number of red cells (usually less than 20/mm^3) and mild pleocytosis may be detected (Bell et al., 1960; Baker, 1983; Gibson et al., 1988; Fernandez, 1990). This is probably a result of diapedesis due to venous dilatation that occurs in low CSF pressure (Baker, 1983).

The aetiology of spontaneous hypoliquorrhoea syndrome remains unclear. In the original paper of Schaltenbrand (1938) three possible mechanisms were proposed:

1 decreased production of CSF;
2 hyperabsorption of CSF; and,
3 leakage of CSF.

No evidence for decreased CSF production has been described in the literature so far. Hyperabsorption has been shown in three cases (Labadie *et al.*, 1976; Kraemer *et al.*, 1987) where lumbar isotope cisternography revealed rapid diminution of radioactivity from the subarachnoid space with rapid appearance of the isotope in the bladder. Leakage mechanisms were found in three other cases. Nosik (1955) documented a dural sleeve tear at L3-4 diagnosed by myelography. Lasater *et al.* (1970) described a collection of protein-rich fluid in the subdural space, and Gibson *et al.* (1988) demonstrated CSF leakage into the epidural space at T5 by radioisotope cisternography. It has been contended that small dural rents may occur during human spinal development and may seal defectively (Lake *et al.*, 1974). Minimal trauma to the intraspinal structures may also create small dural tears (Lasater, 1970).

The course of the disease is benign – usually the headache and associated symptoms subside spontaneously after 2-16 weeks (Bell *et al.*, 1960; Diamond and Baltes, 1973). Bed rest, analgesics and hydration may be of some benefit (Mumenthaler, 1990). In two cases with evidence of CSF leakage successful relief of symptoms has been reported with epidural blood patch application (Baker, 1983; Gaukroger and Brownridge, 1987), and in one case with continuous epidural saline infusion (Gibson *et al.*, 1988). Epidural blood patch and epidural saline infusion are well established techniques in the treatment of post-lumbar headache with a success rate of 90-97% (Gibson *et al.*, 1988). Two cases with presumed hyperabsorption as the cause of hypoliquorrhoea associated headache have also been successfully treated with steroids (Kraemer *et al.*, 1987). However, therapeutic trials in the spontaneous hypoliquorrhoea syndrome remain anecdotal. Rando and Fishman (1992) have recently reported two further cases with CSF leaks demonstrated by radionucleotide cisternography. One of the cases responded to conservative treatment after 4 months, and the other responded to epidural saline infusion.

3. CSF as a Reflection of Cerebral Metabolism

The ways to take a direct biochemical approach to the study of the brain are limited to such methods as biopsy and post-mortem specimen analyses, cerebral arteriovenous differences in metabolite concentrations, PET scans or the study of the CSF. While examining the lumbar CSF is methodologically one of the simplest ways to study cerebral metabolism, it is first necessary to consider what assumptions (Moir *et al.*, 1970) are being made in this process.

First of all, it is necessary to have a method of analysis capable of detecting the desired organic compounds at the very low levels found in the CSF. Next one must be sure that the compound being investigated is derived from cerebral metabolism. This involves knowledge of both cerebral and subarachnoid metabolic pathways and products, as well as of the barrier and non-barrier regions bordering the CSF-containing compartments. Knowing that will help evaluate the assumption that the ventricular and lumbar CSF metabolite concentrations reflect the concentration in the adjacent regions of the brain.

Next, one must be aware that gradients of metabolites exist between ventricular (VCSF) and lumbar (LCSF) cerebrospinal fluid, and the assumption that LCSF will reflect VCSF must be evaluated. While it is hoped that LCSF will ultimately reflect cerebral function, it should be noted that a biochemical abnormality affecting cerebral metabolism is likely to affect metabolism in the spinal cord as well (Garelis *et al.*, 1974). Finally, the effects of diseases and drugs upon cerebral metabolism, metabolite transport, and resulting brain metabolite concentrations needs to be appreciated.

We will focus the discussion of these assumptions around the metabolites of three neurotransmitters – serotonin (5-HT), dopamine (DA), and norepinephrine (NE).

Each of these biogenic amines appears to have its own particular distribution in the brain and spinal cord. For example, in the spinal cord, neurons containing 5-HT and NE are more common than DA-containing neurons.

The pathways and products of 5-HT, DA and NE metabolism are outlined in Figs 3-1 and 3-2. Homovanillic acid (HVA), 5-hydroxy indoleacetic acid (5-HIAA), and 3-methoxy,4-hydroxymandelic acid (VMA) are acid metabolites of DA, 5-HT and NE, respectively. VMA does not appear to be the major product of CNS NE metabolism. However, MHPG, the alcohol metabolite of NE, may be. MHPG can be excreted either in its free form or as MHPG-sulfate. MHPG-sulfate is the major CNS NE metabolite in the rat, guinea pig, rabbit, and green monkey, while free MHPG is predominate in the cat, rhesus monkey and man (Wolfson and Escriva, 1976).

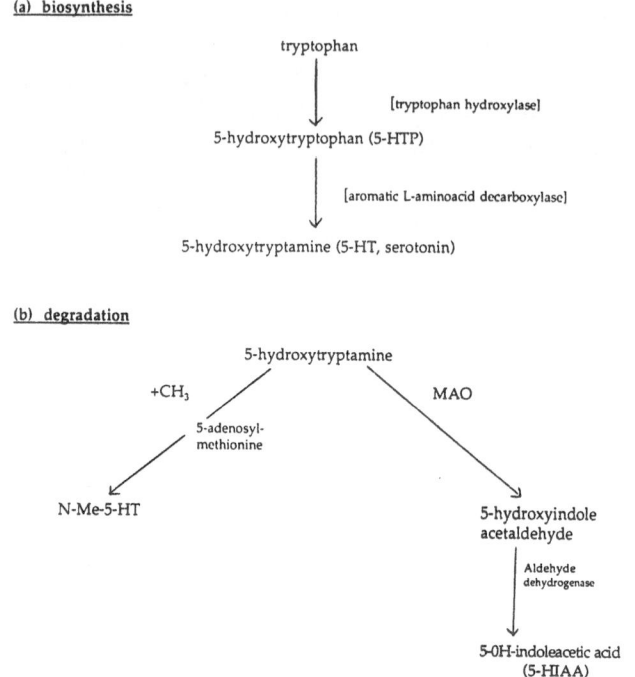

FIG. 3.1. Serotonin biosynthesis and degradation pathways.

After establishing metabolic pathways, one must be sure that the substance present in the CSF reflects metabolic activity of the CNS and not the rest of the body. If the substance does not readily pass the blood-brain or blood-CSF barriers, then the most likely source of the substance found in neuronal ECF and CSF is CNS metabolism. It is hoped that concentrations of these metabolites will provide an index of the turnover of the parent compound, in this case the monoamines, in the CNS. This has been established for the products HVA and 5-HIAA, by administering the labeled substance intravenously into cats and dogs and monitoring the brain and CSF levels of the compound. For the product MHPG, however, no relationship was found between concentrations in the urine and CSF, indicating they may be derived from different sources (Garelis et al., 1974; Moir et al., 1970).

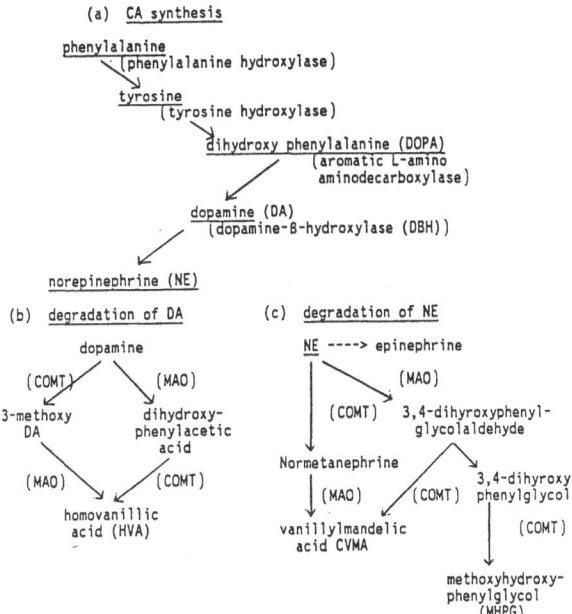

FIG. 3.2. Catecholamine biosynthesis and degradation pathways.

From the previous discussion of the brain-CSF interface, it seems likely that ventricular CSF concentrations would reflect concentrations of products in the adjacent brain. This has, in fact, been shown for the acid metabolites HVA and 5-HIAA from experiments with tryptophan, chlorpromazine, and enzyme inhibitors, and in patients with Parkinsonism (Garelis *et al.*, 1974; Moir *et al.*, 1970). In one canine experiment, the ratio of the concentrations of 5-HIAA or HVA in the caudate nucleus to the corresponding concentrations in the VCSF was constant, even after chlorpromazine treatment when the absolute concentrations were elevated (Moir *et al.*, 1970). Thus, providing no alteration occurs in the transport process for these organic acids, VCSF concentrations appear to reflect those in the adjacent brain tissue.

The critical point in the use of the CSF to evaluate cerebral processes comes in the use of the easily obtained LCSF to reflect VCSF. If both the brain and the spinal cord are affected by the same disease, such as a biochemical abnormality, it seems likely that any effect the spinal cord would have on the LCSF would be to further emphasise the changes in concentrations already effected by the brain. But how well will LSCF reflect changes in the brain without concomitant changes in the spinal cord?

An important issue is how much physical mixing there is between the ventricular and LCSF. Mixing between the cerebral and spinal CSF does occur with the oscillation of the CSF resulting from the arterial pulse and other factors influencing CSF pressure such as coughing, sneezing and physical movement in general. In the absence of physical movement, there is little evidence in man for a net flow of CSF along the spinal subarachnoid space, but motor activity can result in increased levels of metabolites in the lumbar CSF (Garelis et al., 1974). Bulat (1977) found in working with cats that, if precautions are taken so that changes in pressure and CSF flow do not occur, even a gradient of labelled 5-HIAA in cisternal CSF 100 times that of LCSF is not enough to result in labelled 5-HIAA appearing in the LCSF during the course of five hours.

Even though, and perhaps because activity is not always controlled prior to a study, ventricular metabolites do seem to end up in the LCSF. The mechanisms may include diffusion, physical mixing, and perhaps some bulk flow. Evidence for this has come from the study of gradients of the monoamine metabolite concentrations in the CSF between ventricular, cisternal and lumbar levels in control, CSF blockage and precursor loading studies. Moir et al. (1970) found the ventricular to lumbar (V/L) gradient for 5-HIAA to be 4.5:1 and for HVA to be 9:1 in man. These gradients are reduced by probenecid, a drug that inhibits organic acid transport systems that are present in the choroid plexus. While the steep gradient of HVA has been confirmed by other studies, the size of the 5-HIAA gradient is controversial (Sjostrom et al., 1975). MHPG and VMA have not been found to have a significant gradient. In addition to ventricular/lumbar gradients, Jakupcevic et al. (1977) reported that the fluid in the lumbar sac itself is not homogeneous for HVA and 5-HIAA. The site of lumbar puncture and the volume of CSF withdrawn during the procedure may affect these concentrations (Nordin et al., 1982).

Studies of humans with spinal lesions resulting in blockage of CSF flow have been used to try to separate spinal and cerebral metabolite contributions to the LCSF (Garelis and Sourkes, 1973). These studies present evidence that the majority of the HVA in the CSF originates primarily at the level of the lateral ventricle probably from the bordering caudate nucleus, while 5-HIAA appears to have both a significant cerebral and spinal cord origin. Some 23-37% of 5-HIAA in LCSF appears to be contributed by the spinal cord. The work of Sjostrom et al. (1975) on consecutive LCSF samples supports this conclusion. Their results suggest that lumbar levels of HVA reflect cerebral DA activity but that 5-HIAA, MHPG and VMA reflect 5HT and NE secreting neurons in both the brain and spinal cord. These findings correlate well with the known distribution of the various neurotransmitter containing neurons.

In order to answer completely the question of whether lumbar CSF reflects ventricular CSF, one must know all the means of ingress and egress for the compound in question. For the metabolites under consideration, 5-HIAA and HVA are both organic acids that are actively removed from the CSF by a saturable transport process located, in man, in the region of the fourth ventricle (Moir *et al.*, 1970). This transport process appears to be inhibited by probenecid and is probably located in the choroid plexus. The clearance of HVA and 5-HIAA from the CSF varies widely depending on the species studied (Garelis *et al.*, 1974). Studies on spinal subarachnoid perfusions of rhesus monkeys were performed to study the spinal transport of HVA (Kessler *et al.*, 1976 *a,b*). Despite its polar nature, HVA was found to enter capillaries within spinal tissue throughout the spinal cord, and this transport mechanism was largely insensitive to inhibition by probenecid. In another study, HVA was found to be released into the CSF by rhesus monkey spinal cord. Although the spinal cord was once considered to have little DA, more recent studies have shown that DA containing neurons are present and that HVA is produced by the spinal cord, although in quantitatively small amounts.

Bulat and Zivkovic (1978) measured HVA concentrations from cisternal and lumbar fluid in cats, collecting both by open drainage under slightly negative pressure. They found that, even with maximal flow of CSF, approximately 75% of HVA is lost from CSF during its course from the cisterna magna to the lumbar area. The low concentrations of HVA normally found in LCSF, they suggest, reflect the low levels of DA activity in the spinal cord.

Contrary evidence suggesting that lumbar fluid HVA is mainly derived from brain DA metabolism is provided by studies of Garelis *et al.* (1974) and Curzon (1975) wherein little or no HVA was detectable in LCSF when the CSF flow was blocked from above and little or no DA was found in the spinal cord. Stanley *et al.* (1985) also found concentrations of HVA in the cerebral cortex at autopsy to correlate positively with their CSF levels in the same individual, indicating that CSF may devive from cerebral DA metabolism.

Currently most of the HVA in CSF is considered to originate from brain parenchyma adjacent to the lateral ventricles, where the highest concentrations of DA are found (Wood, 1980*b*).

While 5-HIAA does not cross the blood-CSF or blood-brain barriers under normal physiologic conditions, its transport from CSF and CNS to blood is dependent upon an active transport system which can be blocked by probenecid (Moir *et al.*, 1970; Vogt, 1975). When this transport mechanism is blocked by probenecid, 5-HIAA then becomes capable of crossing the blood-CSF and blood-brain barriers. The active transport mechanisms thus serve to counteract these barriers (Wood, 1982*a*).

The relative contributions of brain and spinal cord to LCSF 5-HIAA levels are widely debated. The lumbosacral cord is rich in 5-HIAA which may diffuse into the adjacent CSF. Studies of patients with a partial or complete block of CSF circulation (Garelis and Sourkes, 1973) have provided evidence for a spinal cord origin for 23-37% of the 5-HIAA in LCSF. These figures, though assume that if HVA diffuses from the ventricular to the lumbar CSF then 5-HIAA should do so as well. They also assume that the egress of both compounds out of the CSF is the same, that the circulation of the CSF affects them the same, and that the difference in gradients reflects the spinal cord contribution to 5-HIAA. It is unknown, though how conditions below a spinal block alter CSF dynamics, with respect to these compounds.

Since no significant metabolism of labeled 5-HIAA infused into CSF pathways is thought to occur, Weir *et al.* (1973) performed experiments with anesthetised cats with labelled 5-HIAA to assess the relative cerebral component of LCSF 5-HIAA. The cats were perfused from the cisterna magna to the lumbar sac with an artificial CSF containing labelled 5-HIAA. Using this method they estimated that 40-70% of the 5-HIAA in LCSF was derived cerebrally. Others (Bulat, 1977) have criticised this technique as inducing an artificial craniocaudal flow and so increasing the cerebral component in LCSF.

Bowers (1970) studied changes in 5-HIAA concentrations in rabbit brain and cisternal CSF after administration of various agents affecting serotonin concentrations. The cisternal fluid levels clearly reflected the concentrations of 5-HIAA in brain tissue and they thus concluded that CSF levels of 5-HIAA reflect brain 5-HT metabolism. Bulat (1974) has also shown that changes in 5-HIAA concentration in spinal cord is reflected in the spinal fluid that bathes the cord.

Are determinations of 5-HIAA concentrations in clinically accessible lumbar fluid useful to gauge brain 5-HT metabolism, or do these determinations only reflect spinal cord metabolism for this substance? Bulat and Zivkovic (1971) and Bulat *et al.* (1974) demonstrated that there is little or no equilbration of 5-HIAA concentrations between the cisternal and spinal compartments either acutely (up to 7 hours after intracisternal injection of 5-HIAA) or chronically (up to 21 days after spinal cord injury in cats). Bulat *et al.* (1974) thus maintain that lumbar samplings of 5-HIAA reflect only 5-HT metabolism in adjacent lumbosacral cord. It would thus follow that it is not possible to obtain insight into the biochemistry of brain 5-HT by analyzing the lumbar fluid in this fashion. The studies of Weir *et al.* (1973) and of Garelis and Sourkes (1973), discussed above, however, suggest that it is possible to calculate the percentages of 5-HIAA in LCSF derived from spinal cord and brain, respectively. Stanley *et al.* (1985) have also found that concentrations of 5-HIAA simultaneously measured in brain and CSF at autopsy correlate positively for the same individual and suggest that CSF 5-HIAA may thus reflect brain metabolite levels. This debate is important in considering the use of LCSF as a diagnostic tool reflecting cerebral metabolism. If the site of the altered 5-HT metabolism is not uniform throughout the CNS but is remote from the lumbar sac, and there is little mixing of the CSF, LCSF 5-HIAA may not be of value in evaluating the lesion.

In contrast to the acid metabolites, MHPG clearance from the brain is not blocked by probenecid and lacks a specialised transport mechanism. It has been estimated, in cats, that one-third of the MHPG is cleared from the brain by bulk clearance of the CSF, and two-thirds by diffusion through the CSF and tissues to the capillaries (Wolfson and Escriva, 1976). The latter mechanism is rapid, cannot be blocked by probenecid, and may make lumbar levels of MHPG a poor index of NE metabolism.

Labelled MHPG administered intravenously does not, however, enter the LCSF in significant quantities (Gordon et al., 1975). This observation, along with the fact that levels of MHPG in LCSF correlate with NE concentrations in the same fluid, suggests that MHPG may reflect central noradrenergic activity (Wood, 1982a; Ziegler et al., 1979a,b). Whether or not MHPG follows a rostrocaudal gradient in CSF as does NE remains controversial. Ziegler et al. (1977) reported that the concentrations of MHPG and NE in LCSF progressively increase as additional CSF was removed from the lumbar puncture needle. However, earlier reports by Sjostrom et al. (1975) found MHPG to be evenly distributed throughout the CSF. Ruckebusch and Sutra (1984) also found similar levels of MHPG and NE in ventricular, cisternal and lumbar samplings of anaesthetised sheep.

MHPG has been very useful technically in measuring changes in adrenergic activity, since its concentrations in CSF are about 40 times greater than those of NE, which is at the lower limits of sensitivity with the fluorescent methods available (Fishman, 1980; Ziegler et al., 1976). Kopin et al. (1983) have shown that plasma and CSF concentrations of MHPG are highly correlated. CSF levels are maintained higher than plasma levels due to CNS production of MHPG, even in the presence of an adrenal tumour causing markedly increased peripheral synthesis (Kopin et al., 1983).

Since MHPG is a neutral metabolite of NE, its concentrations in CSF should not be affected by probenecid, a drug which interferes with the active transport of acidic metabolites from the CSF and into the blood. However, large doses of probenecid will result in a 60% increase in MHPG levels in the CSF (Ziegler et al., 1980). Probenecid administration also has been shown to increase plasma and CSF levels of NE (Lake et al., 1978). The probenecid-induced increases in CSF MHPG are thus more likely a result of the increased turnover of NE rather than due to changes in the clearance of MHPG (Ziegler et al., 1980; Lake et al., 1978).

Post et al. (1984a) have summarised the arguments for and against NE, MHPG and VMA reflecting brain or spinal cord NE metabolism (see Table 3-1).

TABLE 3-1. *Does NE, MHPG or VMA in lumbar CSF reflect brain or spinal cord norepinephrine metabolism? (modified from Post et al., 1984).*

Arguments for

Little i.v. labelled NE or MHPG enters CSF in patients

Large plasma-CSF dissociation in phaeochromocytoma

MHPG decreased in patients with cord transections

$MHPG-SO_4$ probenecid sensitive in rat and rabbit

VMA may be sensitive to probenecid blockade

MHPG in urine and CSF do not correlate

Locus coeruleus projects both rostrally and caudally (to spinal cord)

Locus coeruleus stimulation increases spinal cord NE and MHPG

50% of spinal cord MHPG is derived from the locus coeruleus projection

Plasma, not CSF, NE increased following dorsal column stimulation

CSF NE elevated following cerebellar stimulation

CSF NE decreased following caudate stimulation

CSF MHPG increased 50% in rat ventricular-cisternal perfusate following activation of the locus coeruleus

34% of CNS MHPG released into CSF; CSF MHPG reflects central NE turnover and locus coeruleus activity

Arguments against

No ventricular-lumbar MHPG gradient; MHPG and VMA higher in 4th ventricle

MHPG appearance higher after ventricular-cisternal than lumbar-cisternal perfusion

MHPG released from cord and exchanged with CSF

$MHPG-SO_4$ not sensitive to probenecid blockade in humans

No MHPG differences in patients with and without blocks in CSF flow

They conclude that there is still substantial ambiguity in the interpretation of LCSF NE metabolites but that CSF NE and metabolites may reflect a spinal cord source of NE with a contribution coming as well from neurons in the brainstem projecting from the locus coeruleus, which also projects to the forebrain. Concentration of spinal cord NE may thus parallel noradrenergic activity in part of these forebrain structures (Post *et al.*, 1984).

Last of all, in the use of LCSF to reflect CNS metabolism, one must have an understanding of how disease and drugs can alter CSF metabolite concentrations both directly, by altering metabolism, and indirectly, by altering transport functions in the CNS. For example, in parkinsonism, the low HVA levels in the CSF directly reflect the low DA levels in the brain. But drugs such as phenelzine, reserpine, and probenecid, as well as the disease state of hydrocephalus, are believed to alter CSF metabolite concentrations secondarily via an inhibition of the organic acid efflux system, in addition to any direct cerebral effects they might have (Moir *et al.*, 1970). We will look at some of the effects of disease states on LCSF composition in Chapters 6, 7 and 8.

4. Lumbar Puncture

The actual technique of lumbar puncture has not changed markedly since Quincke's description of the procedure in 1891. Prior to Quincke's lumbar puncture, Corning had performed the first dural puncture, injecting cocaine into the subarachnoid space at T11/12 – a dangerously high level – and Wynter had used a drainage procedure making an incision in the skin of a patient with tuberculous meningitis in the lumbar region to drain off CSF. Morton also used the method described by Wynter to treat tuberculous meningitis in 1891. While these early attempts at lumbar puncture were an improvement over trephining the skull, previously the only means of obtaining CSF, the method of Quincke using direct percutaneous puncture in the lumbar region was a vast improvement over his predecessors, both in terms of its simplicity and of its safety (Levinson, 1923). There have been few modifications of his procedure over the ensuing 100 years.

This chapter describes the indications, contraindications, technique, and complications of lumbar puncture. The techniques of cisternal and lateral cervical puncture and methods of ventricular fluid collection are performed less frequently by neurologists and psychiatrists and are thus not described here. The interested reader is referred to the reviews of Fishman (1992) and of Brumback (1989b) for descriptions of these techniques.

Indications for lumbar puncture (LP)

Lumbar puncture has its primary role in neurology and psychiatry as a diagnostic procedure. There are also however several important therapeutic indications for the procedure. Prior to the advent of antibiotics, CSF drainage using lumbar puncture was widely used in the treatment of meningitis. With antibiotics, lumbar puncture is no longer used, although it still is occasionally useful for symptomatic relief of back pain and headaches in patients with chronic meningitis. Similarly, lumbar puncture has been used in the treatment of benign intracranial hypertension. Lumbar puncture is currently used for intrathecal therapy, particularly the administration of intrathecal antibiotics for fungal infections and intrathecal chemotherapy for malignancy (see review of Herndon, 1989b). Lumbar puncture also has a therapeutic role in spinal anaesthesia and analgesia (see review of Lee *et al.*, 1985) and intrathecal baclofen has been reported to be effective in the treatment of spasticity (Penn and Kroin, 1987).

There are a growing number of indications for lumbar puncture as a diagnostic tool. Until the advent of CT and MRI scanning, lumbar puncture was widely used for ventriculography, pneumoencephalography, and isotope cisternography. One of the most common diagnostic indications of LP is that of myelography, which, with the use of newer water-soluble contrast agents and combined with CT scanning, has become a safer and more sensitive radiological procedure. Chapters 6, 7 and 8 of this volume deal with many of the current and potential indications for LP as a diagnostic tool in neurology and psychiatry.

Currently the major indication for lumbar puncture is in the diagnosis of meningitis. Lumbar puncture has both a high sensitivity and high specificity in the diagnosis of bacterial, tuberculous and fungal meningitis. Conditions where lumbar puncture is indicated and has a high sensitivity in diagnosis, but only a moderate specificity, include viral meningitis, subarachnoid haemorrhage, multiple sclerosis, neurosyphilis, inflammatory polyneuropathy, benign intracranial hypertension, and paraspinal abscess. Analysis of CSF is very specific for meningeal malignancy but is not a very sensitive test. LP may be considered to be both moderately sensitive and specific in the diagnosis of intracranial haemorrhage, viral encephalitis and subdural haematoma (Health and Public Policy Committee, American College of Physicians, 1986), but certainly intracranial haemorrhage and subdural haematomas are more appropriately diagnosed with neuroimaging.

Although CT scanning is clearly the procedure of choice in the diagnosis of acute subarachnoid haemorrhage, LP is a more sensitive diagnostic procedure than CT scanning and is indicated in cases where the CT is normal but clinical suspicion remains high. LP is a valuable adjunct to CT and MRI scanning, and electrodiagnostic tests in the diagnosis of multiple sclerosis, Guillain-Barré syndrome, and in CNS malignancy with meningeal involvement. In psychiatry, the use of LP is still primarily for the purpose of excluding neurological conditions. Its use as a research tool has however provided many valuable insights into the biochemistry of psychiatric disorders and these are discussed along with the various potential clinical indications in Chapter 7. Marton and Gean (1986), the Health and Public Policy Committee of the ACP (1986), and the ANN (1993) have recently reviewed the indications for, and cost effectiveness of, LP in clinical medicine. These are discussed further in Chapter 9.

Contraindications of lumbar puncture (LP)

The only absolute contraindication to LP is local infection and suppuration of the skin and deeper tissues in the lumbar area. In these cases, if analysis of CSF is essential, one should consider other techniques of obtaining CSF (e.g. lateral cervical puncture).

Lumbar puncture has, in animal models, been shown to cause bacterial meningitis in the presence of bacteraemia. There is also a number of case reports in the literature of patients developing meningitis following lumbar puncture in the presence of bacteraemia. The occurrence of meningitis resulting from lumbar puncture in a bacteraemic patient, however, is probably uncommon enough that bacteraemia should not be considered a contraindication to lumbar puncture. Indeed bacteraemia may often be considered an important indication for lumbar puncture to rule out concomitant meningitis (Eng and Seligman, 1981).

There are a number of important relative contraindications to lumbar puncture and one must carefully consider the risk/benefit ratio in any given patient. Evidence of increased intracranial pressure with focal neurological signs, is certainly one of the most important of these, due to the risk of transtentorial and foramen magnum herniation which may be fatal. Certainly any signs of progressive herniation should be considered an absolute contraindication to lumbar puncture. A careful neurological examination, with particular attention to any evidence of papilloedema, is important prior to the procedure. In centres where CT scanning is readily available it is ideal to obtain a CT scan prior to LP. Papilloedema in and of itself is not an absolute contraindication to lumbar puncture, as the overall incidence of serious complications in patients with papilloedema due to various causes is only about 1.2% (Korein *et al.*, 1959).

It is important to consider the cause and nature of the increased intracranial pressure when assessing the risk in an individual patient. CT scanning has greatly reduced the need for LP in subarachnoid haemorrhage, haematomas, angiomas, and infarction. Certainly LP is a safe procedure in patients with papilloedema due to benign intracranial hypertension, but should be considered dangerous if the papilloedema is related to an intracranial mass, particularly in the posterior fossa. Gower *et al.* (1987) have suggested CT scanning guidelines for lumbar puncture, suggesting that all patients have enhanced and unenhanced scans prior to LP and that evidence of unequal intracranial pressures be considered contraindications to lumbar puncture, specifically:

1) CT evidence of unequal pressures across the midline (*falx cerebri*), noted by shift of midline structures (septum pellucidum, third ventricle) or

2) CT evidence of unequal pressures between supratentorial and infratentorial compartments – downward or upward herniation.

Evidence of increased supratentorial pressure may be manifest by loss of suprachiasmatic and circummesencephalic cisterns. Evidence of a posterior fossa mass is the most critical contraindication to LP and is often difficult to pick up on CT. Evidence suggesting this includes a shift, compression or obliteration of the fourth ventricle, symmetrical obstructive hydrocephalus or upward transtentorial herniation of the cerebellar vermis. Obliteration of the superior cerebellar cistern and quadrigeminal plate cistern caudal to the midbrain may also be indirect evidence of upward herniation (Gower *et al.* 1987). MRI scanning may often be necessary to delineate posterior fossa lesions.

Other important relative contraindications to lumbar puncture are the presence of a bleeding disorder, the use of anticoagulants, and the presence of a low platelet count below 50 000 / mm^3. CSF bleeding occurs in up to 20% of patients who have undergone LP, usually a result of a puncture of one of the spinal venous plexi. Certainly in most patients such bleeding produces no symptoms but in patients with coagulation deficits, there is a markedly increased risk of serious complications of haemorrhage. Ruff and Dougherty (1981) reported an incidence of 6.7% of serious complications included paraparesis, severe radicular pain and spinal haematomas in patients given anticoagulants after a lumbar puncture. Those who received anticoagulants within one hour of the lumbar puncture were clearly at the greatest risk of bleeding complications. Anticoagulants should clearly then not be administered within one hour of LP. Due to the risk of subarachnoid haemorrhage and epidural spinal haematomas with compression of the cauda equina, lumbar puncture should be performed in patients with low platelet counts only for critical indications. The administration of a platelet transfusion prior to lumbar puncture (as well as after if symptoms develop) should be considered in patients with counts below 20 000 /mm^3 if lumbar puncture is considered to be essential in individual patients. Similarly, in patients on heparin, one should consider discontinuation of heparin or administration of protamine, prior to LP. Patients taking coumadin may have the risk of haemorrhagic complications minimised with administration of vitamin K or fresh frozen plasma prior to LP.

Complications

The overall complication risk of disabling or persistent symptoms has been estimated to be between 0.19% and 0.43% (Wiesel *et al.*, 1985). The most serious complications of haemorrhage, herniation, and infection (discussed above) can be minimised with appropriate consideration of indications and contraindications for the procedure, neurological examination and CT scanning prior to LP, and careful monitoring after the procedure for high risk patients.

Another potentially serious complication of LP is the iatrogenic development of CNS tumours. Reports in the literature suggest that the use of unstyletted needles in the procedure of LP carries the risk of introducing a viable fragment of skin into the spinal canal, causing an epidermoid tumour to develop some years later (Manno *et al.*, 1962; Shaywitz, 1972; Batnitzky *et al.*, 1977; Gardner *et al.*, 1989). The significance of this risk clinically is still debated (Fishman, 1980; Herndon and Brumback, 1989*b*) and the evidence is largely correlational. Epidermoid tumours occurring with a previous history of lumbar puncture appear to be less likely to be multiple, intramedullary, associated with the cauda equina or associated with congenital spinal abnormalities as compared to epidermoid tumours occurring with no previous history of lumbar puncture (Manno *et al.*, 1962). Although some paediatricians will use unstyletted butterfly needles or standard venepuncture needles in neonates to simplify the procedure of lumbar puncture, there is no evidence that this reduces the incidence of traumatic or unsuccessful lumbar puncture. Due to the possible risk of implantation of epidermoid tumours, this practice should be avoided (Halliday, 1989). The implantation of malignant cells by lumbar puncture in acute leukaemia has also been suggested as a potential complication of the procedure and it has been recommended that one wait until the peripheral blood is cleared of blast cells (Brown, 1976). There is however no clear evidence to support this happening clinically (Fishman, 1992).

The most common complication of lumbar puncture is that of post lumbar puncture headache (PLPH). The reported incidence of the PLPH varies between 0.4% and 70% (Cook *et al.*, 1989) with most reporting an incidence of 15-30%. August Bier, who pioneered spinal analgesia and worked at the same hospital as Quincke at Kiel, first reported headache and vomiting as features of convalescence in his first six patients. To investigate this further Bier and his assistant, Hildenbrandt, performed the procedure on each other. Bier's procedure was unsuccessful as the syringe did not fit the needle properly. The success of spinal analgesia in his assistant was evidenced by a series of excruciating tests, including a sharp blow with an iron hammer on the shin. Bier, however, developed typical symptoms of PLPH, and was nursed for several days afterwards by his chief's wife (Lee *et al.*, 1985). He thus was able to give a very accurate first hand account of PLPH with a clear description of the postural accentuation. His assistant was also ill for several days afterwards with vomiting. This possibly related to a lack of sterility in the original procedure, with tap water used to dissolve the cocaine crystals. Bier postulated that his headache was related to leakage of cerebrospinal fluid.

Bier's hypothesis of continued CSF leakage occurring after LP has since been substantiated by direct observation during laminectomy and with radio-isotope myelography, myeloscopy, and autopsy studies (Olsen, 1987). It is thought that this leakage, which may exceed 40 ml, causes a state of decreased CSF volume and pressure which, in turn, produces a downward "sagging" effect on the brain leading to a stretching of pain-sensitive vessels and dura (Fernandez, 1990). Although reduced CSF pressure has been observed following lumbar puncture, there is no clear relationship between the degree of CSF hypotension and the occurrence of headache. Grant *et al.* (1991) studied intracranial CSF volume with MRI imaging in 20 patients before and 24 hours after LP. They found CSF volume decreased in 19 of 20 patients, largely from cortical sulci. With the exception of two patients with headaches who had a large decrease in intracranial CSF volume, there was no apparent relationship between the occurrence of headache and the change in intracranial CSF volume. Patients with PLPH tended to have slightly lower volumes than those without PLPH but this was not statistically significant. They found no evidence of "brain sagging", although their scans were done with the patients in the recumbent position.

An alternative mechanism proposed to explain post lumbar puncture headaches is that of vasodilatation caused by a difference between intravascular and extravascular pressures. This may relate to the decrease in CSF volume causing activation of adenosine receptors resulting in vasodilatation. This is supported by: (1) the reciprocal CSF volume changes as measured by MRI in response to cerebral vasodilatation brought on by hypercapnia and the similarities between PLPH and headache induced by CO_2 inhalation; (2) the direct observation that veins, but not arteries, undergo dilatation after CSF drainage through the cisterna magnum using cranial windows in cats; (3) the exacerbation of PLPH by jugular compression; and (4) the efficacy of caffeine and theophylline in PLPH which cause intracerebral arterial constriction, perhaps due to blockade of brain adenosine receptors (Forbes and Nasor, 1935; Fernandez, 1990; Raskin, 1990; Grant et al., 1991).

Kaplan (1967) has suggested a psychogenic aetiology of PLPH. They performed a double-blind study on 100 prison inmates and found a similar incidence in headache occurring after both diagnostic lumbar puncture and sham lumbar puncture and a much higher incidence of PLPH in those with anxiety about headaches prior to LP. The incidence of headache was recorded only by visits to the sick-bay physician after the procedure. This study is flawed by the lack of description of the headache occurring after lumbar puncture and by the possible compounding factor of increased drug-seeking behaviour in inmate populations. Vandam and Dripps (1956) in their study of over 10 000 patients receiving spinal anaesthetics, gave spinal anaesthetics to 100 persons who had been anaesthetised first with general anaesthetics without telling the patients that the spinal anaesthetics had been administered. They found the same percentage occurrence of typical postural headaches as in their series at large. This then argues strongly against a significant role for a psychogenic aetiology of PLPH.

The most likely mechanism then of PLPH at this time, appears to be through a volume compensation, accommodated by cerebral venous drainage pathways, resulting in venous vasodilation. This may be mediated by adenosine receptor activation. A direct effect of CSF hypotension and decreased volume causing tension on pain sensitive structures by a "sagging" effect of the intracranial contents is suggested by the exacerbation of PLPH in the upright posture with the effect of gravitational forces diverting CSF into the spinal subarachnoid space.

While the study of Grant *et al.* (1991) argues against a direct "sagging" effect, they did not control for postural or gravitational effects. Further imaging studies and the measurement of cerebral blood flow before and after LP should help to elucidate the relative roles of decreased CSF volume and pressure and venous vasodilatation in the pathogenesis of PLPH.

PLPH usually begins within two days of lumbar puncture but may be delayed for up to one to two weeks. It is described as a dull ache or throbbing sensation affecting predominantly the occipital and frontal areas and is often associated with nausea, low back pain, neck pain, and blurred vision. Such headaches are exacerbated by standing, Valsalva manoeuvre and jugular pressure, and will rapidly improve by lying flat. Decrease in CSF volume may occasionally cause labyrinthine dysfunction resulting in hearing loss or tinnitus (Raskin, 1990). The headache usually lasts three to four days, but may occasionally persist for weeks or even for months. It is twice as common in women as in men, and occurs less frequently in children and in the elderly (Vandam and Dripps, 1956). It is less common when performed for spinal anaesthesia than for diagnostic LP. This is most likely related to the restoration of volume with fluid, the better technique of anaesthesiologists, the smaller needles used, and perhaps the use of the anaesthetic agent itself (Fernandez, 1990).

Brocker (1958) in a study of 894 patients using an 18 gauge needle, found an incidence of less than 0.5% of PLPH in patients placed in the prone position after LP, compared to 36.5% in those kept supine. Handler *et al.* (1982) was not able to replicate these findings, finding no difference between his supine and prone position groups after LP. A number of investigators have suggested 24 hours supine bed rest following LP for prevention of PLPH, but recent studies have not shown this to be necessary (Carbaat and van Crevel, 1981; Cook *et al.* 1989). There is even some evidence to suggest that, at least after spinal anaesthesia, early mobilisation may actually have a beneficial effect on both the incidence and intensity of PLPH (Thornberry and Thomas, 1988). The removal of the needle with the patient prone and the foot of the examining table raised has also been suggested to prevent PLPH. Keeping the patient in this position for 30 min after the procedure may allow time for sealing of the dural hole with the resultant negative hydrostatic pressure in the lumbar subarachnoid space (Easton, 1979). The efficacy of this procedure however needs further study (Hilton-Jones *et al.*, 1982; Raskin, 1990). Both increased and decreased fluid intake have also been proposed in the prevention of PLPH but there is no clear evidence to suggest that the incidence of PLPH is related to the patient's fluid intake or state of hydration (Dieterich and Brandt, 1988). The use of intravenous fluids has also been suggested but its efficacy has not yet been adequately studied.

The most conclusive method of preventing PLPH has been with the use of smaller calibre needles. Vandam and Dripps (1956) studied over 10 000 patients undergoing spinal anaesthesia and found the incidence of PLPH reduced by 50% and 66% using 22 and 24 gauge needles respectively, compared to the use of 16 gauge needles. Flatten *et al.* (1989) found the incidence of PLPH using 26 gauge needles to be 6.7% and found no headaches using 29 gauge needles in their series of 149 patients. Although the use of smaller needles for spinal anaesthesia does clearly decrease the risk of PLPH, their use in diagnostic LP is not optimal due to the slow return of fluid and a lack of reliability in assessing pressure dynamics. For diagnostic LPs a 20-22 gauge needle is thus generally preferable.

The orientation of the needle is also important for prevention of PLPH. Although cadaver studies have not demonstrated any difference in the size of the dural hole made by different bevel orientations, Norris *et al.* (1989) and others have shown that orienting the bevel of the needle parallel to the longitudinal dural fibres significantly diminishes the incidence of PLPH clinically following spinal anaesthesia.

Most cases of PLPH may be treated with oral analgesics and usually subside over a few days. However there are occasional patients who become severely debilitated and in whom the headache may last for weeks or months. Intravenous caffeine and epidural blood patches or saline are all effective in treatment of these patients. Sechzer and Abel (1988) showed a dramatic effect of intravenous caffeine using a single 500 mg dose in a double-blind study with 75% of their patients improving after one dose. This success rate increased to 85% when a second dose was given two hours later. Theophylline, which also probably acts on adenosine receptors, may also be an effective oral treatment (Raskin, 1990). In those patients who do not respond to intravenous caffeine, the use of an epidural blood patch has been shown in a number of studies to be effective in the treatment of PLPH, including one recent double-blind trial (Seebacher *et al.*, 1989). While usually a very safe and effective procedure, it does have potential complications of back pain, occurring in up to one-third of patients, with less common complications of paraesthesiae and meningismus. Epidural saline may also be useful when other methods are ineffective (see reviews of Raskin, 1990 and Fernandez, 1990).

Back pain is another common important complication of lumbar puncture and minor local backache is frequently reported. Rarely actual disc herniation may occur and the spinal cord itself may be injured if LP is attempted at too high a level. This is a particularly important complication to be aware of in children, where the cord descends more caudally than in adults. Irritation of the roots of the cauda equina resulting in radicular pain and dysaesthesia may also occur in up to 13%, and a painful root syndrome may be caused by entrapment of a lumbar nerve root in the lumen of the spinal needle tip or by entrapment of a nerve filament in the lumen by the insertion of the stylet (Dripps and Vandam, 1951; Brown, 1976). Young and Burney (1971) have reported one case of nerve filament entrapment by insertion of the stylet causing backache and leg pain. Trupp (1977) reported two cases of lumbar nerve root aspiration causing severe pain and requiring laminectomy which he felt was due to failure to reinsert the stylet prior to withdrawal of the needle.

Other possible complications of lumbar puncture include the subdural injection of contrast medium into a subdural collection of CSF from a previous lumbar puncture, and the occurrence of arachnoiditis due to spinal anaesthesia and myelography. Chronic adhesive arachnoiditis is more likely to occur as the result of myelography when there is subarachnoid blood. In the past, a traumatic tap was therefore reason to postpone myelography unless an urgent study was required, but this is no longer necessary with the use of water-soluble contrast agents (Fishman, 1992).

Technique of lumbar puncture

The procedure should first be adequately explained to the patient and informed consent obtained, particularly in high risk lumbar punctures. A blood glucose should be drawn immediately prior to the procedure ideally with the patient in a fasting state for at least four hours to allow for the equilibrium between blood and CSF glucose values, so that the CSF glucose may be appropriately interpreted. The patient is positioned lying on his/her side with the knees drawn up to the chest and the head slightly flexed. If the physician is right handed, it is usually most comfortable to have the patient lie on his/her left side and conversely on the right side if the physician is left handed. The table should be a firm flat surface and be at a comfortable level for the physician, ideally at eye level. If the LP cannot readily be performed with the patient lying on their side, it may also be done with the patient in the sitting position, but pressure measurements are more difficult to interpret in this position. If the sitting position is used, and if pressure measurements are desired, it is usually easier to reinsert the stylet once puncture of the dura has been achieved and assist the patient to the conventional lying position for manometric measurements. An assistant for reassuring and positioning the patient is extremely valuable.

A history of any related allergic reaction to iodine should be obtained, and if positive other antiseptics used in its place. The patient's back should be washed in concentric circles with iodine-soaked sponges beginning at the site of the LP and working out 2-3 times, and the area should then be cleaned with alcohol-soaked sponges, washing off all of the iodine. Gloves should be changed at this point to avoid the introduction of iodine into the subarachnoid space, taking care not to contaminate the needle with the powder from the inside of the gloves. The patient should be covered with a sterile drape, but drapes with a hole in the middle should be avoided as this may prevent proper visualisation of the patient's back.

The physician should have all equipment ready prior to introducing the needle. This is usually provided for in commercially available disposable lumbar puncture trays, and should include a 20 or 22 gauge LP needle, a stopcock attached to a manometer, and three or four sterile test tubes with stoppers. The L3-L4 interspace may be located by imagining a line connecting the superior iliac crests on each side. The physician should identify the L3-L4 interspace by palpation along the midline of the back. The spinal cord ends at L1 in 90% of adults but may extend as low as L2-L3. The needle may thus be inserted safely at L3-L4 or alternatively at L4-L5 or L5-S1. The L5-S1 interspace is often difficult to reach from the midline because the spine of the 5th lumbar vertebra gets in the way and a paramedian approach may be easier if this interspace needs to be used (see Lee *et al.* 1985).

The area of lumbar puncture should be anaesthetised with a 1 or 2% solution of lignocaine, producing a small wheal at the site with a short 26 gauge needle. The addition of adrenaline is not necessary. One may also inject the deeper layers of the dermis but there is no need to inject deep into the muscle tissue. A 20 gauge spinal needle is used in most instances. The needle must have a properly fitting stylet. The needle should puncture the wheal of local anaesthetic a few millimetres from the entry point of the anaesthetising needle. This is to avoid contamination with blood that might be beneath this site. The needle is inserted in the midline, midway between the chosen spinous processes and angled to a point 10-15 degrees cephalad (more or less directed toward the umbilicus). The bevel of the needle is oriented so that the fibres of the dura mater and the ligamentum flavum are split rather than cut, i.e. parallel with long axis of the spinal cord. The needle is advanced slowly in steps of 3-4 mm at which point the stylet is removed between each advancement to check for the flow of CSF. When the needle has passed through the ligamentum flavum, there is often a slight "give" or "pop" sensation felt. The needle will then have usually reached the subarachnoid space and CSF will appear when the stylet is removed. This is usually at a depth of 4-4.5 cm.

If no fluid appears when the stylet is removed, it should be reinserted and the needle rotated 90 degrees, with the bevel pointing cephalad and removal of the stylet at that point will usually result in the appearance of CSF. If there is still no CSF obtained, one may advance the needle a few millimetres further and again withdraw the stylet, taking care not to introduce the needle too far as puncture of the venous plexus anterior to the cord is the most common cause of a traumatic tap. If, with further advancement, there is still no flow of CSF, the needle should be taken out almost to the skin surface and then re-directed. Fluid should not be aspirated with a syringe.

After the first drop of CSF is obtained to assure CSF flow, the manometer with the stopcock are placed onto the needle as quickly as possible to measure the opening pressure. Pulsation synchronous with the pulse (2-5 mm) and synchronous with respiration (4-10 mm) will normally be observed. In measuring the pressure one must be sure that the craniovertebral axis is horizontal. The normal range is generally from 70-180 mm CSF. The patient should uncurl when measuring the pressure to decrease the intra-abdominal pressure. The patient should be asked to relax and also not to hyperventilate as this may spuriously lower the CSF pressure by decreasing $PaCO_2$. One may assure that there is free unobstructed flow of CSF by asking the assistant to apply firm pressure on the patient's abdomen. This should produce a quick rise in the pressure, followed by a rapid fall after cessation. If the CSF pressure is found to be above 200 mm, one should wait for a couple of minutes and be sure that the patient is adequately relaxed as tension may also spuriously increase CSF pressure. If the patient is using a respirator, this should be briefly disconnected if possible, as positive pressure will also cause a false elevation of CSF pressure.

If the CSF pressure is clearly found to be elevated some authors state that the pressure should be observed for several minutes and the procedure terminated with only the fluid within the manometer used for diagnostic analysis (Tourtellotte and Shorr, 1982; Wood, 1985). Others suggest that the stopcock be turned frequently to monitor the falling CSF pressure and that the CSF be drained very slowly with no more fluid removed when the CSF pressure has fallen to one-half of the initial pressure (Fishman, 1980). Brumback (1989b) suggests that once lumbar puncture is undertaken that there is no reason not to collect sufficient CSF as this represents only a small portion of the fluid that may be lost by leakage after needle removal. Now that micro-techniques are available for cell counts and total protein determination, the fluid in the manometer should usually be sufficient for most diagnostic tests. It is thus prudent to minimise the amount of CSF collected under these circumstances even though this is a comparatively small amount relative to that which may be lost after removal of the needle.

If the CSF pressure is elevated above 400 mm then no CSF should be collected until the pressure has been reduced with intravenous mannitol (1.5-2.0 g/kg over a 30 min period) with the needle still in place. An alternative is the very slow removal of CSF (1-4 drops/min) (Wolpow, 1978), if mannitol is not readily available.

If a patient is noted to have very low CSF pressure, and if any signs of spinal cord involvement are present, one should consider the possibility of a spinal subarachnoid block. Large amounts of protein in the CSF in such patients may cause a yellow or orange tinge in the first few millimetres of CSF (e.g. Froin's syndrome). This may be associated with clot formation of CSF after removal. No fluid should be removed if a LP is performed on a patient who turns out to have a spinal subarachnoid block. Rather the needle should be left in place with the stylet and urgent myelography performed, as it may be very difficult to re-enter the lumbar subarachnoid space after the initial LP. If a spinal block is found, one should consider intravenous mannitol until definitive therapy for the block can be arranged, as this may help to minimise the risk of deterioriation in neurological function which may be precipitated by lumbar puncture where spinal block results from a mass lesion (Brumback, 1989*b*).

The Queckenstedt test is used to detect the presence of a spinal subarachnoid block during lumbar puncture. Due to the use of myelography, CT scanning, and MRI scanning this test is no longer indicated except in a few circumstances, e.g. in patients with chronic meningitis to assess whether patients may be developing a partial or complete spinal block. It may be useful in a variety of patients with arachnoiditis, meningeal lymphoma and carcinoma, sarcoidosis, and patients receiving therapy for fungal and tuberculous meningitis (Fishman, 1992). In these patients repeated myelograms are not indicated and the Queckenstedt test may give a useful guide to the progress of his/her meningeal disease.

The test consists of 10 sec of manual compression of the jugular veins bilaterally. With jugular compression, the CSF pressure will rise 10-30 cm above the baseline pressure and fall to the baseline pressure within 10 sec of release. The neck should be kept in the neutral position (neither flexed nor extended) during the test. The use of a paediatric sphygmomanometer is preferable to manual jugular compression and may be inflated to 20 mm for a period of 10 sec and then abruptly released to zero. The CSF pressure will normally rise to twice the baseline value. A partial spinal block may cause a slow or partial rise or fall in the recorded pressure. No rise in the lumbar CSF pressure with jugular compression indicates a complete spinal block. If the jugular compression test indicates either a partial or complete spinal block, the needle should be left in place and an urgent myelogram performed.

The Tobey-Ayer Test consists of manual compression of the jugular vein unilaterally, which should normally produce only a slight change in CSF pressure unless there is obstruction of one of the lateral venous sinuses. These tests are only valid if one is using a spinal needle that is 20 gauge or larger. (See Fishman 1992 for review.)

The fluid from the lumbar puncture should be collected into at least three sterile tubes with 2-3 ml of CSF in each tube. The first tube is often used for protein and glucose analysis and for microscopic examination. The second tube is often used for culture and sensitivities, and the third for cell count and serology. If blood is obtained during lumbar puncture, it is useful to obtain cell counts in three separate tubes to differentiate between traumatic puncture and subarachnoid haemorrhage. After the desired amount of fluid has been obtained, the closing pressure is recorded. This gives an indication of the volume of the CSF reservoir. A large decrease in the closing pressure compared to the opening pressure is indicative of a small reservoir of fluid, e.g. spinal block. A large reservoir of fluid, on the other hand, will cause only a small decrease in pressure, e.g. in hydrocephalus. After measurement of the closing pressure, the needle should be removed. As discussed earlier there is some controversy concerning the reinsertion of the stylet before removal of the needle. It is probably prudent, however, to remove the needle without replacement of the stylet to avoid entrapment of nerve roots.

After removal of the needle, the area should be vigorously rubbed with an antiseptic to obliterate the needle track and appropriately dressed. In patients who have undergone high risk lumbar puncture, and particularly in patients where the CSF pressure was found to be elevated, one should observe closely for evidence of neurological deterioration after LP and hyperosmolar agents administered if there is any evidence of this. After the procedure care should be taken for the CSF samples to be delivered immediately to the laboratory for analysis. This is particularly important as the total white cell count may decrease as much as 50% in the first half hour if a CSF specimen is allowed to sit at room temperature, due to cell adherence and lysis. Polymorphonuclear leukocytes are more susceptible to lysis than lymphocytes, and the cell count does not therefore decrease proportionally (Meena *et al.*, 1989). Following the procedure, the LP should be clearly documented with the opening and closing pressures and the amount of CSF withdrawn stated. Although increased fluid intake and bed rest are frequently recommended for patients following LP, their efficacy in preventing PLPH has not been clearly substantiated (see discussion above).

Lumbar puncture in infants and children

LP in children is often a difficult procedure and in neonates up to half of lumbar punctures attempted may be unsuccessful. The main indication for lumbar puncture in a neonate is in the diagnosis of meningitis. It may also be useful in suspected subarachnoid haemorrhage where the ultrasound scan or CT is normal, but clinical suspicion is high. There is however, considerable controversy in the paediatric literature as to the indications for lumbar puncture in a neonate or infant even in confirming the diagnosis of meningitis (see Addy, 1987; Neville, 1988; and Halliday, 1989). The sitting position may be easier in many infants, and it may be preferable to have the neck extended rather than flexed. Although some authors (Greensher *et al.*, 1971) have advocated the use of unstyletted butterfly needles for lumbar puncture in neonates, this should be avoided because of the risk of epidermoid tumours (Halliday, 1989). The lowest possible interspace should be used in infants as the conus medullaris extends much lower in the spinal canal. As the distance that one must advance the LP needle in children may vary, Bonadio *et al.* (1988) have devised a formula based on body surface area (m^2) to predict the depth of the LP, in order to minimise the rate of traumatic puncture: depth of LP = 0.77 cm + 2.56 (m^2). In most infants, the depth of lumbar puncture should not exceed 2.5 cm.

The Quality Standards Subcommittee of the American Academy of Neurology (1993) have recently outlined the indications for lumbar puncture in children and these are detailed in Chapter 9.

5. Composition of CSF

Introduction

Many clinicians still consider the chemical make-up of CSF much in the same way that Halliburton (1917) conceived of it, i.e. as a "modified tap water" perhaps with just a dash of sugar and protein. He/she will routinely look at the CSF only for general appearance, cell count, protein, glucose, and bacterial cultures. Le Wontin *et al.* (1984) has compared the study of CSF and other body fluid composition in schizophrenia with the Roman augurs' examination of animal entrail, whereas Thompson (1988) refers to the CSF as a "Cinderella fluid", speaking of the recent surge of interest focused on its composition.

While it is true that 99% of the CSF is composed of water, one must consider that this fluid is in dynamic equilibrium with the ECF of the brain and spinal cord and thus may reflect the activity of the CNS. The composition of the remaining 1% can thus provide a vast amount of information for the clinician. Normal values for some of the main CSF constituents are shown in Table 5-1. Alterations in the concentrations of many CSF constituents which are not currently used in routine clinical practice may someday prove as valuable as many of the numerous laboratory tests now used for the analysis of blood. It is the purpose of this chapter to look at the major constituents of CSF and investigate their role in health and disease.

Various Factors Affecting the Composition of CSF

Developmental changes in CSF composition in infancy and childhood

Age is an important variable to take into account in assessing and interpreting CSF findings. Childhood normal ranges appear to differ significantly from adult ranges, although the most significant variation is seen in the first few months of life (Trotter and Rust, 1989). The differences involve cell count, glucose levels, proteins, and marked developmental changes in blood-brain barrier function. Normal values are presented.

Cell count
In a study of preterm infants between 26 and 40 weeks Rodriguez *et al.* (1990) found a decrease in the mean CSF leucocyte count from the 26th week ($6\pm 10/mm^3$, range 0-44) to the 34th week ($4\pm 3/mm^3$, range 1-11).

TABLE 5.1. Normal values for various CSF constituents (from Lentner, 1981).

Lumbar CSF unless otherwise stated		Amount of substance				Mass			
		unit	mean	s	(Extreme range)	unit	mean	s	(Extreme range)
Inorganic substances									
Bicarbonate									
Chloride	37 subjects	mmol/l	123.3	2.5	-	g/l	4.37	0.089	-
	100 subjects	mmol/l	125	3.0	119-131	g/l	4.43	0.11	4.21-4.65
Phosphorus		μmol/l	-	-	(542-649)	mg/l	-	-	(7.3-20.1)
total	70 subjects	μmol/l	520	74	(442-694)	mg/l	16.1	2.3	(13.7-21.5)
inorganic	47 subjects	μmol/l	433	74	(371-668)	mg/l	13.1	2.3	(11.5-20.7)
Lipid phosphorus		μmol/l	7.1	1.3	-	mg/l	0.22	0.04	-
Sulphur inorganic									
Fluoride		μmol/l	5	-	-	mg/l	0.1	-	-
Bromide		μmol/l	29	-	(18-48)	mg/l	2.3	-	(1.4-3.8)
Iodine		nmol/l	16	-	-	μg/l	2	-	-
Thiocyanate		μmol/l	-	-	(5.2-50)	mg/l	-	-	(0.3-2.9)
Potassium	37 subjects	mmol/l	2.84	0.17	-	mg/l	111	6.6	-
	102 subjects	mmol/l	2.96	0.17	-	mg/l	116	6.6	103-129
	15 subjects	mmol/l	2.8	0.2	-	mg/l	109	7.8	-
Suboccipital CSF, 15 subjects		mmol/l	2.5	0.2	-	mg/l	98	7.8	-
Sodium	37 subjects	mmol/l	147.0	2.6	-	g/l	3.38	0.060	-
	102 subjects	mmol/l	145	3.9	137-153	g/l	3.33	0.090	3.15-3.51
	15 subjects	mmol/l	145	3.6	-	g/l	3.33	0.082	-

TABLE 5.1. Cont.

Lumbar CSF unless otherwise stated	Amount of substance unit	mean	s	(Extreme range)	Mass unit	mean	s	(Extreme range)
Suboccipital CSF, 15 subjects	mmol/l	146	2.5	-	g/l	3.36	0.057	-
Calcium 37 subjects	mmol/l	1.32	0.12	-	mg/l	52.9	4.8	-
50 subjects	mmol/l	1.19	0.08	1.02-1.34	mg/l	47.7	3.2	41.3-54.1
Magnesium 37 subjects	mmol/l	1.12	0.07	-	mg/l	27.2	1.7	-
81 subjects	mmol/l	0.89	0.17	0.55-1.23	mg/l	21.6	4.1	13.4-29.8
11 subjects	mmol/l	1.12	0.09	-	mg/l	27.2	2.2	-
Iron 23 subjects	µmol/l	0.8	0.4	(0.3-1.5)	µg/l	45	22	(17-84)
Copper (a) 30 children	µmol/l	-	-	(0.28-0.24)	µg/l	-	-	(18-27)
(b) 15 subjects	µmol/l	0.25	0.06	-	µg/l	16	4	-
Manganese	nmol/l	-	-	(15-27)	µg/l	-	-	(0.83-1.50)
Zinc 30 children	µmol/l	-	-	(0.37-0.61)	µg/l	-	-	(24-40)
2 subjects	µmol/l	-	-	(0.35-0.92)	µg/l	-	-	(23-60)

TABLE 5.1. Cont.

Lumbar CSF unless otherwise stated		Amount of substance				Mass			
		unit	mean	s	95% range (Extreme range in brackets)	unit	mean	s	95% range (Extreme range in brackets)
Lipids									
Total lipids	138 y.a.					mg/l	12.5	2.43	7.66-17.4
Neutral fat* (triglycerides)	138 y.a.	μmol/l	4.71	2.73	0-10.2	mg/l	4.17	2.42	0-9.01
Cholesterol	138 y.a.	μmol/l	10.2	2.30	5.6-14.8	mg/l	3.95	0.88	2.19-5.71
	41 subjects	μmol/l	12.0	4.0	4.0-20.0	mg/l	4.63	1.54	1.55-7.71
Phospholipids*	138 y.a.	μmol/l	5.21	0.90	3.41-7.01	mg/l	4.03	0.70	2.63-5.43
	41 subjects	μmol/l	7.09	2.20	2.69-11.5	mg/l	5.49	1.70	2.09-8.89
Fatty acids*									
total	17 subjects	μmol/l	26.1	–	–	mg/l	7.36	–	–
free		μmol/l	70	14	–	mg/l	20	4	–
Cerebrosides		μmol/l	3.5	–	–	mg/l	1.0	–	–
		μmol/l	0.87	–	–				
Prostaglandins									
PGE	19 subjects	nmol/l	1.31	2.09	–	ng/l	460	737	–
PGF	19 subjects	nmol/l	1.98	1.88	–	ng/l	701	667	–
Vitamins									
Thiamine (a)	45 subjects	nmol/l	–	–	(49-64)	μg/l	–	–	(13-17)
(b)	36 subjects	nmol/l	15	–	(11-45)	μg/l	4	–	(3-12)
Vitamin B$_6$		nmol/l	–	–	(0-4.4)	μg/l	–	–	(0-0.75)
Nicotinic acid		μmol/l	–	–	(0.8-4)	mg/l	–	–	(0.1-0.5)

TABLE 5.1. Cont.

Lumbar CSF unless other-wise stated		Amount of substance			95% range (Extreme range in brackets)	Mass			95% range (Extreme range in brackets)
		unit	mean	s		unit	mean	s	
Folic acid (a)	30 subjects	nmol/l	53.5	24.9	(28.5-152)	µg/l	23.6	11.0	(12.6-67)
(b)	23 adults	nmol/l	71.6	-	(34-122)	µg/l	31.6	-	(15-54)
(b)	62 subjects	nmol/l	-	-	45-113	µg/l	-	-	20-50
Biopterin	27 specimens	nmol/l	1.7	0.89	(1.1-3.0)	µg/l	0.4	0.21	(0.25-0.7)
	19 specimens	nmol/l	8.0	2.4	-	µg/l	1.9	0.57	-
Vitamin B$_{12}$	62 subjects	pmol/l	16	5.7	(6-26)	ng/l	21.3	7.7	(5.9-36.7)
	15 subjects	pmol/l	13	5.7	-	ng/l	17.8	7.7	(8.0-35.6)
Pantothenic acid	103 subjects	µmol/l	2.37	-	(0.46-7.8)	mg/l	0.52	-	(0.10-1.7)
Ascorbic acid		µmol/l	-	-	(17-119)	mg/l	-	-	(3-21)
Nitrogen-free substances									
Galactose	12 subjects	µmol/l	166	99	-	mg/l	29.9	17.8	-
Fructose	3 specimens	µmol/l	-	-	(220-260)	mg/l	-	-	(40-47)
Mannose	3 specimens	µmol/l	-	-	(56-72)	mg/l	-	-	(10-13)
Sialic acid									
total	28 subjects	µmol/l	38.8	18.4	-	mg/l	12.0	5.7	-
free	28 subjects	µmol/l	11.9	7.1	-	mg/l	3.7	2.2	-

TABLE 5.1. Cont.

Lumbar CSF unless otherwise stated	Amount of substance				Mass			
	unit	mean	s	95% range (Extreme range in brackets)	unit	mean	s	95% range (Extreme range in brackets)
Polyols (polyhydric alcohols)								
Glycerol — 3 specimens	μmol/l	-	-	(11-16)	mg/l	-	-	(1.0-1.5)
Erythritol — 3 specimens	μmol/l	-	-	(29-45)	mg/l	-	-	(3.5-5.5)
Ribitol — 3 specimens	μmol/l	-	-	(20-23)	mg/l	-	-	(3.0-3.5)
Arabitol — 12 subjects	μmol/l	19.0	6.3	-	mg/l	2.89	0.96	-
Mannitol — 12 subjects	μmol/l	4.8	2.0	-	mg/l	0.87	0.36	-
Sorbitol — 12 subjects	μmol/l	17.2	4.6	-	mg/l	3.13	0.84	-
Myoinostol — 3 specimens	μmol/l	-	-	(19-38)	mg/l	-	-	(3.5-7)
— 12 subjects	μmol/l	174	31	-	mg/l	31.3	5.6	-
— 3 specimens	μmol/l	-	-	(200-270)	mg/l	-	-	(36-49)
1.5-Anhydro-sorbitol — 65 adults	μmol/l	-	-	(11-95)	mg/l	-	-	(1.8-16)
— 3 specimens	μmol/l	-	-	(146-323)	mg/l	-	-	(24-53)
Acids								
Acetic acid — 21 subjects	μmol/l	116	55	(19-210)	mg/l	6.99	3.33	(1.14-12.6)
Propionic acid — 21 subjects	μmol/l	2.8	3.2	(trace-13)	mg/l	0.21	0.24	(trace-0.94)
Isobutyric acid — 21 subjects	μmol/l	-	-	(0-3.6)	mg/l	-	-	(0-0.32)
Butyric acid — 21 subjects	μmol/l	-	-	(0-2.8)	mg/l	-	-	(0-0.25)
Isovaleric acid — 21 subjects	μmol/l	-	-	(0-2.7)	mg/l	-	-	(0-0.28)
Caproic acid — 21 subjects	μmol/l	-	-	(0-trace)	mg/l	-	-	(0-trace)

TABLE 5.1. Cont.

Lumbar CSF unless otherwise stated		Amount of substance			95% range (Extreme range in brackets)	Mass			95% range (Extreme range in brackets)
		unit	mean	s		unit	mean	s	
Lactic acid (a)	25 children	mmol/l	1.59	0.33	-	mg/l	143	30	-
(a)	23 subjects	mmol/l	1.62	0.19	-	mg/l	146	17	-
(b)	81 men	mmol/l	1.34	0.37	0.60-2.08	mg/l	120	33	54-186
(b)	133 women	mmol/l	1.20	0.25	0.70-1.70	mg/l	108	23	62-154
(a)	15 subjects	mmol/l	1.63	0.34	-	mg/l	147	31	-
(a) suboccipital CSF,	15 subjects	mmol/l	1.45	0.27	-	mg/l	131	24	-
Pyruvic acid (a)	10 children	mmol/l	0.136	0.029	(0.085-0.184)	mg/l	12.0	2.6	(7.5-16.2)
(b)	23 subjects	mmol/l	0.115	0.017	-	mg/l	10.1	1.5	-
α-Oxoglutaric acid		μmol/l	-	-	(6.1-8.3)	mg/l	-	-	(0.8-1.1)
Succinic acid		μmol/l	-	-	(24-33)	mg/l	-	-	(2.8-3.9)
Citric acid	15 subjects	μmol/l	176	50	-	mg/l	33.9	9.6	-
Ketone bodies (as acetone)	16 subjects	μmol/l	117	65	-	mg/l	6.8	3.8	-
Acetoacetic acid	11 subjects	μmol/l	26.2	12.3	(15.8-53.5)	mg/l	2.67	1.26	(1.61-5.46)
β-Hydroxybutyric acid	11 subjects	μmol/l	46.4	23.9	(23.7-94.1)	mg/l	4.83	2.49	(2.47-9.80)
Nitrogenous substances									
Total nitrogen		mmol/l	13.2	-	(11.2-15.7)	mg/l	187	-	(157-220)
Nonprotein nitrogen		mmol/l	-	-	(17.9-14.3)	mg/l	-	-	(110-200)
Urea	106 subjects	mmol/l	4.16	-	(2.30-6.06)	mg/l	250	-	(138-364)

TABLE 5.1. Cont.

Lumbar CSF unless otherwise stated	Amount of substance				Mass			
	unit	mean	s	95% range (Extreme range in brackets)	unit	mean	s	95% range (Extreme range in brackets)
Creatinine — 37 subjects	mmol/l	4.10	1.12	-	mg/l	246	67	-
37 subjects	μmol/l	64.8	27.6	-	mg/l	7.33	3.12	-
Guanidinosuccinic acid — 10 specimens	μmol/l	-	-	(57.5-92.8)	mg/l	-	-	(6.5-10.5)
Ammonia (a) — 15 subjects	μmol/l	15.5	5.93	< 8.6	mg/l	0.264	0.101	< 1.5
(b) — 20 subjects	μmol/l	11.9	1.76	-	mg/l	0.202	0.030	-
α-Amino nitrogen 8 children, <5years	mmol/l	0.78	0.12	(0.66-0.81)	mg/l	10.9	1.7	(9.2-11.4)
42 adults	mmol/l	0.88	0.08	(0.66-0.81)	mg/l	12.3	1.1	(9.6-14.7)
Ventricular CSF, 8 adults	mmol/l	0.81	0.09	(0.69-0.97)	mg/l	11.3	.1.3	(9.7-13.6)
Amino acids — 10 subjects	mmol/l	1.76	0.34	-				
Choline — 22 specimens	μmol/l	8.3	1.7	(7-13)	μg/l	1.0	0.2	(0.8-16)
Acetylcholine — 16 subjects	nmol/l	103	33	-	μg/l	16.8	5.4	-
Polyamines								
Histamine	nmol/l	87	-	(18-270)	μg/l	9.7	-	(2-30)
3,4-Dihydroxphenyl-acetic acid (Dopa) — 10 subjects	nmol/l	2.9	0.5	-	ng/l	490	80	-
Catecholamines								
Norepinephrine	nmol/l	1.4	-	-	ng/l	240	-	-
Epinephrine	nmol/l	0.24	-	-	ng/l	44	-	-
Serotonin — 48 subjects	nmol/l	5.90	1.08	3.74-8.06	μg/l	1.04	0.19	0.66-1.42
Indoxylsulfuric acid — 50 subjects	μmol/l	4.7	0.9	2.9-6.5	mg/l	1.0	0.2	0.6-1.4

TABLE 5.1. Cont.

Lumbar CSF unless otherwise stated		Amount of substance			95% range (Extreme range in brackets)	Mass			95% range (Extreme range in brackets)
		unit	mean	s		unit	mean	s	
Bilirubin (a)	34 newborn	μmol/l	4.1	1.7	-	mg/l	2.4	1.0	-
	adults	μmol/l	-	-	(<0.2)	mg/l	-	-	(<0.1)
Porphyrins Uric acid	61 men	μmol/l	22	7.7	6.6-37	mg/l	3.7	1.3	1.1-6.3
	57 women	μol/l	16	5.9	4.2-28	mg/l	2.7	1.0	0.7-4.7
Hypoxanthine + xanthine	35 subjects					mg/l	1.3	0.6	(0.25-1.50)
						mg/l	0.97	-	
Cyclic adenosine monophosphate	22 children	nmol/l	22.4	2.8	-	μg/l	7.37	0.92	-
	23 subjects	nmol/l	21	8	-	μg/l	6.9	2.6	-
	14 subjects	nmol/l	8.7	8.3	-	μg/l	2.9	2.7	-
Cyclic guanosine monophosphate	23 subjects	nmol/l	2.4	0.5	-	μg/l	0.83	0.17	-
	14 subjects	nmol/l	3.4	4.0	-	μg/l	1.2	1.4	-
	16 subjects	nmol/l	1.94	0.68	-	μg/l	0.67	0.23	-

y.a. + young adults; *Factors for conversion into mg triglycerides, 0.865; phospholipids, 0.77; fatty acids, 0.282.

A subsequent increase in the mean leucocyte count up to 9 ± 9 cells/mm³ occurred at 40 weeks.

In term neonates the normal range of the CSF leucocyte count is 7-11 cells/mm³ with more than 32 cells/mm³ being considered pathological (Sarff *et al.*, 1976). The high percentage of polymorphonuclear cells (up to 60% in the term neonate) appears to reflect the differential WBC count in the blood (Fishman, 1980). In the first week of life CSF cell count decreases in the term neonate (Sarff *et al.*, 1976), but increases in the preterm infant (Rodriguez *et al.*, 1990).

In the age group between six weeks and twelve months the total WBC count decreases, with a mean of 2.63 ± 2.45 cells/ul between six and twelve months (Portnoy and Olson, 1985).

Neonates may demonstrate a cellular polymorphism consisting of exogenous cells, eosinophils, basophils, plasma cells, bone marrow cells, histiomonocytic cells, cell aggregates and free cells (Dalens *et al.*, 1982). Macrophages may be prominent in the neonatal CSF (Pappu *et al.*, 1982). CSF cytology in the neonate is often difficult to evaluate and the clinical indications for LP, particularly in the first week of life, are controversial (Schwersenski *et al.*, 1991).

Glucose levels

CSF glucose content is proportionally higher in relation to blood glucose in neonates than in older children and adults, being about 81% of blood glucose levels in term and 74% in preterm infants (compared to 50%-65% in adults). However, analogous to serum glucose levels, absolute CSF glucose values are significantly lower in the neonatal age group than in adults with a mean 52 mg/dl (Sarff *et al.*, 1976), compared to 90 mg/dl in adults.

Protein

Total protein values in newborn infants (mean 90 mg/dl), especially in the preterm infant (mean 115 mg/dl), are significantly higher than in the CSF of children or adults (Wenzel and Felgenhauer, 1976; Maurer and Rieder, 1978; Sarff *et al.*, 1976).

Childhood normal values for CSF immunoglobulins have been reviewed by Eeg-Olofsson *et al.* (1981), Statz and Felgenhauer (1983) and by Rust *et al.* (1986). CSF IgG is elevated in the fetal period and decreases significantly until the age of six months when levels are lowest and then slightly increases after the age of one year (Statz and Felgenhauer, 1983). The CSF IgG index showed no age-related differences in a study by Eeg-Oloffson (1981), nor did the IgG synthesis rate. However, Rust *et al.* (1986) report a slight decline in the IgG index between the age of two months until the age of 18 years. The higher values seen in infancy may relate to a selective permeability to IgG during development. IgM could not be detected in the CSF of term neonates, and IgA only in a few cases with a high range of normal IgA serum levels (Statz and Felgenhauer, 1983). IgA is found in the CSF of preterm infants, even with low serum IgA levels, reflecting a more permeable blood-brain barrier. CSF total protein, IgG and albumin concentrations tend to increase with age through adulthood (Tibbling *et al.*, 1977).

The increased CSF protein and low serum/CSF albumin ratios in pre-term and term neonates indicate an immaturity of the blood-brain barrier which has considerable clinical implications for the paediatrician. Alpha-fetoprotein in the CSF during fetal development is another marker for an immature blood-brain barrier suggesting an increased permeability (Seller and Adinolfi, 1975). Data on the increase of the serum/CSF albumin ratio during infancy and childhood confirm a continuous development of the barrier function with the greatest rate of maturation during the third month of life (Statz and Felgenhauer, 1983).

Other age-related changes in CSF
The concentrations of many amino acids are elevated in the neonatal period and with advanced age. Acid-base parameters in the neonate are similar to those of adults after 26 weeks gestation and do not vary with gestational age (Hermansen and Ellison, 1982). Various neurotransmitters, cyclic nucleotides and hormones in the CSF also vary with age (Wood, 1980; Wood, 1982; Hare *et al.*, 1982b; Ollat and Sebban, 1983; Ballenger *et al.*, 1983). The CSF production rate is also decreased in healthy aging. This along with the ventricular dilatation that may occur with aging may influence the concentrations of many substances in the CSF (May *et al.*, 1990). The clinician and researcher must be aware of these normal variations in CSF studies.

Pregnancy

Davis (1979) sampled CSF from pregnant women undergoing spinal anaesthesia for delivery and reported normal opening pressure, cell count and protein concentration. Increased CSF levels of prolactin, human placental lactogen and human chorionic gonadotrophin have also been demonstrated in pregnancy (Assies *et al.*, 1978; Jordan *et al.*, 1979; Berkowitz *et al.*, 1981; Peake *et al.*, 1983). Steinbrook *et al.* (1982) reported that, unlike plasma levels, CSF beta-endorphin-like immunoreactivity does not change over the course of pregnancy or during labour. Decreased CSF glucose (reflecting decreased fasting serum levels due to increased circulating insulin) and decreased uric acid (also reflecting reduced serum levels) have also been reported in pregnancy (Meeks *et al.*, 1983).

Iatrogenic changes in CSF composition

The process of lumbar puncture may result in several changes in CSF cytology. The CSF sample may become contaminated by peripheral blood, epithelial, cartilage or vertebral bone-marrow cells and make interpretation of the data difficult (Kruskall *et al.*, 1983). A traumatic tap causing blood to enter the CSF may result in a white cell pleocytosis which may last up to 20 days following the tap (Bickerstaff, 1980). The number of red blood cells contaminating the fluid specimen correlates directly with the observed white blood cell count, total protein, and IgG content (Reske *et al.*, 1981). The CSF glucose is unaffected by artificial blood contamination.

CSF concentrations of 5-HIAA and HVA may be altered by the volume of CSF withdrawn during lumbar puncture and even by the site of lumbar puncture (Nordin *et al.*, 1982). These variables are probably related to the ventriculospinal gradients of 5-HIAA and HVA. A time lag between lumbar puncture and laboratory analysis of the specimen may result in a lower cell count, increased protein (due to cytolysis), decreased glucose, and increased pH (Reske *et al.*, 1981).

The procedure of pneumoencephalography or the accidental introduction of air during lumbar puncture may also cause pleocytosis. The mononuclear count, in particular, will rise during the process of pneumoencephalography. Only the very first part of the fluid may thus be used for cytological examination during this procedure (Bickerstaff, 1980). Care must also be taken in the use of probenecid in the study of CSF as, in the cat, it has been found to allow peripherally administered 5-HIAA to enter the CSF, although this point is controversial (Garelis *et al.*, 1974; Vogt, 1975). Although probenecid induced increases in acid metabolites have been used widely as an indicator of central turnover rates of biogenic amines, recent studies suggest that this may not be an accurate interpretation of probenecid studies (Cowdry *et al.*, 1983). The technique of using probenecid may not adequately control for CSF metabolite transport as a source of variance. Probenecid levels must be adequately controlled for in such studies.

The physician must also be careful in using local anaesthetics during lumbar puncture. Many local anaesthetics will react with the agents used to determine protein concentrations in the CSF (Shealy, 1969). Injudicious use of procaine, tetracaine or other local anaesthetics may thus cause a falsely elevated reading of the protein content.

Post-mortem changes in CSF

Shortly after death the CSF pressure drops to zero while both the cell count and total protein usually rise (Tourtellotte and Shorr, 1982). Paulson and Stickney (1971) studied the cisternal CSF composition of 150 adult cadavers. They noted increases in potassium, chloride, β-glucuronidase, acid phosphatase, CPK, magnesium, phosphorous, and iron levels. The concentrations of sodium, carbon dioxide, and glucose tended to decrease after death. Changes in the colour, temperature, pressure, electrophoretic pattern and pH were also noted. Coe (1977) has reviewed the changes seen in these and other CSF constituents after death. CSF levels of potassium, aminonitrogen, nonprotein nitrogen, creatine, ammonia, inorganic phosphorous, and others may be useful in determining the post-mortem interval (Coe 1977, 1979; Schoning and Strafuss, 1980; Moar, 1982). Endo *et al.* (1990) found the concentrations of 3, 4-dihydroxyphenylacetic acid (DOPAC) to increase in parallel with the increment of the post-mortem interval, suggesting DOPAC may also be useful in the determination of the post-mortem interval.

Other factors causing alterations in CSF composition

The CSF concentrations of biogenic amines, cyclic nucleotides and other constituents may be greatly affected by the time of day the sample is obtained (Udayakumar *et al.*, 1982; Perlow and Lake, 1980). Foods or diet supplements rich in amino acid precursors (e.g. tyrosine, tryptophan, glutamine) may markedly affect the CSF concentrations of neuro-transmitters and their metabolites (Wood, 1980*b*; Danguir *et al.*, 1982). Height and weight may also affect the composition of CSF for some substances (Banki and Molnar, 1981*a*). Various hormones, biogenic amines and amine metabolites may also be affected by sleeping and feeding times, by REM sleep, by number of hours slept the night prior to lumbar puncture, by changes in light-dark conditions, by stress, and by the time of year of CSF sampling (Ballenger *et al.*, 1983; Mens *et al.*, 1982; Udayakumar *et al.*, 1982; Danguir *et al.*, 1982; Schwartz *et al.*, 1983; von Knorring *et al.*, 1983; Benson *et al.*, 1983*a*; Losonczy *et al.*, 1984; Csernansky *et al.*, 1988). Differences in gender are also very important, particularly in the measurement of CSF proteins (Ahonen *et al.*, 1978).

Handling of the CSF samples is also an important variable, particularly in determining the CSF cell count. The various assays used and storage conditions greatly affect biochemical measures in the CSF.

One must also take into account the effects of disease states (discussed in the next section) and drugs on the concentrations of CSF constituents. Antiemetics, hypnotics, sedatives, antiparkinsonism agents, anaesthetics, analgesics, antipsychotics, and anticonvulsants in particular may have a significant impact on CSF composition (Wood, 1980*b*, 1982*a*). In meningitis, the CSF concentration of penicillin increases. This effect is generally attributed to an increased permeability of the blood-brain and blood-CSF barriers. However, data presented by Lorenzo and Spector

(1976) also suggests that the organic acid efflux system is partially inhibited in meningitis. The change in CSF penicillin levels during inflammation and resolution correlated well with the ability of isolated choroid plexus of *Haemophilus influenzae* innoculated rabbits to take up penicillin (Lorenzo, 1977). Another anionic drug, methotrexate, is found in much larger concentrations in the CSF of patients who have leukaemia with meningeal involvement (Domer and Kaiser, 1977). The researcher must be aware of these variables in studies of the CSF.

Some of the main variables affecting biochemical measurements in the CSF are summarised in Table 5-2.

TABLE 5.2. *Some variables affecting CSF composition.*

Clinical factors
Age
Sex
Height and weight
Activity level/bedrest/hours slept prior to LP
Inpatient vs. outpatient status
Stress
Diet
Drugs
Disease state – diagnosis, severity, stage and duration of illness
Genetic, environmental and experiential conditions

Procedural factors related to lumbar puncture
volume, aliquot of CSF (gradients of metabolites)
site of LP
position – sitting vs. lying
use of local anaesthetics
occurrence of "traumatic" LP
time of day and time of year of LP
   (diurnal and seasonal variations of metabolites)
size of needle used (important for pressure measurements)

Methodological factors
handling of CSF sample – delay to analysis
probenecid levels and duration of blockade
storage conditions
   – time before freezing
   – temperature frozen
   – thawing and freezing
   – storage time
assay used (sensitivity, specificity)

Appearance

The normal clear and colorless appearance of CSF can be altered by various disease states to become cloudy or pigment-tinged.

A scale ranging from 0 to 4+ is commonly used to grade the turbidity of CSF (Krieg, 1979):

0 – clear

1+ – faintly cloudy

2+ – cloudy, but newsprint easily read through collection tube

3+ – very cloudy – cannot easily read newsprint through tube

4+ – unable to see newsprint through tube.

The presence of erythrocytes, leukocytes, microorganisms, contrast media and epidural fat (aspirated during lumbar puncture) may all contribute to the turbidity (Krieg, 1979).

After collection, the CSF specimen should be spun down and its appearance compared with an identical tube of water using daylight rather than artificial light when possible against a white background. One should look vertically down the entire length of the tube (Meena et al., 1989).

Visual inspection of a fluid specimen can accurately be used to detect CSF pleocytosis. The fluid becomes "snowy" in appearance when exposed to direct light with as few as 50 cells/mm^3. This is due to the "Tyndall Effect" where the light is scattered by the suspended particles (Simon and Abele, 1978). A fluid specimen will just become cloudy at counts of between 200-400/mm^3 and may be xanthochromic or pink-tinged at counts of 500-6000/mm^3 (Fishman, 1992; Lee et al., 1975). Grossly bloody specimens are not observed unless the count exceeds 6000/mm^3.

A bloody specimen caused by a traumatic tap must be differentiated from one due to subarachnoid haemorrhage. In the former, the pressure is usually normal or low, earlier tubes are more bloody than those tubes filled later, the blood may clot, and the specimen will not be xanthochromic (except in the case of severe jaundice or hypercarotinaemia). The CSF in subarachnoid haemorrhage may have pigment changes out of proportion to the protein level, will have a uniform mixture of blood or xanthochromic pigment within the fluid, and may be under increased pressure (Wallach, 1980). Computed tomography is also a valuable tool in excluding sub-arachnoid haemorrhage.

The combined use of spectrophotometry and cytology have a high diagnostic reliability in determining whether blood-stained fluid is due to traumatic puncture or haemorrhage (Buruma et al., 1981). Quantitative CSF spectrophotometry is a quick and sensitive technique for detecting compounds of haemorrhagic and non-haemorrhagic origin and in the diagnosis of intracranial vascular disorders (Kjellin, 1983).

There are three major pigments observed in CSF which derive from erythrocytes. Bilirubin, derived from haemoglobin, may be detected in CSF in both free and conjugated forms in severe jaundice, giving a yellow tint to the fluid. Its presence may be detected by spectrophotometry or by the van den Bergh reaction (Fishman, 1992; Kjellin *et al.*, 1974). Oxyhaemoglobin (pink-red) and methaemoglobin (dark yellow-brown) are the two other main pigments found in CSF and may be identified by spectrophotometry or by the benzidine (oxyhaemoglobin) or potassium cyanide (methaemoglobin) tests. Methaemoglobin is characteristically found in intracranial haematomas while oxyhaemoglobin and bilirubin are responsible for the xanthochromia seen in subarachnoid haemorrhage (Kjellin, 1983). Urobilinoids and carotenoids are other pigments which are infrequently detected in CSF (Fishman, 1992; Kjellin *et al.*, 1974). Xanthochromia may also occur with rifampin therapy (Liggett *et al.*, 1982), with an increased concentration of CSF protein, with melanin in LCSF due to meningeal melanosarcoma, and in normal premature infants due to elevated CSF protein, hyperbilirubinaemia, and immaturity of the blood-CSF barrier (Krieg, 1979).

Cells in the CSF

The cell count of CSF should be done as quickly as possible after obtaining the specimen. Allowing the specimen to sit in a test tube at room temperature will decrease the total WBC count by up to 50% in the first half hour (Meena *et al.*, 1989). This is because the cells will become clumped or enmeshed in fibrin and will lyse and deteriorate rapidly on standing, complicating interpretation (Bauer, 1982; Shah, 1982). PMNs are more susceptible than lymphocytes to this disintegration. In the case of traumatic tap or suspected subarachnoid haemorrhage several tubes should be sent to the lab for serial cell counts.

The CSF is virtually free of cells normally, containing 0-5 WBCs/mm^3 in adults (Heilman *et al.*, 1977). A count of 5-10/mm^3 is considered a borderline pleocytosis and a count of > 10/mm^3 is consistent with disease of the CNS or meninges. The presence of any cells in the CSF other than lymphocytes and monocytes is always abnormal (Tourtellotte and Shorr, 1982), with a few exceptions (Kolmel, 1977; Kjeldsberg and Krieg, 1984). The normal differential count consists of 65 (+ 17.7)% large lymphocytes, 17 (+ 15.1)% small lymphocytes, and 16(± 9.5)% monocytes (Tourtellotte and Shorr, 1982).

Any case of haemorrhage into the CSF will alter the white count dramatically. An approximation of the white count in blood-contaminated fluid may be obtained by the following formula:

$$\text{Corrected WBC count (CSF)} = \text{WBC (CSF)} - \frac{\text{WBCs (blood)} \times \text{RBC (CSF)}}{\text{RBC (blood)}}$$

Normally there is about one WBC added per 700 RBCs (Bauer, 1982). The total protein of the CSF may similarly be corrected by subtracting about 1 mg/dl for every 1200 RBC/ml (Kjeldsberg and Krieg, 1984), or by the formula:

$$\text{Protein actual} = \text{Protein}_{CSF} - \frac{\text{Protein}_{serum} \times (1\text{-Hct}) \times RBC_{CSF}}{RBC_{blood}}$$

It is important that the protein and cell count measurements be performed on the same sample tube in traumatic LPs (Mehl, 1986). Such corrections assume normal haematocrit, normal serum protein, an accurate CSF RBC count, measurements performed on the same tube, and that all RBCs present are due to traumatic tap (Kjeldsberg and Krieg, 1984). Clotted specimens will result in inaccurate calculations and heparinisation of a very bloody specimen at collection may allow more accurate interpretation.

Mehl (1986) prospectively studied the usefulness of formulae for calculating WBC counts, neutrophil percentage, and protein using an experimental model for traumatic LP by adding blood to clear CSF. He found a wide range of variance in the observed to expected ratios and points out some of the limitations of interpreting results from traumatic LPs. Bonadio *et al.* (1990) on the other hand, found that CSF abnormalities are rarely obscured by blood contamination from a traumatic LP, reviewing the CSF findings in 92 children with traumatic lumbar punctures.

The types of leukocytes observed in the CSF samples in cases of suspected meningitis are important in arriving at a rapid diagnosis in order to institute prompt therapy. A predominance of polymorphonuclear cells (PMNs) indicates an acute infection (or an exacerbation of a chronic infection) by a pyogenic bacteria (De Jong, 1979). The inflammation may directly involve the meninges or be in close proximity (e.g. mastoid cells, CNS tissue). The presence of a lymphocytosis in CSF suggests a viral infection (e.g. encephalitis, meningitis, rabies, polio), fungal or tuberculous infection (especially if markedly elevated), CNS tumour, or other chronic inflammatory processes of the meninges or ependyma. Toxic meningitis, aseptic meningitis, cerebrovascular disease, postinfectious encephalitis, trauma, polyneuritis, carcinomatous meningitis, parasitic infections, lymphocytic choriomeningitis, and many other CNS inflammatory diseases may also be associated with a lymphocytic pleocytosis (De Jong, 1979; Fishman, 1980; Bauer, 1982). A subacute meningeal inflammatory process (e.g. late tuberculous meningitis, influenzal meningitis, or aseptic meningitis with brain abscess) frequently results in an increase in both PMNs and lymphocytes (a "mixed" pleocytosis) (De Jong, 1979).

Mollaret's meningitis, a benign recurrent form of meningitis of uncertain aetiology is characterised by a predominance of mononuclear cells in the CSF with a variable number of neutrophils. It is associated with fever, myalgia and meningeal signs and may represent a recurrent viral infection. There may be epithelioid or endothelial cells present. Neutrophils may occasionally be the dominant cell type. When examined by electron microscopy, the lymphocytes and neutrophils are seen to contain unusually large quantities of glycogen granules (Herndon and Brumback, 1989a).

Increased numbers of plasma cells, monocytes and/or pia-arachnoid mesothelial cells are also frequently seen as part of a mixed pleocytosis (Kjeldsberg and Krieg, 1984). Plasma cells may be seen with syphilis, tuberculosis, sarcoidosis, parasitosis, subacute sclerosing panencephalitis, collagen disease, Guillain-Barré syndrome, subarachnoid haemorrhage, and CNS tumours (Tourtellotte and Shorr, 1982). Eosinophils in the CSF are seen in parasitic or fungal infections and in foreign body and allergic reactions (Labadie, 1980). Kuberski (1979) has reviewed the various causes of eosinophils appearing in the CSF.

Other types of cells seen in the CSF include various types of macrophages, choroidal cells, ependymal cells, arachnoid cover cells, cartilage cells, glial cells, bone marrow and various tumour cells (Oehmichen, 1976). The interested reader is referred to the atlases of den Hartog Jager (1980), Kolmel (1977), and Oehmichen (1976) and to the reviews of Bigner and Johnston (1981b), and Herndon and Brumback (1989a).

Inorganic Constituents

Calcium

Calcium has perhaps received the most attention of the ions in the CSF. The concentrations of both total and ionised calcium vary little with respect to changes in plasma level (Goldstein et al., 1979). Values range from 2.2 to 3.4 mEq/l (DeJong, 1979) compared to plasma levels of 4-5.5 mEq/l (Rosenberg, 1990). This is thought to be due to the secretion by the choroid plexus of a fluid with near-constant composition with the BBB remaining impermeable to calcium ions (Bradbury and Sarna, 1977). Calcium enters the CSF largely by carrier-mediated transport systems with only minor quantities entering by passive-diffusion (Goldstein et al., 1979; Wood, 1982a). The ionised fraction of calcium is somewhat higher in CSF because of the lower protein content, although some does bind to lactate and to citrate (Goldstein et al., 1979; Wood, 1982a). Ventricular fluid concentrations have been reported as being somewhat higher than that of lumbar samplings (Lowenthal, 1972), although some contend that LCSF levels reflect VCSF levels (Jimerson et al., 1980; Wood, 1982a).

Extracellular unbound calcium levels are generally higher than intracellular concentrations in the CNS. In anoxia, calcium levels fall in the extracellular space while potassium concentrations rise. Calcium may enter the cell either by agonist-operated channels activated by excitatory neurotransmitters or by a change in voltage across the membrane accompanying depolarisation (Rosenberg, 1990).

Calcium has been shown to alter the synthesis, transport, release, and receptor activation of various neurotransmitters (Jimerson et al., 1980). Low concentrations of calcium in the ECF will result in an increased excitability of neurons. Changes in calcium concentrations have thus been implicated in affecting changes in mood, cognition, and behaviour (Carmen, 1981). A study of electrolytes in CSF by Jimerson et al. (1979) found CSF calcium, while not differing significantly from controls, to be positively correlated with the severity of symptoms in depressed patients. Jimerson et al. (1979) also noted that symptom remission from acute psychosis in schizophrenic patients was accompanied by increased CSF calcium levels. The occurrence of seizures in patients with severe hypocalcaemia has implicated calcium in the pathogenesis of epilepsy. Jimerson et al. (1979, 1980) reported lower CSF calcium in some patients with refractory generalised or complex-partial seizures receiving anticonvulsant therapy. Low CSF calcium is also seen in tetany and with tumours of the diencephalon (DeJong, 1979). Elevated CSF calcium has been reported in purulent meningitis, in the presence of increased total protein in CSF, and with elevated blood calcium as in hyperparathyroidism (Lowenthal, 1972; DeJong, 1979).

Magnesium

Magnesium is the only major cation found in greater (about 30% higher) concentrations in CSF than in plasma (Lowenthal, 1972).

Like calcium, its CSF levels remain constant despite alterations in plasma levels. This is attributed to secretion by the choroid plexus of a near constant concentration of Mg^{++} in the face of a relatively impermeable BBB (Bradbury and Sarna, 1977). Ventricular fluid levels are usually higher than lumbar concentrations (Wood, 1982a).

Though hypomagnesaemia may result in seizures and many other neurological problems and hypermagnesaemia in paralysis, the CSF Mg^{++} levels remain unchanged with blood fluctuations. CSF Mg^{++} has been shown to be correlated with CSF protein and will drop to near serum levels in purulent meningitis or ischaemic brain disease (Heipertz et al., 1979a; Fishman, 1980; Krieg, 1979).

Cohen et al. (1982) found lower CSF levels of Mg^{++} in patients with liver cirrhosis both in comatose and postcomatose conditions, with levels decreasing to serum levels in the former group. This was probably due to impairment of the blood-CSF barrier in hepatic coma. A strong linear correlation was also found between CSF and serum Mg^{++} levels in the postcomatose group. Slightly decreased levels are also seen in tuberculous meningitis (DeJong, 1979). Elevated CSF Mg^{++} has also been reported in patients with intracranial haemorrhage, probably related to cell necrosis (Heipertz et al., 1979a), and in anticonvulsant-treated seizure patients (Jimerson et al., 1980).

Zinc

Zinc is an essential trace element for the body. It plays an important role in protein synthesis, stabilisation of biological membranes, DNA replication and repair, and enzyme function (Potkin et al., 1982). There are over 70 enzymes known to require zinc for their participation in a variety of metabolic processes. Zinc may also play an important role in neuronal function (Hesse, 1979).

There have been few studies of zinc in the CSF. Bogden and Troiano (1978) found low CSF zinc concentrations in withdrawing alcoholics who developed delirium tremens or a prolonged hallucinatory state. They suggest that zinc deficiency may be a contributing factor to the neurological consequences of alcoholism. Mildly diminished CSF zinc concentrations have also been found in ex-heroin addicts (Potkin et al., 1982).

Palm and Hallmans (1982) and Palm et al. (1982a) found CSF zinc levels increased in patients with Guillain-Barré syndrome, malignant brain tumours and subarachnoid haemorrhage. They also found CSF zinc concentrations to correlate with CSF protein and CSF albumin levels. Others (Bogden et al., 1977) have not found any relation between protein and zinc concentrations in the CSF.

Normal CSF zinc concentrations have been noted in zinc deficiency, in patients on oral contraceptives or corticosteroid therapy and in both drug-free schizophrenics and schizophrenics undergoing neuroleptic therapy (Palm and Hallmans, 1982; Palm et al., 1982a; Potkin et al., 1982).

CSF zinc concentrations do not vary between sexes and do not correlate with age but are significantly higher in blacks than in whites (Potkin et al., 1982).

Phosphorus

Inorganic phophorus levels in CSF are about 60% those of plasma and remain relatively stable despite alterations in plasma concentration (Wood, 1982a; Goldstein et al., 1979). Phosphorus levels in the CSF increase parallel to the increases of total protein found in poliomyelitis, measles, encephalitis, and viral and bacterial meningitis. They are also increased in degenerative neurological illness and in tetany (Lowenthal, 1972; DeJong, 1979).

Sodium

As in plasma, sodium is the major cation of the CSF, present in concentrations of about 138 mEq/l in both fluids (Wood, 1982a). It is actively secreted across the blood-CSF barrier and will reach a maximum level about 1-2 hours after an acute elevation of plasma sodium. This active transport mechanism is unidirectional and is modified by osmotic forces (Fishman, 1992; Maren, 1977). Because of the effects of proteins, which are negatively charged, on the flow of ions across a semi-permeable membrane (the Donnan equilibrium), there exists about a 5mV electrical potential in CSF with respect to blood. A theoretical 6-17% excess of sodium in plasma relative to CSF because of this effect is prevented by the active transport of sodium into the CSF (Fishman, 1992; Wood, 1982a). The CSF sodium concentrations parallel changes in plasma levels in normal states as well as in hyponatraemia and hypernatraemia, though the changes may be less marked than those seen in the plasma sodium level (Krieg, 1979). Tracer studies with ^{24}Na have shown CSF and plasma levels are closely related, with an exchange time from blood to brain of about two hours. Sodium transported into the CSF is slowed by the carbonic anhydrase inhibitor acetazolamide (Rosenberg, 1990).

CSF sodium levels have been found to be elevated out of proportion to the plasma levels in encephalomalacia and tuberculous meningitis (Lowenthal, 1972). CSF sodium may also be elevated in hypertension (DeJong, 1979).

Potassium

The concentration of potassium in CSF is remarkably stable even with severe and prolonged plasma level alterations. The concentration is low when compared to plasma and brain intracellular levels (Bradbury and Sorna, 1977; Goldstein, 1979). The CSF K$^+$ content generally stays within the range of 2.5 to 3.5 mEq/liter with an average value of 3 mEq/litre (DeJong, 1979). The half-time of exchange for K$^+$ across the BBB is about 24 hours (Rosenberg, 1990). There is a tendency for the CSF concentration to deviate from the plasma concentration as the fluid passes from ventricle to cisterna magna to cortical subarachnoid space. The ECF of the brain thus has a lower concentration of K$^+$ than that found in newly formed CSF (Davson et al., 1987).

Active transport mechanisms for K$^+$ homeostasis have been postulated to exist in the brain capillary endothelial cells and in the astrocytic component of the BBB (Bradbury and Sarna, 1977; Goldstein, 1979). The efficiency of these active transport mechanisms in removing K$^+$ from the CSF is illustrated by the fact that subarachnoid haemorrhage, despite haemolysis of RBCs with the subsequent release of K^+, does not result in increased CSF concentrations of K^+ (Fishman, 1992). Goldstein (1979) suggests that brain capillaries act similarly to renal tubules in that they possess ouabain sensitive K^+ transport carriers which depend on oxidative metabolism. The active transport systems of the choroid plexus are also important in K^+ homeostasis in newly formed CSF acting with K^+-Na^+ activated ATPase. Sodium is exchanged for potassium when potassium levels are increased in the CSF and ouabain interferes with this exchange by inhibiting ATPase (Rosenberg, 1990). Elevated CSF potassium levels have been found in neonatal haemorrhage and aspiration pneumonia, in experimental and spontaneous seizure disorders, after cardiac arrest, and in the post-mortem period (Krieg, 1979; Lowenthal, 1972).

Chloride

Chloride is the major CSF anion and exceeds the plasma level by 15-20 mEq/l. CSF levels passively reflect changes in plasma concentrations. The higher levels in the CSF are favoured by the blood-CSF electrical potential (Wood, 1982a). Chloride levels decrease in the face of conditions in which total protein is increased (e.g. infection, haemorrhage) and in alkalotic states, varying inversely with the CSF bicarbonate concentration (Sorensen, 1971). Low CSF Cl^- used to be considered almost pathognomonic of tuberculous meningitis, although this is clearly no longer the case (Schoen, 1984). Rather, the low CSF levels of Cl^- seen in tuberculous meningitis, are probably a non-specific indicator of infection and a reflection of hypochloraemia secondary to prolonged vomiting.

Although CSF chloride levels generally reflect serum levels in both hypochloraemic and hyperchloraemic states, the absolute changes are much . less in the CSF. Radioisotope studies of chloride transport indicate that its transport is closely coupled to sodium transport (Sorensen, 1971). Since both sodium and chloride transport are dependent on carbonic anhydrase (as well as Na^+-K^+ activated ATPase) their transport into CSF is inhibited by acetazolamide (Fishman, 1992; Sorensen, 1971). This effect, however, does not alter the rate of secretion of chloride by the choroid plexus (Fishman, 1992). Both choroidal and extrachoroidal mechanisms may thus play a role in the regulation of CSF chloride concentrations.

Acid Base Balance

The acid-base status of the CSF does not necessarily parallel that of the blood. The pH of the CSF-ECF compartment must be optimal for the enzyme activity necessary to maintain neurotransmission. The pH is normally about 7.32 in the CSF and varies, as in all body fluid compartments, according to the Henderson-Hasselbach equation (Lowenthal, 1972; Wood, 1982a):

$$pH = pKi + \log (HCO_3/sP_{CO2})$$

where pKi is the dissociation constant of carbonic acid, "s" is the CO_2 solubility coefficient and P_{CO2} is the partial pressure of carbon dioxide.

Acid-base balance in the CSF, however, differs from that of blood in that the CSF lacks significant protein and phosphate buffer systems. The pH and bicarbonate concentration (HCO_3) in the CSF are usually lower than arterial values, while the P_{CO2} reflecting the tension of adjacent tissues is some 8-10 mm Hg higher (Fencl, 1971). The pH of the CSF may move in the opposite direction to that of the blood in certain clinical situations, such as with haemodialysis in uraemic patients and with $NaHCO_3$ treatment of patients with metabolic acidosis (Arieff, 1989).

The P_{CO2} in the lumbar CSF will reflect the tissue CO_2 tension of the lumbar region. It is generally somewhat higher than the simultaneously measured cisternal P_{CO2} which is a reflection of the brain P_{CO2} (Fencl, 1971). Bicarbonate concentrations are, however, about the same in the LCSF and cisternal CSF. The pH of the LCSF is thus generally more acidic than cisternal values (Plum and Posner, 1968).

The main factors accounting for the maintenance of a stable pH in the CSF in the face of acid-base changes in the blood are: (1) alterations in respiratory rate, (2) regulation of CSF HCO_3^- concentration, (3) alterations in cerebral blood flow and (4) the buffering capacity of the brain tissue itself (Fishman, 1992).

Alterations in respiration will affect blood and CSF P_{CO2}. The H^+-sensitive chemoreceptors in the respiratory centre of the brainstem regulate respiration, stabilising the pH in response to changes in P_{CO2}.

Variations in the P_{CO2} will have a significant effect on the pH since there is essentially no buffering capacity for CO_2 in the CSF (Fencl, 1971). CO_2 is transferred readily across the BBB, which is relatively impermeable to H^+ and HCO_3^-. Adaptive changes seen in CSF HCO_3^- concentrations due to alterations of central P_{CO2} tend to restore the $[HCO_3^-]/P_{CO2}$ ratio to achieve stabilisation of pH. This is more complete than in the blood (Leusen et al., 1983).

The P_{CO2} depends primarily on the cerebral blood flow, neural CO_2 production, and the arterial-CSF gradient. States of respiratory acidosis will, because of the changes in P_{CO2}, have profound effects on the CSF pH, approaching the variations seen in blood. Metabolic acidosis, on the other hand, may have little or no effect on the pH of the CSF (Lowenthal, 1972).

The primary mechanism behind this relative constancy of the CSF pH with respect to systemic changes involves the regulation of CSF bicarbonate levels via active transport processes in the choroid plexus. The cerebral blood flow may also participate in the clearance of CO_2 and H^+ (Fishman,

1992). Its regulation is pH-dependent. Brain tissue cells also exert an important influence on the pH of the CSF and ECF. The physicochemical buffering of glial cells with their carbonic anhydrase system, in particular, appear to be important (Leusen *et al.*, 1983). The glial cells may be capable of actively transporting HCO_3^- from the CSF.

Metabolic changes in CNS tissues may cause a CSF acidosis with little or no changes observed in the systemic arterial pH. This is seen in head injury, meningitis, subarachnoid haemorrhage and cerebral ischaemic insult. Gordon and Rossanda (1968) monitored blood and CSF pH in 18 unconscious patients with various brain lesions. They noted the blood pH to be elevated because of a tendency for hyperventilation in these patients, while the CSF pH was markedly reduced. They suggest that monitoring the CSF acid-base parameters may be the best guide to determining the settings of the respirator in the treatment of these patients. Arieff (1989) points out, however, that the CSF plays a role more of a passive sink for blood and brain and that the CSF pH does not necessarily reflect CNS acid-base status. Brain pH may actually be closer to arterial pH than that of CSF in many clinical circumstances.

Leusen *et al.* (1983) and Arieff (1989) have reviewed the regulation of acid-base balance in the CSF and central nervous system.

CSF anion gap

It has been suggested that the anion gap (calculated as the sum of the values for Na^+ and K^+ minus that for Cl^- and CO_2) may be of value in monitoring CSF acidosis as it is in systemic acidosis. Olson and Arnoldi (1982) measured the anion gap in children with suspected meningitis. They found the CSF anion gap to be markedly elevated in bacterial meningitis when compared to aseptic meningitis and to other systemic and local bacterial or viral infections. They did not, however, find this a useful guide in deciding therapy for these children, since only 76% of those with bacterial meningitis had an increased anion gap, and all of these had CSF cell counts, sugar, protein and gram stain findings indicating a bacterial aetiology before the anion gap was known.

Organic Constituents

Lactate and pyruvate

The CSF and CNS levels of lactate are largely independent of blood concentrations since it exists in an almost completely ionized form in the range of normal physiological pH (Weyne and Leusen, 1975). Normal levels are in the 9.0 to 26.0 mg/dl range (1.13 to 3.23 mmole/l). Neonates have higher levels (10-40 mg/dl; mean 24.7), approaching adult levels at 11 to 20 days of age (Kjeldsberg and Knight, 1986). CSF lactate also increases with increasing age (Yesavage *et al.*, 1982).

Studies of lactate transport across the BBB have yielded many conflicting results and some exchange between the compartments may occur via carrier-mediated transport mechanisms (Weyne and Leusen, 1975). CSF levels are, however, generally thought to normally depend directly on CNS lactate production by anaerobic metabolism and thus to reflect CNS levels (Krieg, 1979). Lactate levels are affected primarily by CNS energy metabolism, acid-base balance, hypoxia, and P_{co_2}. Unlike other CSF metabolites, lactate is cleared at a very slow rate from CSF and may, in cases of increased CNS production (e.g. hypoxia), reach high levels (Cutler, 1980). Lactate and pyruvate transport are easily saturated and are thought to be linked to ketone transport mechanisms (Cutler, 1980).

Changes in lactate levels make an extensive contribution to the acid-base balance in the brain. Lactate thus plays an important role in the regulation of cerebral blood flow and metabolism and pulmonary ventilation (Weyne and Leusen, 1975).

Increased lactate levels in CSF have been found in seizures, CNS cancers, traumatic brain injury, Kearns-Sayre Syndrome, ischaemia, subarachnoid haemorrhage, hydrocephalus, low blood pressure, hypocapnia, low arterial PO_2, multiple sclerosis, alcohol withdrawal seizures, and comas of nervous origin as well as in meningitis and other CNS infections where they find their chief diagnostic utility (Controni *et al.*, 1977; D'Souza *et al.*, 1978; Komorowski *et al.*, 1978; Brook *et al.*, 1978; Krieg, 1979; Jordan *et al.*, 1983; Dwivedi and Reddy, 1983; Kuriyama *et al.*, 1984). Busse and Hoffman (1983) found CSF lactate to be a good indicator of oedema due to cerebral infarction. Decreased levels of CSF lactate are seen in barbituric coma and poliomyelitis (Lowenthal, 1972). Levels may be readily measured in the CSF using either enzymatic or gas-liquid chromatographic techniques (Kjeldsberg and Knight, 1986). The use of CSF lactate in the differential diagnosis of meningitis is discussed further in Chapter 6.

Increased pyruvate levels, normally similar to serum levels, are found in infections, hepatic coma, and vitamin B1 deficiency (Lowenthal, 1972). The lactate/pyruvate ratio is a reflection of the CNS redox potential. It depends on the activity of the enzyme lactate dehydrogenase. Any alteration in the brain glycolytic pathway may result in an increase of the lactate/pyruvate ratio. This is seen in ischaemia, subarachnoid haemorrhage, hypoxia, seizures, and meningitis (Fishman, 1992; Wood, 1982*a*).

Glucose

Glucose is another substance that possesses a bidirectional transport system. The concentration of glucose within the CSF is normally maintained within narrow limits, about 60% of the plasma concentration. The normal range is 50-80 mg/dl in adults and 45 to 100 mg/dl in children (Kjeldsberg and Knight, 1986).

The transport of glucose from blood to CSF is believed to be by both simple and facilitated diffusion. Carrier-facilitated diffusion is quantitatively more important and many times faster than simple diffusion and specific glucose transporter proteins have recently been identified (Fishman 1992). Glucose may be transported via a carrier mechanism more avidly when blood glucose levels are low (Rosenberg, 1990). The transport of glucose from CSF to blood is more controversial. Studies of nascent rabbit CSF showing the glucose concentration to be 60% that of plasma, indicate that the choroid plexus may secrete glucose at a lower concentration than it absorbs it. Metabolism of the glucose by the tissues of the CNS has been proposed as a way of lowering the CSF glucose concentration. Finally the transport of glucose from CSF to blood by an uphill carrier process has been proposed (Lorenzo, 1977). The glucose that is rapidly taken up *in vitro* by the choroid plexus has been found to be used for metabolic processes of the choroid plexus (Lorenzo, 1977). Other studies using isolated perfused sheep choroid plexus found a carrier-mediated, partially Na^+ - dependent uphill transport process for the transport from CSF to blood for glucose, galactose, and 3-0-methylglucose (Deane and Segal, 1976). Preliminary work with horse choroid plexus suggests that the CSF to blood transport is an active process (Cserr, 1975b). Work with the frog choroid plexus found sugar transport across the choroid plexus to be by facilitated diffusion, stereospecific, insensitive to anoxia and independent of the external cation composition (Pollay, 1974). Thus it appears that the transport process for glucose may vary in different species. In humans the major mechanisms for removal of glucose from CSF are (1) glucose utilisation by neural, glial, ependymal and neuronal cells and (2) bulk flow of CSF into the venous system (Fishman, 1992). Bulk flow is less important for maintaining a CSF/plasma ratio less than 1.0.

CSF concentrations of glucose generally parallel plasma levels with approximately a 1 1/2 to 2 hour time lag. A state of equilibrium is reached in approximately 4 hours. Within the CSF a rostrocaudal gradient has been noted (Cutler, 1980; Wood, 1982a). The mechanism for this is also a point of controversy.

Since CSF glucose lags several hours behind plasma levels it is best measured in relation to plasma levels with the subject in the fasting state. Low CSF glucose may be masked by hyperglycaemia. Low levels are seen in many illnesses including subarachnoid haemorrhage, hypoglycaemia, neoplastic or inflammatory infiltration of the meninges, and in tuberculous, bacterial, fungal, amebic, syphilitic, chemical or rheumatoid meningitis

(Fishman, 1992; Olson *et al.*, 1974; Wood, 1982*a*). CSF glucose may remain decreased for 2-3 weeks following resolution of acute meningitis. An increased lactate level, caused by increased anaerobic glycolysis, is usually found concomitantly with a hypoglycorrhachia (except in hypoglycaemia). An increased CSF glucose concentration usually is a reflection only of hyperglycaemia and of no clinical significance, although it may also be seen in acute encephalitides (De Jong, 1979).

Glucose oxidase test strips have been used for the diagnosis of CSF rhinorrhoea and otorrhoea. They have, however, limited diagnostic value in determining CSF leakage in these conditions, as normal secretions usually contain glucose as well in the absence of CSF leakage. CSF rhinorrhoea and otorrhoea are better evaluated by radioisotope cisternography or by the demonstration of an extra band of transferrin located in the β-2 fraction of protein electrophoresis (Kjeldsberg and Knight, 1986). Quantitative analysis of glucose in rhinorrhoea, if done quickly, may also be clinically useful with values over 40mg/dl suggestive of the fluid being CSF.

Proteins

The subject of protein regulation in the CSF has a great potential for aiding diagnosis, and for evaluating therapy and prognosis. Normally, the CSF has very low levels of total protein (about 28 mg/100 ml) compared to those in plasma (of about 7000 mg/100 ml) (Milhorat, 1976). Protein levels in the CSF have been found to be high in human fetuses and neonates. Adinolfi *et al.* (1976) provide evidence that the human blood-CSF barrier is not fully developed during early life.

CSF proteins differ from those in plasma in having (1) a more prominent prealbumin fraction on electrophoresis, (2) the presence of the tau fraction not seen in serum, (3) the presence of only very small amounts of glycoprotein and lipoprotein, and (4) a proportionately lower fraction of gamma globulin (Fishman, 1980).

The CSF protein consists primarily of albumin (56-76%) but also contains significant fractions of prealbumin (2-7%), α-1-globulin (2-7%), α-2-globulin (3.5-12%), β-globulins (8-18%) and gamma-globulin (5-12%) (Bauer, 1982). Immunoelectrophoresis has identified several proteins within each of these major classes seen as "peaks" on electrophoresis. α-1 Globulins include α-1-antitrypsin, α-1-lipoprotein and α-1-glycoprotein. α-2 Globulins include haptoglobulin, coeruloplasmin, erythropoietin, α-2-macroglobulin and α-2-lipoprotein. Transferrin, tau fraction, plasminogen, complements, β-lipoprotein, β-trace protein and haemopexin are all β-globulins. They are present in higher concentrations in CSF than in serum and in higher concentrations in ventricular than in lumbar fluid (Fishman, 1980). Gamma globulins include the various immunoglobulins discussed later.

TABLE 5.3. *Interrelationship of CSF and serum protein concentrations with the molecular radii of the proteins as measured by (a) column chromatography and (b) exclusion gel electrophoresis (derived from Felgenhauer, 1974).*

Protein	Molecular weight	Radius (A)		Concentration (mg/l)				Serum/ CSF
		a	b	Serum	N	CSF	N	
Prealbumin	61 000	31.5	33.6	238	29	17.3	40	13.8
α_1-Antitrypsin	45 000	33.5	32.0					
α_1-Antichymotrypsin	45 000		34.2					
Hemopexin	80 000		35.0					
Albumin	69 000	37.4	35.5	36 600		155.0	52	237
α_2-HS-Glycoprotein	49 000	37.9	34.1	479	28	1.7	24	282
Transferrin	81 000	35.7	37.3	2040	30	14.4	30	142
Acid α_1-Glycoprotein	44 100	36.4		664	28	3.6	37	185
Plasminogen	143 000	42.0	43.4	156	26	0.25	**	622
Coeruloplasmin	152 200	47.6	45.5	366	28	0.97	26	377
Immunoglobulin G	150 000	51.8	57.0	9870	30	12.3	90	802
Immunoglobulin A	150 000	56.3	96.0	1750	30	1.3	54	1346
α_2-Macroglobulin	798 000	108.0		2220	30	2.0	90	1111
Fibrinogen	340 000			2964	27	0.65	**	4550
Immunoglobulin M	800 000	121.0		700	30	0.6	22	1166
β-Lipoprotein	2 239 000		122.0	3728	25	0.59	**	6322

** = Equal amounts of seven cerebrospinal fluids are pooled and the protein content was determined after concentrating up to 100-fold. The values are means from six concentrates.

Proteins in the CSF can result from *de novo* synthesis by the nervous tissue, but plasma has been found to be the predominant source. Studies utilising ventriculo-cisternal perfusion and acetazolamide suggest that 50% of radioiodinated serum albumin (RISA) enters the CSF via the choroid plexus and 50% extra choroidally (Levin and Tradatti, 1976). Pial blood vessels have a permeability similar to choroidal capillaries, and, along with the cerebral capillaries, provide extrachoroidal sources of plasma proteins.

Table 5-3 shows the various proteins that can be measured in the CSF and the relationship of their CSF concentrations to their molecular size. Their plasma: CSF concentration ratios can be correlated better to their hydrodynamic radii than to their molecular weights (Felgenhauer, 1974). The quantitative amounts of CSF proteins relative to serum are useful in determining their percentage transfer and degree of intrathecal synthesis. Proteins which demonstrate 500% transfer (i.e. are approximately 5-fold higher in CSF than serum) are considered to be synthesised primarily intrathecally. These include β-trace, gamma-trace, tau, myelin basic and glial fibrillary acidic proteins. ß-trace is the most abundant CSF protein after albumin and may be synthesised by astrocytes and/or oligodendrocytes (Thompson, 1988). Proteins that demonstrate 100% transfer include β2-microglobulin and enolase and for these proteins the brain is probably a source equivalent to other tissues. Prealbumin, lysozyme, eosinophil cationic protein, complement C'9, lactoferrin and ferritin are probably partially synthesised intrathecally. Most other proteins demonstrate less than 1% transfer and are mainly derived from the plasma pool (see Thompson 1988 for review).

Within the CSF there are several protein concentration gradients, as seen in Table 5-4. This suggests that there may exist selective protein transport functions within the blood-CSF barrier. From the ventricular to the lumbar region the concentrations of albumin increase 2.2 times while IgG levels increase 2.6 times and pre-albumin decreases by 0.7 (Weisner and Bernhardt, 1978).

CSF total protein is non-specifically increased in a large variety of diseases. It is a reliable index of increased endothelial cell permeability and of defects in protein absorption. It may increase proportionately with an increase in cell count or it may increase independently of cell changes (albuminocytological dissociation). The latter case occurs with specific alterations in permeability and with blockage of the CSF circulation. Increased total protein is seen in cases of neurosyphilis, neoplasia, intracranial haemorrhage, seizures, cerebral trauma, cerebral thrombosis, endocrine conditions (myxoedema, diabetic neuropathy, hyperadrenalism, hypoparathyroidism), metabolic states (uraemia, hypercalcaemia, de-hydration), toxic conditions (ethanol, isopropanolol), obstruction of CSF circulation (tumour, abscess), with increased CNS synthesis of immunoglobulins (meningitis, Guillain-Barré syndrome, multiple sclerosis, collagen-vascular disease), and with increased plasma protein levels (Krieg, 1979). The CSF:serum concentration ratios for albumin, IgG, α-2-macroglobulin and other proteins may be used as parameters to discriminate between different blood-CSF barriers (Keir and Thompson, 1986).

TABLE 5.4. *Ventricular, cisternal, and lumbar CSF gradients of total protein and protein fractions (determined by immunological methods) (from Weisner and Bernhardt, 1978).*

Protein	Ventricular			Cisternal			Lumbar		
	n	x̄ (mg/l)	SD	n	x̄ (mg/l)	SD	n	x̄ (mg/l)	SD
Total protein	27	256	59	33	316	58	127	420	55
Albumin	27	83	25	33	127	41	127	186	66
IgA	27	<8	–	33	8	–	127	8	–
IgG	27	9	4	33	14	5	127	23	10
IgM	27	<11	–	33	<11	–	127	11	–

Albuminocytological dissociation can occur in diptheric polyneuritis, in Guillain-Barré Syndrome, poliomyelitis, seizures, cerebral infarction, sarcoidosis, myxoedema, and with tumours of the CNS, especially those of the cerebellopontine angle (Tourtellotte and Shorr, 1982).

As discussed earlier, a falsely elevated total protein may also be seen with the injudicious use of local anaesthetics during lumbar puncture (Shealy, 1969).

Protein levels are decreased in benign intracranial hypertension, hyperthyroidism, leukaemia, in acute water intoxication, after pneumoencephalography, following a stroke or seizure, and in normal young children (Fishman, 1992; Lowenthal, 1972; Tourtellotte and Shorr, 1982).

Many specific protein changes in CSF have also been studied. These include albumin, prealbumin, α-1 globulins, α-1-microglobulins, beta globulins, gamma globulins, myelin basic protein, trace proteins, interferon, eosinophil cationic protein, "14-3-3" protein, S-100 protein, and ferritin (Lowenthal, 1972; Krieg, 1979; Fishman, 1992; Trotter and Brooks, 1980; Kobatake *et al.*, 1980; Panitch *et al.*, 1980a; Sindic *et al.*, 1981; Hallgren *et al.*, 1982, 1983; Sindic *et al.*, 1982; Boston *et al.*, 1982; Killingsworth, 1982; Itoh *et al.*, 1983; Weisner and Roethig, 1983).

The interested reader is referred to the excellent reviews of Lowenthal *et al.* (1984), Einstein (1982) and Thompson (1988).

Immunoglobulins

The study of CSF proteins was greatly advanced by Elvin Kabat in 1942, first separating out the various proteins with the technique of electrophoresis into the prealbumin, albumin, alpha, beta and gamma globulin fractions discussed earlier. With the use of radioimmunoassay and immunochemical assays the alpha, beta and gamma globulin fractions have been further separated into their various protein constituents. The gamma globulin fraction represents about 12% of the total CSF protein (vs. about 18% of the serum protein). The major immunoglobulins IgG, IgA, and IgM are all present in normal CSF as well as very small amounts of IgD and IgE. CSF gamma globulin normally originates from plasma, but intrathecal synthesis has been demonstrated in a variety of inflammatory disorders. The most studied of the immunoglobulins in the CSF is IgG, which is present in much greater concentrations than IgA or IgM. It represents about 5-12% of the total CSF protein (vs. 15-18% of the total serum protein) and consists of two types of polypeptide chains – two "heavy" and two "light" chains. The "light" chains are further divided into "kappa" and "lambda" chains. An increased ratio of kappa:lambda light chains is seen in a number of inflammatory diseases affecting the CNS, particularly multiple sclerosis (Fishman, 1980).

A number of formulae have been devised to distinguish between the increased CSF IgG concentrations seen in multiple sclerosis and other inflammatory conditions as deriving from plasma or from local CNS production. The IgG index (the ratio of CSF/serum IgG to CSF/serum albumin) compensates for the influence of serum levels on CSF IgG. An increased IgG index (above 0.7) indicates CNS production of IgG although false increases may occur with moderate or severe blood-brain barrier damage (Link, 1987).

The qualitative and quantitative changes of IgG and other immunoglobulins seen in multiple sclerosis and other disease states are discussed further in Chapter 6. Link (1987), Thompson (1988), and Trotter and Rust (1989) have reviewed some of the recent advances in the study of CSF immunoglobulins.

Enzymes

CSF enzymes may originate from contamination by peripheral tissues, from CNS tissue, or from other cellular elements, such as lymphocytes, in the CSF. Table 5-5 shows the main enzymes studied in the CSF. There have been over 50 enzymes identified in CSF. These have been extensively reviewed by Banik and Hogan (1983) and by Einstein (1982, pp. 173-220). The concentrations of all the enzymes determined in CSF are much lower than their corresponding plasma values. The same methods used to quantify enzymes in serum cannot be used in CSF because of the different ion concentrations, different substrates and the cell count variations in CSF (Lowenthal and Karcher, 1980). Immunological determinations and gas-liquid chromatography may be best for use in the CSF.

TABLE 5-5. *Enzymes detected in the CSF (modified from Fishman, 1980).*

Acetylcholinesterase
Adenylate kinase
Aldolase
Arginine esterase
Arylsulfatase
Aspartate aminotransferase
Catechol-O-methyltransferase
Choline acetyltransferase
Cholinesterases
Creatine phosphokinase
  Isoenzymes
Dehydrogenases
  Iscitric
  Lactic
  Malic
Dopamine beta-hydroxylase
Enolase
β-Galactosidase
Glucuronidase
Leucine aminopeptidase
Lipases
Lysozyme
Phosphatases, acid and alkaline
Phosphohexose isomerase
Phospholipases, A_1, A_2, C
Proteolytic enzymes
Ribonuclease
Transaminases
  Glutamic-oxalacetic transaminase
  Glutamic-pyruvic transaminase

The enzyme lactate dehydrogenase (LDH) originates in CSF from diffusion across the blood-CSF and brain-CSF barriers as well as from cellular elements within the CSF. The measurement of specific LDH isozymes may be useful in distinguishing the predominant source of the enzyme. Increased CSF LDH is seen in meningitis, subarachnoid haemorrhage, leukaemia, lymphoma, carcinoma metastatic to the CNS, hydrocephalus, epilepsy, Huntington's chorea, and the lipidoses. LDH may be of aid in the differential diagnosis of meningitis. The LDH isozymes in viral meningitis are generally LDH 1, 2 and 3 whereas LDH 4 and 5 predominate more in bacterial meningitis. LDH 1 and 2 (of brain tissue origin) in either case are associated with a poor prognosis. The total LDH is also usually higher in bacterial meningitis than in viral meningitis (Krieg, 1979; Banik and Hogan, 1983).

Several enzymes detected in CSF may also be of use as biological tumour markers. These include enolase, adenylate kinase, aldolase, pyruvate kinase, lysozyme, and many others (Schold and Bullard, 1980; Royds et al., 1981a,b; Wasserstrom et al., 1981; Timperley et al., 1982; Hallgren et al., 1982; Vivekanandan et al., 1982) and are discussed in Chapter 6. Adenylate kinase may also be useful in evaluating the progression and/or acuteness of a variety of CNS disorders (Unger et al., 1983).

Enolase (14-3-2 protein) is a glycolytic enzyme which may be useful as both a tumour marker (especially in low grade astrocytoma and fast developing tumours) and as an index of active demyelinization (Lowenthal et al., 1984). It has three distinct subunits (alpha, beta and gamma) and these may be differentiated by an enzyme linked immunosorbent assay (ELISA). Gamma-gamma enolase is present predominantly in neurons and in neuroendocrine cells. It has thus been designated neuron-specific enolase (NSE) and is found significantly increased in Creutzfeldt-Jacob disease, meningeal haemorrhage, thrombosis, Guillain-Barré syndrome, and schizophrenia (Vermuyten et al., 1990).

Amino acids

Since many amino acids are synthesised in the CNS and act as neuro-transmitters (glycine, γ-aminobutyric acid, glutamate, aspartate), the amino acid regulatory mechanism of the CSF is important. The total concentration of amino acids in the CSF is about one-third that of plasma. The individual amino acid concentrations may differ widely from plasma, as with proline (400 times the plasma level), or may not differ at all, as with glutamate (Lorenzo, 1974). CSF levels of individual amino acids appear to be regulated even though the exchange of amino acids between the blood and CSF is rapid (Lorenzo, 1974). Ventriculo-cisternal perfusion and choroid plexus uptake studies provide evidence for active efflux mechanisms operative in the ventricles for arginine, cycloleucine, leucine, gamma aminobutyric acid (GABA), glycine, lysine, tyrosine, and taurine (Lorenzo, 1974). The role of the choroid plexus in this uptake is controversial. The isolated choroid plexus does accumulate amino acids, but does not do so during ventriculo-cisternal perfusion. Lorenzo (1977) states that no accumulation is seen in vivo as the amino acids are rapidly transferred to the circulation.

Extraventricular and extrachoroidal sites for amino acid absorption are believed to include the pia-arachnoid membranes, particularly the pial blood vessels (Wright, 1971). It is not known whether the influx and efflux systems for amino acids are linked. Large neutral amino acids such as tryptophan, alanine, or α-methyl-dopa compete with each other for uptake (Markovitz and Fernstrom, 1977). The activity of some transport systems implicated in amino acid regulation may vary with age and development of the CNS barrier system.

TABLE 5.6. *Concentrations of amino acids in CSF and their relation to plasma levels (derived from McGale et al., 1977).*

Amino acid	CSF concentration Mean ± SD (μmol/l) n = 37		Male CSF concentration Mean ± SD (μmol/l) n = 17		Female CSF concentration Mean ± SD (μmol/l) n = 20		Plasma concentration Mean ± SD (μmol/l) n = 37	
Phosphoserine	4.2	1.7	3.8	1.4	4.5	1.8	8.3	5.7
Taurine	7.6	2.1	6.5	1.3	8.5	2.3	77.2	26.1
Phosphoethanolamine	5.4	2.3	6.2	2.2	4.6	2.0	5.1	3.3
Threonine	35.5	8.9	35.6	9.6	35.4	8.5	165.5	61.4
Serine	29.5	6.5	28.4	6.9	30.4	6.1	139.7	51.6
Asparagine	13.5	4.6	13.7	3.4	13.1	5.4	111.7	52.1
Glutamic acid	26.1	18.9	25.3	22.7	24.0	16.3	61.3	30.8
Glutamine	552.0	79.0	543.0	97.0	552.0	67.0	641.0	93.0
Glycine	5.9	1.8	6.3	1.9	5.6	1.7	323.7	256.0
Alanine and citrulline	34.3	8.2	36.2	8.2	32.6	8.1	282.7	101.6
2-Aminobutyric acid	3.5	1.4	3.6	1.6	3.5	1.2	488.5	192.1
Valine	19.9	4.1	21.3	4.1	18.7	3.8	29.8	12.2
Methionine	2.5	0.9	2.8	1.1	2.2	0.8	308.6	116.0
Isoleucine	6.2	1.4	6.7	1.5	5.8	1.2	123.7	50.0
Leucine	14.8	3.9	16.6	4.2	13.0	2.8	27.7	11.7
Tyrosine	9.5	2.6	9.6	3.0	9.1	2.2	76.7	29.8
Phenylalanine	9.9	2.0	10.6	2.1	9.4	1.6	155.3	58.6
Ornithine	3.8	0.9	4.1	0.8	3.6	0.9	73.0	26.3
Lysine	20.8	4.0	22.1	4.2	19.9	3.6	64.0	24.2
Histidine	12.3	2.2	12.6	2.0	12.0	2.3	73.5	25.8
Arginine	22.4	4.2	23.1	3.5	21.9	4.8	170.7	64.2

The major amino acids that have been identified in the CSF are shown as they relate to plasma levels in Table 5-6 (McGale *et al.*, 1977). The CSF levels of 13 of these amino acids relate directly to the plasma concentrations (McGale *et al.*, 1977). These concentrations vary greatly with differences in age and sex. Various concentration gradients within the CSF have been described (Szilagyi *et al.*, 1974), which generally show a caudocranial increase in concentration.

The total amino acid level in CSF increases in meningitis and in CSF blocks and decreases in multiple sclerosis and benign intracranial hypertension (Lowenthal, 1972). Changes in the concentrations of specific amino acids in the CSF have been noted – in hepatic coma, hyperammonaemia, Tay-Sachs, PKU, and various amino acidopathies (Lowenthal, 1972). Various abnormalities of CSF amino acid levels have also been reported in depression (Goodnick et al., 1980) and in Parkinsonism (Chase, 1980). Glutamine levels are found increased in epilepsy, narcolepsy, and in various liver diseases (Lowenthal, 1972). The excitatory amino acids glutamate and aspartate have been found elevated in the CSF in amyotrophic lateral sclerosis suggesting a role for excitotoxicity in the pathogenesis of this disorder (Rothstein et al., 1990). Excitatory and inhibitory amino acids have been suggested to play a role in epilepsy and a variety of neuropsychiatric disorders, but CSF studies have been somewhat contradictory (Pitkanen et al., 1989; Olney, 1989). Concentrations of the amino acid GABA have been found to vary in many neurological and psychiatric illnesses. These findings are described in the neurotransmitter section of this chapter and further in Chapters 6, 7, and 8.

Peptides and hormones

The CSF may play an important role in transport of hypophysiotropic peptides to target areas of the brain (Knigge et al., 1975). Such peptides may enter the portal circulation from CSF via specialised ependymal cells called tanycytes (Cutler and Spertell, 1982; Knigge et al., 1975; Oliver et al., 1975). Studies with radioactively labelled thyrotrophin-releasing hormone (TRH) indicate that TRH is capable of crossing the median eminence from CSF into hypophyseal portal blood and stimulating the release of thyrotrophin (Oliver et al., 1975). Many other peptides have also been shown to produce physiological actions following intraventricular injection (Knigge et al., 1975; Cutler and Spertell, 1982).

These hormones may be directly secreted by neurons in the perivascular space of the portal capillaries, or they may reach the portal circulation via ependymal structures in the median eminence after direct secretion or diffusion into the CSF of the third ventricle (Knigge et al., 1975). The control of these releasing and inhibiting hormones involves neurotransmitters and other neuropeptides. Table 5-7 shows the effects of intraventricular injection of neurotransmitters and neuropeptides on the release of pituitary hormones.

Endorphins are a class of endogenous opioid neuropeptides found in CSF which have received a lot of attention recently. The major compounds in this class are the encephalin pentapeptides and beta-endorphins. They are believed to be involved in learning, memory, reward behaviour, posture,

TABLE 5.7. *Effect of intraventricular administration of neurotransmitters and brain peptides on pituitary hormone release (from Wood, 1982b).*

Neurotransmitter or peptide	Prolactin	GH	TSH	FSH	LH	ACTH
Acetylcholine	-	+	-	+	+	+
γ-Aminobutyric acid	+,-	+	-	0	+	+
Norepinephrine	?+	+	+		+	-
Dopamine	-	+	-		+,-	0
Serotonin	+	+	0		+,-	+
Melatonin	+				-	
Histamine	+				?+	
Somatostatin	0	+	-	-	-	
Cholecystokinin	+	+	-	0	-	
Gastrin	-	+	-	0	-	
Vasoactive intestinal peptide	+	+	0	0	+	
Substance P	?+	+	0	0	+	
Neurotensin	-	+	0	0	-	
Opioids	+	+	-	0	-,0	

Abbreviations: +, stimulation; 0, no effect; -, inhibition; GH, growth hormone; TSH, thyrotrophin; FSH, follicle-stimulating hormone; LH, luteinizing hormone; ACTH, adrenocorticotrophin.

locomotor activity and pain mechanisms (Bloom and Segal, 1980). Intraventricular injection of β-endorphin will produce analgesia and electrical stimulation of the thalamus and periacqueductal grey causes release of β-endorphin into the VCSF of patients with chronic pain (Rossier *et al.*, 1979; Cutler and Spertell, 1982). It is thus thought to play a key role in centrally mediated suppression of pain (Bloom and Segal, 1980), and patients with neurogenic and phantom pain have been found to have low CSF endorphin levels (Wood, 1980b; Terenius and Wahlstrom, 1979). That CSF endorphins (fraction I) increase after acupuncture also suggests a role in pain perception and may illuminate the physiology of acupuncture (Sjolund *et al.*, 1977).

The β-endorphin present in CSF seems to be primarily of CNS origin since CSF concentrations are greater than and do not correlate with plasma levels (Krieger, 1982). The fact that normal levels of β-endorphins are seen in both hyper- and hypopituitarism suggests that it originates in the brain rather than pituitary tissue (Terenius and Wahlstrom, 1979).

The effect of β-endorphin given intraventricularly is to elevate blood pressure and cause hyperglycaemia, akinesia, analgesia, hypothermia, respiratory depression and electroconvulsive activity (Wood, 1982b). Opioids will also stimulate prolactin and GH release and suppress TSH and LH secretion (van Kammen *et al.*, 1985b). CSF endorphins and encephalins may be measured by radioimmunoassay (RIA), radioreceptor assay (RRA) and by high-pressure liquid chromatography (HPLC) and electrophoresis (Terenius and Wahlstrom 1979; Post *et al.*, 1982; Nyberg *et al.*, 1983).

Lindstrom *et al.* (1978) have implicated endorphins in the pathophysiology of some psychotic states. They found elevated levels of endorphins in the CSF of patients with manic-depressive psychosis, puerperal psychosis and schizophrenia. Levels were also found to revert to normal in some of these patients following treatment with neuroleptics, propanolol, and/or electroconvulsive therapy (ECT). Geschwind (1977) has suggested that higher levels of endorphins may explain why some psychotic patients show a relative insensitivity to pain. The role of CSF endorphins in various neuropsychiatric disorders is discussed further in Chapters 6, 7 and 8; CSF and serum studies have recently been reviewed (Frecsa and Davis, 1991).

Low concentrations of the sex steroid hormones (testosterone, oestradiol, and progesterone) as well as cortisol are also present in the CSF (Marynick *et al.*, 1980). The CSF levels of these hormones correlate well with their free plasma concentrations (Cutler and Spertell, 1982). Their significance in CSF is unclear. Extremely variable results have been obtained by different investigators studying CSF cortisol levels in patients with affective disorders and with schizophrenia (Post *et al.*, 1983).

The anterior pituitary hormones – growth hormone (GH), thyrotrophin (TSH), lutenizing hormone (LH), follicle-stimulating hormone (FSH) and prolactin – are all present in CSF in lower concentrations than those in plasma (Table 5-8). These are generally thought to originate primarily from plasma with somewhat restricted transport across the blood-CSF barriers because of their high molecular weight (Cutler and Spertell, 1982). The adenohypophysis and brain may also be capable of secreting these hormones directly into the CSF. Suprasellar extension of pituitary tumours results in direct secretion into the CSF, causing an increased CSF/plasma ratio. Posttreatment measurements of CSF adenohypophyseal hormones may thus be useful in determining the efficacy of therapy in these patients (Jordan *et al.*, 1976). Elevated CSF concentrations of pituitary hormones (with no change in CSF:plasma ratio) are seen in pituitary tumours without extension. Elevated CSF levels of prolactin are seen in pituitary prolactinomas, but may also be seen in pregnancy (Jordan *et al.*, 1979). Similarly growth hormone is elevated in acromegalics and adrenocorticotrophin (ACTH) is increased in Nelson's Syndome (Cutler and Spertell, 1982; Jordan *et al.*, 1976).

ACTH has attracted much attention since it is suspected of having psychoactive properties. CSF ACTH levels undergo a diurnal rhythm, are decreased by morphine administration, increased by neurologic stress, and are unchanged in response to hypophysectomy or corticosteroid administration (Hosobuchi, 1982). ACTH is produced by both pituitary and brain tissue, especially the hypothalamus (Hosobuchi, 1982), with the latter probably accounting for the origin of the majority of ACTH in the CSF

TABLE 5.8. *Normal values for hormones detected in human plasma and CSF (from Wood, 1982b, with permission).*

Hormone	Units	Plasma concentration	CSF concentration	CSF:Plasma ratio
Adrenocorticotrophin	pg/ml	65 ± 15	73 ± 11	1.12
		74 ± 10	98 ± 11	1.32
Cortisol	fmol/ml		14.4 ± 0.3	
	μg/ml		14 ± 0.9	
	μg/100 ml		0.68 ± 0.08	
Somatostatin	pg/ml		55 ± 6	
			42.9 ± 1.7	
			130.9 ± 10.8	
			142 ± 8	
Growth hormone	ng/ml	1.95 ± 0.20	0.35 ± 0.03	0.17
		6.7 ± 1.5	0.5 ± 0.1	0.07
Thyrotrophin-releasing hormone	pg/ml		40.2 ± 6.9	
			4.9 ± 0.7	
Thyrotrophin	μU/ml	5.95 ± 0.30	2.65 ± 0.20	0.44
		4.0 ± 0.7	0.1 ± 0.0	0.025
Thyroxine, total	ng/100ml	7400	185(pooled)**	0.025
Thyroxine, free		2.4	5.8	2.4
Triiodothyronine, total	ng/100ml	168	17.4 (pooled)**	0.1
Triidothyronine, free	ng/100ml	0.32	1.77	5.53
Prolactin	ng/ml	25 ± 7	0.4 ± 0.1 (5)**	0.02
		7 ± 0.1	1.2 ± 0.2 (30)**	0.17
	μg/l		1.75 ± 0.23 (18)**	
Lutenizing hormone	mlU/ml		5.7 ± 1.5 (6)**	
	IU/l		2.39 ± 0.13 (17)**	
Follicle-stimulating hormone	mlU/ml		5.3 ± 1.2 (6)**	
	IU/l		1.67 ± 0.10 (17)**	
Testosterone, female	ng/100ml		1.4 ± 0.3 (16)**	
Testosterone, male			11.1 ± 1.1 (9)**	
Oestradiol, female	pg/ml		2.4 ± 0.4 (16)**	
Oestradiol, male			2.2 ± 0.2 (9)**	
Progesterone, female	ng/100ml		4.5 ± 0.8 (16)**	
Progesterone, male			3.9 ± 0.5 (9)**	
Melatonin	pg/ml	63 ± 8	59 ± 12 (8)/	0.94
Arginine vasopressin	pg/ml	2.8 ± 0.2	2.4 ± 0.2 (12)**	0.86
Insulin	μU/ml	38.0 ± 4.5	11.0 ± 1.3 (21**	0.29
Cholecystokinin	pM		14.0 ± 3.2 (10)**//	
Gastrin	pM		3.4 ± 1.0 (10)**//	
Vasoactive intestinal polypeptide	pmol/ml	7.3	49.9 ± 4.9 (14)///	7.3
Calcitonin	pg/ml	89 ± 13	28 ± 3 (27)/	0.31

TABLE 5.8. *Cont.*

Hormone	Units	Plasma concentration	CSF concentration	CSF:Plasma ratio
β-Melanocyte stimulating hormone	ng/l	16.1 ± 1.1	60.1 ± 8.9 (30)**	3.73
Substance P	fmol/ml		7.0 ± 8.9 (30)/	
	pg/ml		1.00 ± 0.13 (14)**	
β-Lipoprotein	pg/ml	78.2 ± 13.7	89.3 ± 16.1 (4)**	1.14
β-Endorphin	pg/ml	5.5 ± 2.3	17.9 ± 2.3 (4)**	3.25
	ng/ml		6.1 ± 0.5 (9)**	
	fmol/ml		22.3 ± 1.1 (5)/	
Methionine-encephalin	pmol/ml		3.12 ± 1.23 (10)/	
	ng/ml		26.8 ± 0.8 (9)**	
	pg/ml	69.3 ± (25)**	13.3 ± (7)**	0.19

* Mean ± standard
** Nonendocrine control patients
/ Normal volunteers
// Personal communication from original source
/// Number of patients in parenthesis

(Wood, 1982b). Unlike the other pituitary hormones, the CSF concentrations of ACTH are similar to that of plasma. There does not, however, appear to be a correlation between CSF and plasma levels; CSF ACTH is thought to be primarily of central origin (van Kammen et al., 1985b).

Antidiuretic peptides (Arginine vasopressin, AVP) have also been detected in CSF (van Kammen et al., 1985b; Wood, 1982b). They are thought to originate from the direct secretion of neurosecretory cells which may be functionally separate from the supraopticohypophyseal tract. Intravenous administration of AVP does not elevate CSF levels, implying a central origin. Their CSF concentrations are moderately increased in the syndrome of inappropriate antidiuresis and in diabetes insipidus. Their physiological significance in CSF is unknown, but they may play a role in memory and learning and in CSF formation (McDonald and Krishnan, 1991). Normal, decreased, and increased levels of CSF AVP have all been reported in depressed patients (Post et al., 1982). Sundquist et al. (1983) studied plasma and CSF AVP in various neurological disorders and noted elevated CSF AVP in cerebrovascular disease and decreased concentrations in dementia and Parkinson's Disease. They also found a lower CSF/plasma gradient in those patients with dementia and Parkinson's disease. Elevated CSF/plasma gradients have also been reported in anorexia nervosa (Post et al., 1982).

Other peptides detected in human CSF include 16 K fragment, beta-lipotrophin, alpha and beta-melanocyte stimulating hormone, calcitonin, neurophysin, angiotensin I and II converting enzymes, substance P, neurotensin, somatostatin, gastrin, cholecystokinin, vasoactive intestinal peptide, bradykinin, bombesin, diazepam-binding inhibitor, thyrotrophin releasing hormone, luteinising releasing hormone, luteinising hormone, insulin, and follicle stimulating hormone (Post *et al.*, 1982, 1983; van Kammen *et al.*, 1985*b*). Table 5-8 shows the CSF and plasma concentrations of the various hormones and peptides detected in the CSF.

The rostro-caudal gradients for the various peptides in the CSF are much less pronounced than for amine metabolites. There have been few studies which have looked at correlations between ventricular and lumbar CSF levels. In general most peptides are relatively evenly distributed throughout the ventriculo-spinal system (see review of Gjerris, 1988*a*). The roles the neuropeptides and hormones play in various neuropsychiatric disorders are discussed in Chapters 6, 7 and 8. They have also been reviewed by Robinson (1983), van Kammen *et al.* (1985*b*) and by Nemeroff (1991*a*).

Vitamins

Vitamin C

Ascorbic acid can be synthesised by many species, but humans are not able to synthesise ascorbic acid because of a lack of the enzyme L-gluconolactone oxidase. In man, the concentration of ascorbic acid is higher in the brain and CSF than in plasma, so that the blood to CSF movement is probably against a concentration gradient (Lorenzo, 1977). There is no significant gradient between cisternal and lumbar CSF concentrations (Degrell and Nagy, 1990).

Vitamin C can exist as two forms. The first, ascorbic acid, is the reduced and largely ionised form (at physiologic pH). The second, dihydroascorbic acid, is the oxidised, nonionic and more lipid soluble form. While evidence suggests that the more prevalent form, ascorbic acid, enters the brain and CSF by an active transport process, dihydroascorbic acid levels in plasma increase in certain disease states like diabetes mellitus, and may influence the relative rates of uptake of both the oxidised and reduced forms (Lorenzo, 1977).

The choroid plexus can accumulate ascorbic acid against a concentration gradient and has been strongly implicated as the predominant site for the transport of ascorbic acid from the blood to the CSF and the CNS. No evidence for a carrier mechanism for the reverse direction has been found. Lorenzo (1977) points out that a special transport system could maintain ascorbic acid at a constant level within the CNS, and if ascorbic acid enters the CNS primarily through the CSF, the function of a nutritive role of the CSF in this case seems likely. Evidence for this includes the following: (1)

the finding that *in vitro* isolated choroid plexus and brain have active transport systems for ascorbic acid, (2) the fact that ascorbic acid does not easily pass through brain capillaries, (3) the ability of intraventricularly administered ascorbic acid to penetrate into the brain, (4) the *in vivo* entry of ^{14}C-ascorbic acid into first choroid plexus, followed by entry into the CSF and then into brain areas around the CSF and (5) the previously mentioned higher CSF and brain levels of ascorbic acid relative to plasma (Spector and Ellis, 1984).

Brau *et al.* (1984) found CSF levels of ascorbic acid to be lower in patients with increased intracranial pressure, with cerebral tumours, and in head traumatised patients. The ascorbic acid may be consumed by free radicals produced after certain types of injury to the CNS. Ascorbic acid can act as a free radical scavenger and thus may serve a protective function in such conditions, defending against the propagation of free radical reactions. Brau *et al.* thus suggest that vitamin C may be useful in the management of such patients. Decreased levels of ascorbic acid in CSF are also found in tuberculous meningitis and in other infections (Lowenthal, 1972).

Folate and vitamin B12

In plasma, CSF, and other body fluids, 5-methyl-tetrahydrofolic acid (MeTHF) is the major form of folic acid (FA). The concentration of MeTHF in the CSF and brain is greater than that in plasma, and, since the CSF level falls more slowly than the plasma level, in deficiency states, it has been suggested that a regulatory mechanism functions to maintain MeTHF in the CSF. Lorenzo (1977), postulates that there are two important transport mechanisms for folate in the CNS. One is specific for MeTHF and carries it from the blood to the CSF. The other system is specific for folic acid and transports it in the opposite direction, from the CSF to the blood. As the CNS lacks dihydrofolate reductase, which converts FA to MeTHF, and only MeTHF is active, these mechanisms make physiologic sense.

Methotrexate is a folic acid analog that does not penetrate the blood-CNS barriers well. In addition, methotrexate appears to be removed from the CSF, in part, by the organic acid transport system inhibited by probenecid (Domer and Kaiser, 1977). Methotrexate and folic acid are both concentrated by the isolated choroid plexus, and it can be speculated that both compounds have similar regulatory mechanisms.

Vitamin B12 is unique among the water-soluble vitamins in that the serum levels greatly exceed the CSF levels by a factor of about 20 (Fishman, 1980). Both vitamin B12 and folate are increased in multiple sclerosis (Lowenthal, 1972). Botez *et al.* (1982*a*) noted that patients with B12 deficiency and with folate deficiency (with folate responsive neuropsychiatric symptoms) had concomitant decreased levels of CSF 5-HIAA. They suggest that deficiencies of these vitamins may produce their CNS effects by diminishing serotonergic metabolism.

Van Tiggelen *et al.* (1984) found decreased CSF levels of B12 in 11 of 13 patients with neurasthenic symptoms and in six of 13 geriatric patients with dementia associated with normal serum B12 levels. An additional three geriatric patients had decreased levels of B12 in both serum and CSF. They thus suggest that measurement of CSF B12 levels should be done in the evaluation of patients with organic mental symptoms, as many B12 deficiency states may otherwise go undetected and thus untreated. Similarly, Regland *et al.* (1992) found low CSF B12 levels and CSF/serum B12 ratios in their group of 42 patients with non-specific dementia compared to controls. They suggest that use of the CSF/serum B12 ratio may be a better indicator of central B12 transport function than either CSF or serum values alone.

Other vitamins

Thiamine and inositol, a carboxylic hexitol, are also believed to be regulated in the CSF. Thiamine appears to possess a carrier-mediated transport system for the CSF to blood transfer, but not for the reverse (Lorenzo, 1977). Inositol appears to be unique among the water soluble vitamins in that there is evidence for a carrier system for this compound that is bidirectional between the CSF and the blood. CSF levels are about five times that of plasma levels. Inositol levels are increased in tuberculous meningitis, diabetes, senile dementia, Alzheimer's disease, and bacterial meningitis (Lowenthal, 1972). Botez *et al.* (1982*b*) found that three of five patients with low CSF thiamine also had decreased CSF levels of the serotonin metabolite 5-HIAA. Both CSF thiamine and 5-HIAA levels increased after treatment with thiamine.

Lipids

The analysis of the lipid constituents of the CSF has been difficult because of their susceptibility to oxidation, their propensity to form complexes with carbohydrates and because of the minute quantities present. The total lipid concentration is but 1/700 of the serum level (Lumsden, 1972). The more recent use of gas chromatography has made for more accurate quantification of the various lipid components possible. CSF lipid concentrations are generally independent of serum levels.

Abnormalities in the various lipid constituents have been detected in a number of neurological diseases. Increased total cholesterol levels have been noted in trauma, cerebral infarction, CNS tumour, and multiple sclerosis (MS) (Lumsden, 1972). The esterified component is particularly increased in MS (Pedersen, 1974). CSF phospholipids are increased in a variety of neurological illnesses including tumours, haemorrhage, infection, amyotrophic lateral sclerosis, spondylosis, polyneuritis, Tay-Sach's Disease, Niemann-Pick Disease, retrobulbar neuritis and multiple sclerosis (Lumsden, 1972; Lowenthal, 1972; Fishman, 1980). Alterations of CNS lipids are probably responsible for the abnormal lipid profiles seen in the CSF in Tay-Sachs and retrobulbar neuritis, whereas breakdown of the BBB may be responsible for the abnormalities in CSF lipids in other disorders, especially in meningitis and with tumours (Tourtellotte and Shorr, 1982). Fatty acid abnormalities in CSF have been shown in schizophrenia, manic-depressive states, multiple sclerosis, and in strokes (Lowenthal, 1972; Smith and Thompson, 1977; Welch and Meyer, 1980; Neu, 1981a,b). The lipid abnormalities in MS are dealt with in detail in Chapter 6.

Kaye *et al.* (1992) have recently developed an HPLC method of measuring glycosphingolipids in the CSF which promises to have use both in the diagnosis and in therapeutic monitoring of patients with lysosomal storage diseases. Patients with G_{M1} gangliosidosis have increased CSF levels of G_{M1} ganglioside. G_{M2} ganglioside is elevated in Tay-Sachs, Sandhoff's and AB variants of G_{M2} gangliosidoses. CSF sulfatides may be elevated early in the course of metachromatic leukodystrophy and could be useful in monitoring the effectiveness of bone marrow transplantation or other therapies. Patients with Fabry's disease also showed an increase in CSF globotriaosylceramide.

Prostaglandins

Studies of prostaglandin (PG) transport may provide evidence for the physiological role of this efflux system of the CSF (Bito and Wallenstein, 1977). While prostaglandins are produced by the brain, cerebral tissue lacks the enzymes required for their inactivation. Consequently, termination of the actions of PGs may require transport out of the CNS.

Prostaglandins do not diffuse well through cell membranes, but are found to accumulate *in vitro* in the choroid plexus. This uptake of PG against a concentration gradient is saturable and can be inhibited by the organic acid transport inhibitor probenecid. A probenecid-sensitive facilitated transport process for PG, located at the capillary-glial interface, seems likely. Inhibition of the organic acid efflux system with probenecid rendered the brains of rabbits more sensitive to the effects of exogenous prostaglandins applied topically to the brain (Bito and Wallenstein, 1977). Thus inhibition of PG transport increases the effects of exogenous (and presumably endogenous) prostaglandins.

The choroid plexus appears to be highly organ specific for PGE2 in that, of the five naturally occurring PGs (PGA, PGA2, PGE1, PGE2, and PGF2), only PGE2 has a significant effect on the cAMP production

(Feldman et al., 1979). PGE2 will cause a dose related increase in cAMP in rat choroid plexus via activation of adenylate cyclase (Feldman et al., 1979). PGE2 is thought to increase CSF production via this and possibly other mechanisms. CSF levels of PGE2 may be a good index of encephalopathy (White et al., 1983).

Total PGE levels in the CSF have not been found to differ between normal controls, schizophrenics, and depressed or manic patients in a study by Gerner and Merril (1983). Gerner and Merril found higher levels in normal males than in normal females and found no correlation of CSF levels with age. Alterations of CSF PGE concentrations have been reported in patients following strokes, with meningitis, and in other neurological illness (White et al., 1983).

PGF2 - alpha has received a lot of attention recently. Increased CSF concentrations are found in meningitis and in febrile convulsions (Tamai et al., 1983). Aspirin may thus be effective in febrile convulsions by antagonising the effects of PGF2 - alpha. Increased CSF levels are also seen following strokes, with subsequent decreases related to the improvement of symptoms (Tourtellotte and Shorr, 1982).

Abnormalities in CSF prostaglandins have also been observed in meningitis, epilepsy, encephalitis, cerebral arterial spasm, schizophrenia, stroke, and multiple sclerosis (Rosenblum, 1975; Wolfe et al., 1975; van Kammen and Sternberg, 1980; Mathe et al., 1980; Cohen and Allen 1980; Fishman, 1980). The interested reader is referred to the review of White et al. (1983).

Neurotransmitters

The neurochemical analysis of CSF is complicated by many factors. One must consider the concentration gradients of neurotransmitters and metabolites between CSF compartments, and how these gradients alter the distribution and metabolism in the CNS, as well as the intercorrelations among the metabolites (Stanley et al., 1985; Kruesi et al., 1988; Gjerris et al., 1988; Jibson et al., 1990; Degrell and Nagy, 1990). The effects of age, sex, weight and number of hours of sleep prior to lumbar puncture may be important sources of variance for some neurotransmitters and metabolites (Ballenger et al., 1983). The use of age- and sex-matched controls and the selective screening of subjects for various neurological and psychiatric illnesses will reduce individual variations (Wood, 1980b). Although special diets need not be strictly adhered to prior to the study of CSF, the overeating of foods rich in amino acid precursor substances or amino acid supplementation of diets should be controlled. It is also important to restrict physical activity, fluid intake, exposure to stress and medications which may alter neurotransmitter levels prior to CSF sampling. Due to the circadian rhythms of the biogenic amines and other substances, CSF sampling must be done at the same time of day in all subjects (Wood, 1980b) and seasonal variation is also important.

Even with well controlled CSF sampling and accurate analysis, the substance being quantified in the CSF may not precisely reflect its concentrations in CNS tissue. This is discussed further in Chapter 3. Alterations in CSF circulation, absorption, metabolism, contamination from peripheral sources, and alterations in the blood-CNS-CSF barriers may further complicate the issue. Gjerris (1988b) has discussed the many methodological considerations in measuring CSF neurotransmitter metabolites.

Gamma Aminobutyric Acid (GABA)

This amino acid, present in the brain and the spinal cord in large concentrations, serves as a major inhibitory neurotransmitter in both tissues. The sensitive enzymatic-fluorometric assay for GABA in CNS tissue cannot be used to assay GABA content of LCSF because of ionic interferences. Only with the development of a specific radioreceptor assay (Enna et al., 1977a), an ion-exchange fluorometric method (Wood et al., 1978) and mass spectrometric analysis (Faull et al., 1978) has it been possible to accurately identify and quantify GABA in CSF.

CSF concentrations of GABA may be affected by both age and sex. Ballenger et al. (1983) found females under 40 to have lower GABA levels than males under 40. There was, however, no significant sex difference noted for subjects over 40. They also found CSF GABA levels to correlate negatively with age among female subjects but not among males.

There is some dispute over whether or not GABA is capable of passing through the BBB. Parentally administered GABA has been shown to have only minimal central accumulation. No correlation between plasma and CSF levels has been demonstrated (Wood, 1980b). Oral L-glutamine administration, however, was found to increase GABA levels in the CSF of a patient with Huntington's chorea (Berry and Steiner, 1979). A rostrocaudal gradient has been shown for both free and total GABA concentrations by comparing suboccipital and lumbar CSF (Grove et al., 1982a,b). CSF concentrations of GABA correlate highly with brain GABA concentrations but are only minimally affected by peripheral blood concentrations (Bohlen et al., 1979; Grove et al., 1982).

Within the CNS, the highest concentration of GABA is in the hypothalamus, extrapyramidal areas, and cerebellum (Wood, 1980c). Brain concentrations are higher than spinal cord concentrations. Alterations in brain GABA concentrations in response to GABA transaminase inhibitors correlate closely with cisternal CSF levels (Bohlen et al., 1979). Palfreyman et al. (1983) studied CSF total GABA and homocarnosine in relation to brain GABA concentrations in rats after treatment with gamma-vinyl-GABA (a GABA-transaminase inhibitor). They found both indices to correlate with brain GABA, though only CSF GABA provided an accurate assessment of brain concentrations with respect to time after treatment. Perlow and Lake (1980) showed a daily rhythm in CSF levels of GABA with highest concentrations noted at midday.

GABA is thought to act in an inhibitory manner by increasing chloride ion permeability and inducing neural hyperpolarisation (Wood, 1980c). It may act in the regulation of blood pressure and control of various neuroendocrine functions. Alterations in its metabolism have been implicated in a variety of neurological and psychiatric disorders (Enna *et al.*, 1980; Wood, 1980a; Hare *et al.*, 1980). Lumbar CSF levels of GABA are reduced by 50% in patients with Huntington's chorea and also may be low in certain patients at risk for this disease (Butler *et al.*, 1980; Fishman, 1992). Post-mortem analysis of striatal tissue indicates a loss of GABAergic neurons in Huntington's chorea as well as a disturbance of dopaminergic and cholinergic neurons (Butler *et al.*, 1980).

Since the concentrations of glutamic acid decarboxylase (GAD), the primary enzyme in GABA synthesis, in the substantia nigra and globus pallidus are lower in patients with untreated Parkinson's disease, there may be some reciprocal modulation of GABAergic and dopaminergic neurons in these areas. (Hare *et al.*, 1980; Teychenne *et al.*, 1980). GAD levels return to normal following long-term treatment with L-DOPA. Although Hare *et al.* (1980) found low GABA levels in the CSF of six patients with Parkinsonism, the studies of Enna *et al.* (1977b) and of Teychenne *et al.* (1980) did not. Teychenne *et al.* (1980) found no difference in CSF GABA levels between either treated or untreated patients with Parkinsonism or their controls. They postulate that, while GABAergic activity may modulate dopaminergic neurons, there is no evidence of the reverse being true.

Other neurological illnesses in which GABA levels in CSF are diminished include MS, cerebellar cortical atrophy, dementia, amyotrophic lateral sclerosis, and Alzheimer's disease (Enna *et al.*, 1977b, 1980; Hare *et al.*, 1980; Wood, 1980b). Schmidt and Loscher (1982) found similar CSF GABA levels in patients with multiple sclerosis, ischaemic strokes, polyneuropathies, and intracranial tumours. Altered GABA levels in CSF have also been reported in various psychiatric disorders, notably schizophrenia and manic-depressive psychosis (Faull *et al.*, 1978; Hare *et al.*, 1980; Post *et al.*, 1980b). These are discussed further in Chapter 7.

Serotonin (5-hydroxytryptamine, 5-HT)

The midbrain, pons, and substantia nigra contain the highest concentrations of serotonin (5-HT) found in the CNS. Ascending serotonergic tracts travel to almost all areas of the diencephalon and telencephalon, originating in the raphe nuclei of the pons and midbrain. The medulla sends out descending serotonergic fibres to the spinal tracts. Both excitatory and inhibitory roles have been postulated for serotonin as a neurotransmitter (Wood, 1980c).

Serotonergic activity has also been associated with the regulation of several neuroendocrine systems. For example, serotonergic activity increases growth hormone and prolactin serum concentrations (Wehrenberg et al., 1980). It also augments release of ACTH and inhibits both gonadotrophin and ADH release (Wood, 1982b). Reinhard et al. (1979) postulated that serotonergic neurons from the raphe nuclei act with chemoreceptors in the control of the brain microcirculation. Serotonergic tracts may participate in the regulation of vasoconstrictor mechanisms, vascular permeability, and body temperature (Wood, 1980c), as well as in sleep (Bremer, 1977) and pain sensitivity (Akil and Liebeskind, 1975).

Serotonin has been implicated in the pathogenesis of various neurological and psychiatric illnesses including depression (van Praag, 1980a,b), myoclonus (Chadwick et al., 1978), epilepsy (Meldrum, 1978), parkinsonism (Klawans, 1975; Pycock, 1978), and attention deficit disorder associated with hyperactivity (Brase and Loh 1975). These are discussed further in Chapters 6, 7 and 8.

Passive diffusion of serotonin across the BBB can be demonstrated only after intravenous administration of large (nonphysiological) concentrations. Inferences about serotonin concentration are often made by quantification of its metabolic precursors L-tryptophan and L-5-hydroxytryptophan (5-HTP) and of its major acidic metabolite 5-hydroxyindoleacetic acid (5-HIAA) (see Fig. 3-1). Wagner et al. (1982) have described a technique of high-performance liquid chromatography with electro-chemical detection that may be useful for the determination of 5-HT, tryptophan, 5-HTP, and 5-HIAA (as well as of DA, NE, DOPAC, and HVA).

L-tryptophan readily crosses both the blood-brain and blood-CSF barriers and is metabolised by tryptophan hydroxylase, the rate limiting step in 5-HT synthesis. Dietary supplementation with L-tryptophan increases serum and CSF concentrations of tryptophan and increases brain concentrations of serotonin and 5-HIAA (Fernstrom et al., 1974; Moir, 1974; Modigh, 1975). A concentration gradient exists for tryptophan between the CSF in the ventricle and spinal subarachnoid space (Young et al., 1974). The lumbar CSF concentrations reflect primarily spinal sources of tryptophan (Wood, 1980c).

Young et al. (1974) found no correlation between CSF levels of tryptophan and 5-HIAA and suggested that the CNS concentration of tryptophan may not be adequately reflected in the CSF or, alternatively, that CNS tryptophan is not the main factor in controlling serotonin synthesis. Korf et al. (1983) also found no such correlation in their psychiatric patients. In contrast, Modigh (1975) did find a significant correlation between the concentrations of tryptophan and 5-HIAA in rat CSF. They also noted correlations between CSF and brain levels of tryptophan and of 5-HIAA, suggesting that central serotonergic activity may best be monitored by concomitant measurement of both CSF parameters. The value of using CSF tryptophan concentrations to estimate either 5-HT turnover or as an indicator of substrate availability is thus unclear.

After having crossed the BBB tryptophan is hydroxylated to form L-5-hydroxy-tryptophan (5-HTP), which serves as the immediate precursor of serotonin (see Fig. 3-1). 5-HTP in turn is converted by the enzyme L-amino acid decarboxylase to serotonin. This conversion occurs primarily in the extraneuronal glial cells (Wood, 1982b). Since oral administration of 5-HTP elevates CSF metabolites of serotonin, it has been used experimentally in the therapy of patients with myoclonus, depression, and seizure disorders (Trimble et al., 1975; Van Woert and Sethy, 1975).

Serotonin is metabolised rapidly to 5-HIAA in the brain (with a Tl/2 of 5-10 min). The measurement of 5-HIAA in CSF is often used as an indicator of CNS metabolism of serotonin. As discussed in Chapter 3, there is considerable debate about the origin of 5-HIAA in the various CSF compartments. However, 5-HIAA found in the CSF probably originates from the CNS metabolism of 5-HT.

CSF levels of 5-HIAA have been studied in several neurological and psychiatric diseases. These are discussed in Chapters 6, 7, and 8.

Dopamine (DA)

While dopamine is found predominantly in the nucleus accumbens and caudate nucleus, it is also found in the substantia nigra, hypothalamus, and olfactory area of the human brain (Mackay et al., 1978). It is thought to be present in significant quantities in the spinal cord and does not freely cross the blood-CSF or blood-brain barriers (Wood, 1980c). Dopamine, generally considered to be an inhibitory transmitter, has been implicated in the modulation of motor function (via the nigrostriatal pathways) and in the inhibition of prolactin, melanocyte-stimulating hormone (MSH) and thyroid stimulating hormone (TSH) release (via the tubero-infundibular system) (Wood, 1982b; Van Praag, 1980a,b). However, growth hormone (GH) release is stimulated by the dopaminergic infundibular system. A third system of dopaminergic pathways, the mesolimbic (fibers extending from the tegmentum to the limbic system and cortex), is probably involved in mood and impulse regulation (Van Praag, 1980a,b).

Assays that are available for the quantification of DA in brain tissue, have detected acid-hydrolisable conjugates in ventricular CSF. Until recently, current analytical methods have lacked the sensitivity necessary for LCSF determinations. Elchisak et al. (1982) have described a gas-chromatography-mass spectrometry (GC-MS) assay capable of detecting dopamine in ventricular and lumbar fluid samplings.

The decreased brain tissue DA content first found in Parkinson's disease and subsequently reported in Alzheimer's disease and senile dementia prompted studies of DA precursors and metabolites in CSF. Tyrosine and L-DOPA are the major precursors. Dopamine is metabolised in the brain to 3, 4-dihydroxyphenyl-acetic acid (DOPAC) and to HVA.

Tyrosine, the dietary precursor of DA, is taken up and metabolised only by those cells that normally contain tyrosine hydroxylase activity. Though brain tyrosine concentrations correlate highly with brain catechol synthesis (Wurtman et al., 1974), there is no clear relationship between CSF levels of tyrosine and dopamine metabolites.

DA is metabolised in the brain by catechol-O-methyltransferase (COMT) and monoamine oxidase (MAO) to DOPAC and to HVA (see Fig. 3-2). Intravenous administration of radiolabelled L-DOPA results in a rapid appearance in CSF and brain tissue of both radiolabelled HVA and DOPAC (Extein et al., 1974; Wood, 1980c). HVA concentration is more widely used as an index of dopaminergic activity than DOPAC because the DOPAC content of LCSF is only 1% of that of HVA (Wood, 1982a). Conversely, studies of the acid metabolites of dopamine in ventricular and cisternal CSF often use DOPAC concentrations because in these areas DOPAC is found at levels about three times greater than HVA.

Important variables that must be considered in using HVA as an indicator of DA activity include age, sex, exercise, position, stress, and diurnal rhythms (Wood, 1982a). One must also assume, as in the study of any metabolite, that the normal removal mechanisms for HVA play an important role in determining CSF levels. For example, the high levels of HVA found in LCSF in hydrocephalus (Shaywitz et al., 1980; Tabaddor et al., 1978a), meningitis, and encephalitis (Bakke et al., 1974) might be explained either by enhanced DA metabolism or, more likely, by interference with the active transport mechanism necessary for the removal of the acid monoamine metabolites from CSF (Fishman, 1980). These assumptions and the use of CSF metabolite studies as an indicator of central DA activity are further discussed in Chapter 3.

CSF analysis of HVA concentrations have been undertaken in many neurological and psychiatric illnesses where alterations in DA metabolism are implicated. Several investigators have demonstrated low LCSF concentrations of HVA in Parkinsonism, senile and presenile dementia, depressive psychosis, the Shy-Drager syndrome, Creutzfeldt-Jakob disease, Parkinsonian dementia of Guam, Gilles de la Tourette Syndrome, progressive supranuclear palsy, olivoponto-cerebellar degeneration, dystonia musculorum deformans, dominant striatonigral degeneration (Moir et al., 1970; Bowers, 1974a,b; Post et al., 1974; Ouvrier, 1978; Fishman, 1992; Van

Praag, 1980*a,b*), and in a number of psychiatric disorders (see Chapters 6 and 7).

High values of HVA have been noted in hepatic coma, meningitis, encephalitis, and Reye's Syndrome (Curzon, 1975; Bakke *et al.*, 1974; Shaywitz *et al.*, 1980).

Le Witt *et al.*, (1992) have recently developed a new method using a coulometric electrode array with HPLC and GC-MS to simultaneously measure multiple DA metabolites in the CSF, including HVA, 3-O-methyldopa, 3,4-dihydroxyphenylacetate, 3-methoxytyramine, DA, DA-3-sulphate, homovanillol, and levodopa.

Norepinephrine (NE)

Norepinephrine is formed from dopamine by the enzyme dopamine-β-hydroxylase. It is the principal adrenergic neurotransmitter in the CNS (Costa and Neff, 1972). Although a direct and significant relationship exists between plasma and CSF levels of NE, intravenous infusions of labelled NE evoke peak CSF concentrations that are only about 2% that of the peak plasma levels (Ziegler *et al.*, 1977*a,b*). This relationship reminds us that plasma NE crosses the blood-CSF and blood-brain barriers poorly. Further, peripheral sympathetic activity contributes to CSF NE content (Wood, 1982*a*). The origin of CSF NE and its metabolites is discussed further in Chapter 3.

Within the human brain, NE is found in greatest concentrations in the hypothalamus, nucleus accumbens, and mamillary bodies (Mackay *et al.*, 1978). The noradrenergic system is involved in the regulation of cerebral blood flow, permeability of cerebral microvasculature, reinforcement and learning behaviour patterns, as well as consciousness and arousal mechanisms mediated via the locus coeruleus in the rostral fourth ventricle (Wood, 1982*a*). NE also participates in the regulation of pituitary hormones via tegmental fibres to the hypothalamus. These noradrenergic fibres augment TRH, LH, GH, gonadotropic hormones, and prolactin secretion and inhibit ACTH and ADH release (Balestreri *et al.*, 1979; Wood 1980*c*). A rostrocaudal gradient for NE in CSF as well as diurnal variation patterns have been reported (Ziegler *et al.*, 1977*a,b*; Wood; 1980*c*).

NE is metabolised via the monoamine oxidase system to 3-methoxy-4-hydroxyphenylethylene glycol (MHPG) and to lesser quantities of vanillyl-mandelic acid (VMA) (see Fig. 3-2). VMA represents about 8% of NE metabolites in LCSF and about 20% in VCSF (Wood, 1980*b*). MHPG is present in highest concentrations in the pons and hypothalamus. Its use as an indicator of central noradrenergic activity was discussed in Chapter 3.

Dopamine-β-hydroxylase (DBH), the enzyme which synthesises NE from DA, is another valuable indicator of central noradrenergic activity. CSF DBH activity is increased by phenoxybenzamine and physostigmine administration and decreased by clonidine and by MAO inhibitors (Major *et al.*, 1983).

NE and its metabolites have been implicated in various neuropsychiatric disorders (see Chapters 6, 7 and 8).

Acetylcholine

Acetylcholine (ACh) has received much less attention than other neuro-transmitters in CSF studies. This has been in part due to its relative instability in CSF and in part to the lack of sensitivity of the various bioassay methods used (Fishman, 1992). The normal range of concentrations varies greatly depending on the type of assay employed. The recent use of gas chromatography/mass spectrometry (GC/MS) in quantifying both ACh and its precursor and metabolite choline (Ch) may facilitate future investiga-tions of ACh metabolism in CSF.

ACh and Ch levels in CSF have been looked at with varying results in a variety of illnesses including CNS tumours, aneurysms, head trauma, Parkinsonism, Huntington's chorea, epilepsy, meningitis, migraine, and psychoses (Schain 1960; Welch *et al.*, 1976*a,c*; Chase 1980; Fishman, 1992; Flentge *et al.*, 1984). Because of the wide range of assays used in these studies, these data are difficult to interpret. The diagnostic and therapeutic potential of this important central neurotransmitter thus remains elusive.

Acetylcholinesterase (AChE) has also been used as a possible indicator in the CSF of central cholinergic activity. Davis and Goodnick (1983) have reviewed the CSF AChE findings in schizophrenia, mania, depression, anxiety, Huntington's chorea, Parkinson's disease, epilepsy, postconcus-sion syndromes, and dementia. AChE levels have not been found to be consistently increased or diminished in any of these illnesses. This is discussed further in Chapter 6.

Cyclic nucleotides

Cyclic nucleotides are formed by the action of the enzymes adenylate and guanylate cyclase. These enzymes convert ATP (adenosine triphosphate) to cAMP (cyclic adenosine monophosphate) and GTP (guanosine tri-phosphate) to cGMP (cyclic guanosine monophophosphate), respectively. Their synthesis is regulated by the availability of triphosphate, calcium ions, NE, DA, serotonin, histamine, PGs, peptides and other neuromodulators (Daly 1977*a*; Rudman *et al.*, 1977). Cyclic nucleotides are thought to act as "second messengers" in regulating the effects of various neuro-transmitters and hormones. Within the CNS they may be important in the secretion of CSF, the maintenance of the blood-CNS barriers, temperature regulation, hunger and thirst mechanisms, blood pressure control and the regulation of various behavioural functions (Daly 1977*b*). Adenosine is thought to play an important role in regulating cerebral blood flow (Winn *et al.*, 1983).

Since cyclic nucleotides do not readily cross the CNS barrier systems, CSF levels may indicate CNS activity. The CSF concentrations of cAMP and cGMP are both markedly lower than their corresponding plasma values (Daly, 1977a,b). The CSF levels are thought to originate primarily from an active-transport mediated extrusion of intracellular cyclic nucleotides which serves as a major mechanism for their termination of action in addition to their hydrolysis by phosphodiesterase (Rindler et al., 1978; Wood, 1982a). The CSF concentrations may thus reflect the intracellular activity of cAMP and cGMP in the CNS (Bonnet, 1982).

Increased CSF levels of cAMP have been reported in meningitis, schizophrenia, migraine, amyotrophic lateral sclerosis, seizures, and following cerebral infarction (Welch et al., 1975, 1976; Heikkinen et al., 1974; Wood and Brooks, 1980; Brooks et al., 1980; Bonnet, 1982). Rudman et al. (1976) found decreased CSF levels in prolonged coma secondary to trauma and haemorrhage. The cAMP levels had a high negative correlation to the grade of coma. Fleischer et al. (1977) found a similar relationship of cAMP and degree of coma. Papageorgious et al. (1983) noted markedly decreased levels in the CSF of patients with cerebral ischaemia in deep coma and in meningitis. Other investigators have reported no significant variations of cAMP levels in mania, depression, Parkinsonism, Huntington's chorea, dystonia, dyskinesia and spinocerebellar degeneration (Daly, 1977b).

Variable results have been reported in a number of other neurological and psychiatric illnesses. These are discussed in Chapters 6, 7 and 8.

The CSF concentrations of cGMP have not been as extensively investigated. Increased levels have been reported in brain tumours, with increased intracranial pressure, posttraumatic coma, with neuroleptics and in systemic lupus with neurologic involvement (Rudman et al 1976; Trabucchi et al., 1977; Kassan and Kagen 1978; Fleischer et al., 1977; Bonnet 1982).

CSF cGMP levels are decreased in Parkinson's disease and in some cases of amyotrophic lateral sclerosis (ALS) (Belmaker et al., 1978; Brooks et al., 1980; Bonnet, 1982). Trabucci et al. (1977) reported no change in CSF levels in patients with epilepsy or with cerebrovascular disease.

Polyamines

The polyamines spermine, spermidine, and their precursor putrescine, are involved in nucleic acid metabolism and thus are related to cellular division and proliferation and to the process of myelination (Fishman, 1992; Leland et al. 1983). They are thought to be involved in the synthesis of protein in the nuclear cell membrane and in RNA synthesis (Einstein, 1982). CSF concentrations of putrescine are increased in medulloblastomas, myelomeningocele, and hydrocephalus; levels of spermidine are elevated in glioblastomas, astrocytomas, medulloblastomas, myelomeningocele, encephalocele, and hydrocephalus (Leland *et al.*, 1983). CSF polyamines may prove useful in monitoring tumour progression and in evaluating hydrocephalus and disorders of myelination. Fulton *et al.* (1983) have reviewed the clinical role of CSF polyamine levels in CNS tumours, pituitary disease, and subarachnoid haemorrhage (SAH), and these are also discussed further in Chapter 6.

Other constituents of the CSF

Other substances which have been measured in CSF include oxygen, ammonia, urea, procoagulants, creatinine, urate, hypoxanthine, polyhydric alcohols, iron, aluminium, boron, chromium, copper and other trace metals. The interested reader is referred to the excellent reviews of Cutler and Spertell (1982), Fishman (1992), Wood (1980*a*, 1982*a*, 1983), Lowenthal and Karcher (1980), Hochwald (1983), Tourtellotte and Shorr (1982), Davson *et al.* (1987) and Herndon and Brumback (1989*c*).

6. CSF in Neurological Illness

Introduction

As many drugs and pathological conditions affect the composition and dynamics of the CSF, lumbar puncture is increasingly becoming an important tool for the clinician for the diagnosis and treatment of specific disease processes. Table 6-1 summarises the effects of various neurological illnesses on some CSF findings. In this chapter we will examine more in depth the many diagnostic and therapeutic possibilities of the CSF.

TABLE 6.1. *Some CSF findings in neurological illness (from Scheinberg et al., 1983, with permission).*

Disease	Colour	Pressure	Cells	Protein	Sugar
A. *Viral*					
Poliomyelitis	Xanthochromic or Colourless*	N or I N or I	0-500 P,M	20-350	N
Mumps	Colourless*	N or I	0-200 M	20-125	N
Lymphocytic choriomeningitis	Colourless*	N or I	10-200 maybe more,M	20-200	N
Coxsackie	Colourless*	N or I	25-250 M	50-100	N
Echo	Colourless*	N or I	10-4000 P	50-100	N
Herpes simplex	Colourless*	I	(few RBC 100-1000 M or P)	50-200	N
Herpes zoster	Colourless*	N	1-300 (40% of pts.)	20-110	N
E. Equine	Colourless*	N or I	500-3000 P	20-200	N
St. Louis	Colourless*	N or I	10-200 M	20-200	N
Measles	Colourless*	N or I	45-100 M	0-500	N
Rabies	Colourless*	N	5-500 M	50-100	N
B. *Bacterial*					
Meningococcal	Cloudy, pus**	I	25-10 000 P	50-1500	0-40
Pneumococcal	Cloudy, pus	I	25-10 000 P	50-1500	0-40
H. influenziae	Cloudy, pus	I	1000-6000 P	50-1500	0-40
E. Coli	Cloudy, pus	I	25-10 000 P	50-1500	0-40
Staphylococcal	Cloudy, pus	I	25-10 000 P	50-1500	0-40
TB	Opalescent, xanthochromic, pellicle	I	25-1 000 M	45-500	10-45

TABLE 6.1. *Cont.*

Disease	Colour	Pressure	Cells	Protein	Sugar
Brucellosis	May be cloudy	I	5-500	50-500	below 40
C. *Partially treated bacterial meningitis (unknown)*					
	May be cloudy	I	500-1000	50-500	30-50
D. *Parainfectious encephalomyelopathy (viral)*					
	Clear	N or I	5-200 M	15-175	Normal
E. *Fungal meningitis*					
Cryptococcosis	Clear or cloudy	I	10-800 M	100 in 90% up to 500%	below 40 in 55
F. *Sarcoidosis*					
	Clear	I	10-200 M	50-200 gamma-globulin increased	15-40
G. *Subacute sclerosing panencephalitis (Dawson's, Van Bogaert's)*					
SSPE	Clear	N	10-50 M	Normal gamma-globulin increased	Normal
H. *Progressive multifocal leukoencephalopathy*					
	Clear	N	5-10 M	Normal	Normal
I. *Haemorrhagic leukoencephalopathy*					
	Clear	N	10-50 M few RBC in some	Normal	Normal
J. *Rickettsial infections*					
Typhus	Clear	N or I	25-200 M	50-100	Normal
Rocky Mountain spotted fever	Clear	N or I	25-200 M	50-100	Normal
K. *Syphilis*					
Meningo-vascular[+++]	Clear	N or I	10-100 M	50-100	Normal
Tabes dorsalis[+++]	Clear	N	0-75 M	30-70	Normal
General paresis	Clear	N	15-100 M	50-150	Normal

TABLE 6.1. *Cont.*

Disease	Colour	Pressure	Cells	Protein	Sugar
L. *Protozoan diseases*					
Trichinosis	Clear	N	0-50 M	Normal	Normal
Toxoplasmosis	Clear or				
	xanthochromic	I	0-50 M	50-100	Normal
Schistomiasis	Clear	I	0-50 M	50-100	Normal
M. *Chronic infection and complications*					
Cerebral abscess					
Encapsulated	Clear	I or N	0-800 P	45-200	Normal
Ruptured	Purulent	I	20-50 000 P	200	Normal
Subdural					
empyema	Clear	I	25-500 P	75-150	Normal
Dural sinus					
Thrombosis	Turbid, Cloudy	I	5-500 P	50-200	Normal
Spinal epidural					
abscess	Xanthochromic	N or I	5-500	100-1500	Normal
N. *Guillain Barré syndrome*					
	Clear or				
	xanthochromic	N	0	50-1500	Normal
O. Brain and spinal cord tumours					
Brain tumour	Clear or				
	Xanthochromic	N or I	Usually 0, may be 20-100 P or M	50-1000	Normal
Spinal tumour	Clear or				
	xanthochromic	I partial or com- plete block	Usually 0, may be 10-50 M	100-1500	Normal
Carcinomatous					
meningitis	Clear	I	50-500 M tumour cells	50-200	Under 35
P. *Haemorrhagic diseases***					
Ruptured berry aneurysm	Bloody, xantho- chromic	I	RBC up to 5 × 10^6 WBC in proportion	Increased according to blood content	Normal
Cerebral haemorrhage	Bloody, xantho- chromic	I	RBC up to 5 × 10^6	As above	Normal
Subdural haematoma	Clear or xanthochromic	N or I	RBC up to 10 000	N or I	Normal
Epidural	Bloody or xanthochromic	I	RBC up to 10 000 WBC in proportion	Increased	Normal

TABLE 6.1. *Cont.*

Disease	Colour	Pressure	Cells	Protein	Sugar
Intracerebral haematoma	Bloody or xanthochromic	I	RBC up to 10000 WBC in proportion	Greater than appropriate for no. of RBC	Normal
Q. *Head trauma*					
Concussion	Clear	N	0	Normal	Normal
Concussion with oedema	Clear	I	0	Normal	Normal
Cerebral contusion	Bloody	I	RBC-WBC	N or I	Normal
R. *Degenerative diseases*					
Parkinson's disease	Clear	N	0	45-50	Normal
Friedreich's ataxia	Clear	N	0	45-75	Normal
Charcot Marie tooth	Clear	N	0	45-75	Normal
Huntington's chorea	Clear	N	0	45-50	Normal
Alzheimer's	Clear	N	0	45-75	Normal
Syringomyelia	Clear	N or I	0-20 M	10-249	Normal
S. *Demyelinating diseases*					
Multiple sclerosis	Clear	N	0-2- M	45-75 (also increased gamma-globulin)	Normal
Schilder's disease	Clear	N or I	0-20 M	45-75 (also increased gamma-globulin)	Normal
Parainfectious encephalomyelitis	Clear	N or I	15-250 M		Normal
Central pontine myelinolysis	Clear	N	0-20 M	45-75	Normal

* Faint opalescence may be present in any of the viral meningoencephalitides ("aseptic meningeal reaction").

** All purulent fluid may clot.

+ CSF serology positive in all cases, except for late tabes dorsalis. Blood serology almost always positive.

+ + Gammaglobulin elevated.

*** Following initial haemorrhage, the CSF develops a leukocytosis due to an aseptic meningeal reaction.

Note: P = polymorphonuclear; M = mononuclear cell; I = increased.

Multiple Sclerosis

Introduction

Multiple Sclerosis (MS) is a progressive demyelinating disease characterised by acute exacerbations and by spontaneous remissions. It is the leading cause of serious neurological illness in the young and middle-aged population of Europe and the United States. A great deal of information has been compiled on MS since its original description by Charcot in 1868. Still the cause remains unknown; there is no specific treatment, and even the diagnosis of MS is far from clear cut.

There is no specific laboratory test for MS. The diagnosis rests on interpretation of the clinical signs and symptoms aided by visual, auditory and somatosensory evoked responses, CSF data (McLeod, 1982) and magnetic resonance imaging (Kirshner et al., 1985). The diagnosis can be difficult, particularly in early and atypical cases.

The examination of the CSF is essential both for arriving at the diagnosis of MS and for studying its pathophysiology. The examination of CNS tissue in MS shows distinct morphological and biochemical abnormalities but, of course, is not practical from a clinical standpoint. The examination of CSF in MS has been extensively reviewed by Lowenthal (1977), Johnson (1980), Thompson (1977), Bauer et al. (1980), Walker and Thompson (1983), Tourtellotte (1985, 1987), and Trotter and Rust (1989). The main abnormalities seen in the CSF include a mononuclear pleocytosis, increased immunoglobulins and increased protein. The appearance, pressure, and glucose content are almost always normal. CSF abnormalities can now be detected in more than 90% of cases of MS (Johnson, 1980; Tourtellotte, 1985).

Cytological changes

The cell count in MS is usually normal or only slightly elevated. Approximately 90% of patients have cell counts of less than 10 per mm^3. Rarely will cell counts be above 50/mm^3. A CSF pleocytosis is more likely immediately following an acute exacerbation (Perkin et al., 1983). An increased number of mononuclear leukocytes may be seen in the CSF, particularly in the early stages, reflecting cellular infiltration found in the regions of acute and chronic demyelinating plaques (Reunanen and Ilonen, 1982; Sayk et al., 1980). Though there is evidence that they reflect the increased intrathecal immunological activity in MS, their presence does not correlate well with clinical exacerbations and remission (Reunanen and Ilonen, 1982; Tourtellote, 1985). Other investigators have reported on occasion increased numbers of blast-like cells, eosinophils, T-cells, reactive lymphocytes, plasma cells (Lumsden, 1972; Thompson, 1977; Tourtellotte, 1985; Sayk et al., 1980; Walker and Thompson, 1983) and atypical plasma cells (Kraft *et al.*, 1989). There is no correlation, however, between the presence of these cells in the CSF and clinical relapse.

Tourtellotte (1970) and Thompson *et al.* (1983) found an increased total CSF leukocyte count to correlate with an increase in intrathecal IgG synthesis. Since intrathecal IgG is a by-product of the MS inflammatory reaction in the brain, this correlation supports the hypothesis that the CSF cells are an integral part of the multiple sclerosis lesion (Tourtellotte, 1985).

Baumhefner and Tourtellotte (1985) reported a slight increase in B-cells and a lower number of T-cells in the CSF of his patients compared to their peripheral blood. This was, however, similar to their neurological control group. There is evidence for a selective loss of T-suppressor/cytotoxic lymphocytes (Morimoto *et al.*, 1987; Chofflon *et al.*, 1989) and an increased percentage of helper/inducer T-cells (Chofflon *et al.*, 1989) resulting in an increased ratio of T-helper/T-suppressor cells in the CSF, but not in the peripheral blood.

Brinkman and colleagues (1983) found 90 ± 9% of the CSF cells in their MS patients were T-lymphocytes and noted no significant differences between their MS patients and neurological controls in percentage of T-lymphocyte subpopulations. Treatment with cyclophosphamide reduced the percentage of T-helper/inducer lymphocytes and increased that of T-suppressor/cytotoxic lymphocytes, normalising the T-helper/T-suppressor ratios in both CSF and in peripheral blood.

It should be noted that these imbalances of T-cell population are not specific for MS (Brinkmann *et al.*, 1983), and T-subset enumeration is of no clear clinical relevance (Tourtellotte, 1987).

Protein

Total protein and albumin

CSF protein may be mildly or moderately elevated in about one-third of patients with MS (Lumsden, 1972). This increase is largely thought to be due to a breakdown in the blood-CSF barrier secondary to increased endothelial cell permeability. This is supported by the demonstration of focal enhancement of MS plaques by radiocontrast material with computed tomography (Weinstein *et al.*, 1978), the correlation between total protein and albumin concentrations (Tourtellotte, 1970; Walker and Thompson, 1983), and the detection of haptoglobin polymers not normally found in CSF (Takeoka *et al.*, 1983).

Tourtellotte (1970) found that 99.7% of patients have total protein and albumin levels below 108 mg/dl and 65 mg/dl respectively, and that concentrations above these levels should cast doubt on the diagnosis of MS. The CSF albumin levels are of more practical relevance than total protein levels.

Of the protein constituents of the CSF, the immunoglobulins have shown the most specific changes in MS. In particular, the presence of oligoclonal bands or demonstration of an increased IgG synthesis rate in the CSF form the key to the diagnosis of laboratory-supported definite MS. (LSDMS) (Paty *et al.*, 1991).

Immunoglobulins: quantitative changes

CSF immunoglobulin G (IgG) is elevated in about two-thirds of patients with MS (Johnson, 1980). The subclass IgG1, in particular, is significantly elevated in MS, and less so IgG 2, 3, and 4 (Losy *et al.*, 1990; Kaschka *et al.*, 1979). This pattern is less marked in the sera than in the CSF. Alterations in other immunoglobulins in the CSF may also be important in the pathogenesis of MS (Sindic *et al.*, 1980).

The question arises as to whether the elevated IgG originates from local CNS production or from defects in the BBB. The concentration of CSF IgG in normal subjects will follow serum levels, remaining at levels of about 1/300 of the serum value (Fishman, 1980). The CSF levels in MS, however, occur as a rule without changes in the serum concentrations. That this IgG production occurs locally in the CNS is also confirmed by the finding of an increased CSF IgG/albumin ratio, a normal serum/CSF albumin ratio and a high "IgG index", and by the measurement of the activity of radio-labelled IgG in serial CSF and blood specimens following intravenous administration (Al-Kassab and Olsen, 1982; Johnson, 1980; Walker and Thompson, 1983).

The IgG index is thought to be the clearest indication of IgG synthesis occurring within the CNS and has been shown to be elevated most often in patients with the most malignant type of MS (Johnson and Nelson, 1977; Link and Tibbling, 1977; Al-Kassab and Olsen, 1982). Perkin *et al.* (1983) found it to be elevated in 77.7% of their patients with definite MS. It can be calculated by the following formula (Link and Tibbling, 1977):

$$\text{IgG index} = \frac{\text{(CSF/Serum IgG ratio)}}{\text{(CSF/Serum Albumin ratio)}}$$

It should be noted, however, that the IgG index elevation is not specific for MS. An increased IgG index has also been reported (albeit much less frequently) in a variety of other neurological conditions including meningitis, encephalitis, neurosyphilis, cerebrovascular disease, cerebral metastases, tuberculous arachnoiditis, motor neurone disease, and carcinomatous meningitis (Johnson, 1980; Perkin *et al.*, 1983).

The determination of daily intrathecal IgG synthesis is also very useful in the diagnosis of MS. This requires that IgG and albumin be measured by electroimmunodiffusion concomitantly in CSF and in serum. The following formula is employed (Tourtellotte, 1984):

Intra-BBB IgG synthesis =

$$5 \times \left[\ IgG_{CSF} - \left(\frac{IgG_s}{369} - Alb_{CSF} - \frac{Alb_s}{230} \right) \times \left(\frac{IgG_s}{Alb_s} \right) \ \right]$$

Using this formula, Tourtellotte and Ma (1978) have demonstrated elevated IgG synthesis (>3 mg/d) rate in 92% of patients with clinically definite MS. It correlates roughly with the total CSF WBC count and is proportional to cerebral plaque burden detected by MRI if the patient has not received ACTH or steroids for at least three months (Tourtellotte, 1987). Increased intra-BBB IgG synthesis may also be seen in 12% of normals and in 30-50% of patients with various CNS infections. It is also commonly seen in a number of inflammatory diseases of the CNS including SSPE, AIDS, chronic CNS infections, Guillain-Barré syndrome and vasculitides (Tourtellotte, 1987; Paty et al., 1991).

Other calculations using IgG concentrations used in evaluating MS include the CSF IgG/CSF total protein ratio and the CSF IgG/CSF albumin ratio, both of which are found elevated in MS (Tourtellotte, 1984).

Measuring CSF IgG levels is also useful in evaluating the prognosis of MS as well as establishing its diagnosis. High levels of IgG may be associated with relapse and with degree of disability, whereas low levels have been associated with a relatively benign course (Walker and Thompson, 1983). The IgG index may possibly have prognostic significance in determining which patients presenting with optic neuritis will later develop MS (Schipper et al., 1984).

Immunoglobulins: qualitative changes

(1) Oligoclonal bands

Approximately 90% to 95% of patients with clinically definite MS will display oligoclonal IgG bands when concentrated CSF is subjected to agarose electrophoresis or isoelectric focusing (Johnson, 1980; Schmidt and Neumann, 1980). Comparison must be made with the concentration of serum IgG. Even higher rates are achieved using unconcentrated CSF immunoblotting with monoclonal antibodies to IgG subclasses in combination with the double-antibody avidin-biotin- alkaline phosphatase system (Losy et al., 1990). These methods demonstrate unique CSF IgG oligoclonal bands, consisting predominantly of the IgG 1 subclass (Kaschka et al., 1979), but in decreasing frequency also of IgG 3, IgG 2, and IgG 4 -subclasses (Losy et al., 1990). Mattson et al. (1982) contends that most of the oligonclonal antibody in MS may be "nonsense antibody" with perhaps only a small portion directed towards an aetiologic agent. Tourtellotte (1987) has proposed that oligoclonal antibody is produced by a clone or a few clones of plasma cells and that the bands represent antibody to a single antigen. Each patient with MS has his/her own unique pattern of oligoclonal bands which may be genetically determined and comparable to finger prints. Oligoclonal bands are not pathognomonic for MS, and the presence or absence of bands does not relate to functional disability, age of onset, or duration of illness (Rocchelli et al., 1983).

Oligoclonal bands have also been reported in patients with subacute sclerosing panencephalitis, herpes simplex encephalitis, Alzheimer's disease, cerebrovascular disease, idiopathic vertigo, seizure disorders, amyotrophic lateral sclerosis, polyneuropathy, CNS glioma, plasma cell dyscrasias, carcinoma, viral infections, neuroborreliosis and African Burkitt's lymphoma (Miller et al., 1983; Chu et al., 1983; Wallen et al., 1983).

The demonstration of oligoclonal IgG bands is nonetheless the most valuable laboratory test in MS (Tourtellotte, 1985). It is seen in 90% of MS patients and in only about 8% of non-MS CNS disorders. Ebers (1984) compared the frequency of elevated intrathecal IgG synthesis rate, IgG index and unique CSF oligoclonal bands in clinically definite MS cases. He found increased intra-BBB IgG synthesis in 90%, an increased IgG index in 92% and oligoclonal bands in 99% (compared to 9%, 9%, and 7% respectively in controls). The number and pattern of oligoclonal bands does not clearly correlate with intra-BBB IgG synthesis or with cerebral plaque area as demonstrated on MRI (Tourtellotte, 1987).

When studied longitudinally, MS patients rarely change their unique oligoclonal pattern, and they do not go away, except for brief periods of time, during the course of the illness or with treatment (Tourtellotte, 1987). When oligoclonal IgG band patterns are found in the serum in MS they are different than those found in the CSF (Mehta et al., 1984).

The predictive value of oligoclonal bands   CSF IgG levels are useful in the diagnosis and in evaluation of the prognosis of MS. In a prospective study of suspected MS Thompson et al. (1985) showed the presence of CSF oligoclonal banding at presentation to be associated with development of further disease activity. In this study the presence of CSF oligoclonal banding activity demonstrated a stronger correlation than that of abnormal evoked potentials. The IgG index (Schipper et al., 1984) and oligoclonal bands (Stendhal-Brodin and Link, 1983) have prognostic values in determining which patients presenting with optic neuritis will later develop MS. A recent combined clinical, CSF oligoclonal IgG and IgM band, and magnetic resonance imaging (MRI) study (Sharief and Thompson, 1991) indicates that CSF oligoclonal IgG and MRI findings at presentation have less predictive value than oligoclonal IgM. Hartard *et al.* (1988), however, found no significant correlation between CSF oligoclonal bands and progression of MS. In clinically definite MS, CSF Ig G seems not to relate to the severity or duration of the disease process in MS (Thompson *et al.*, 1985; Sand and Sulg, 1990).

(2) Kappa/Lambda ratio

The normal Kappa/Lambda ratio of about 1.0 is increased in the CSF in MS. The increase of free light chains in MS occurs only in the CSF and not in serum and suggests that a specific IgG of unusual structure may be synthesised intrathecally in MS. Lolli *et al.* (1991) confirmed the increase of free kappa or lambda light chains measured by both ELISA and isoelectric focusing. There is no correlation between increased intrathecal IgG production and increased intrathecal systems of free light chains (Lolli *et al.*, 1991), suggesting that these free light chains originate from plasma cells, and not from degradation of whole IgG.

(3) Specific viral antibodies

There have been various reports of different viral antibodies being detected in MS CSF. Norrby *et al.* (1974) in a study of 150 patients with MS found increased levels of CSF antibodies to measles (57%), rubella (19%), and mumps (15%), HSV Type 1 (11%) and parainfluenza Type 1 (3%) viruses, with 71% of the patients demonstrating antibodies to at least one of the viruses. They also found a reduction of the serum/CSF ratio of antibody titers indicating local CNS production of these antibodies. Miyamoto *et al.* (1976) found increased titres of vaccinia antibody which was particularly high in those patients with the "progressive" form of MS. Johnson and Nelson (1977) reported high percentages of CSF antibodies to multiple viruses with the most striking differences being for measles antibodies (found in 72% of their MS patients compared to 5% in controls). Albrecht *et al.* (1983) reported significantly elevated CSF:serum antibody ratios to measles virus, but not to eight other viruses studied, in 50% of their of MS patients. It has also been proposed that the presence of a MS-specific antigen in CNS tissue of MS patients may contain a glycoprotein of a persistent virus such as measles (Rastogi *et al.*, 1983). The significance of the various reports of viral antibody titers in the aetiology and pathogenesis of MS is thus highly controversial.

Schadlich *et al.* (1990) showed that intrathecally synthesised antibodies against measles and/or rubella were increased in 80% of 221 of MS cases but not in controls in a study of 476 cases of inflammatory and non-inflammatory diseases of the CNS. Although the pathogenic role of the intrathecal antiviral response in MS remains unknown, it is still characteristic for MS. They suggest that the demonstration of intrathecally synthesised antibodies against neurotropic viruses not related to respective infections may serve as a helpful test to differentiate between MS and other inflammatory diseases of the CNS.

Myelin basic protein

Since demyelination often occurs during the active phases of MS, it is reasonable to look at the CSF for possible products of this process. The major proteins in myelin are specific to myelin and can be identified by radioimmunoassay. Myelin basic protein (MBP) is the most thoroughly characterised protein of myelin. It comprises about 10% of the dry weight of myelin (Cohen *et al.*, 1978). Warren and Catz (1985) and Kohlschutter *et al.* (1980), among others, have demonstrated that MBP can be used as an index of active demyelination in MS, being elevated in acute exacerbations. Haempel *et al.* (1980) differentiated central and peripheral types of MBP in CSF, finding the former increased in MS.

Barkhof *et al.* (1992) have shown that CSF MBP correlates significantly with Gd-DTPA enhancement of lesions on MRI. They further showed CSF MBP to correlate with the reduction in both Gd-DTPA enhancement and clinical disability after treatment with intravenous methylprednisolone, indicating a reduction in myelin breakdown (as measured by MBP) as well as in inflammation.

Cohen *et al.* (1980a,b) showed MBP to also be elevated in other neurologic diseases where there is a breakdown of myelin, including anoxia, necrosis due to radiation or chemotherapy, and the leukodystrophies as well as in some nondemyelinative diseases.

Antibodies to MBP have also been found by many investigators to be elevated in the CSF in MS, supporting an autoimmune hypothesis (Panitch *et al.*, 1980a,b). Alvord *et al.* (1984a,b) found markedly elevated levels of MBP within the first day of the acute attack of MS, decreasing rapidly thereafter, especially if anti-MBP antibodies were present. Warren and Catz (1986) found all their patients with clinically active MS had elevated levels of anti-MBP antibodies, whereas patients in remission had low or undetectable anti-MBP levels. Antibodies to MBP have also been detected in SSPE and in other neurological diseases.

Anti-MBP antibodies are found predominantly in the free form in acute relapses and in the bound form when the illness is progressing insidiously (Warren and Catz, 1987).

Although elevated CSF anti-MBP antibodies are not specific for MS, they are strongly associated with disease activity and may be involved in the pathogenesis of demyelination in patients with MS.

Anti-autoantigen antibodies

Though some MS patients have anti-autoantigen ab (antibodies to smooth muscle, rheumatoid factor mitochondria and nucleic acids) in higher levels in the CSF than serum, its clinical significances remains uncertain (Tourtellotte, 1985). No association to IgG oligoclonal bands has been established.

Anti-idiotype antibodies

A study by Arnon *et al.* (1979) found no compelling evidence for idiotype-anti-idiotype complexes (< 5% dimer) in MS CSF. Gerhard *et al.* (1981), using hybridised monoclonal antibodies to CSF IgG, identified an idiotype determinant of an IgG population constituting approximately 1% of IgG in the CSF of one MS patient. Interestingly the idiotype persisted for six years. However, the idiotype was not present in three other MS CSF samples.

Warren and Catz (1988) have postulated that various clinical phases of MS are dependent on a specific idiotypic cascade. They demonstrated that CSF from patients in remission has an anti-MBP neutralising ability, whereas inhibition of this neutralisation was observed with CSF from patients with insidiously progressive disease. The anti-MBP neutralising effect, they speculate, could be due to an anti-Id1 antibody, anti-anti-MBP, in patients in remission. A third anti-Id2 antibody, anti-anti-anti-MBP, could then be related to the inhibition of anti-MBP neutralisation.

Myelinotoxins

Tabira *et al.* (1977) found that the injection of CSF from MS patients near the optic nerve of tadpoles would produce lesions in myelin. They found the myelinotoxic activity to correlate with the severity and duration of the illness but not with gamma-globulin or total protein concentrations. Stendahl-Brodin *et al.* (1979) confirmed these results and found this activity to be related to the presence of oligoclonal bands in CSF from patients with optic neuritis. The nature of such a myelinotoxic factor and its role in the pathogenesis in MS remain to be elucidated.

Lipids in the CSF of patients with MS

The CNS contains an exceptionally high concentration of lipids in both white and grey matter. The fact that the myelin sheath is principally composed of lipids has caused many investigators to look at their possible role in the pathogenesis of multiple sclerosis. Myelin is composed of proteins (enzymes and structural proteins), comprising about 20% of the dry weight, and lipids, comprising the other 80% (Yatsu, 1975). The three main classes of lipids are the sterols (primarily cholesterol), sphingolipids, and phospholipids. The only lipids restricted to myelin are the cerebrosides and sulphatides (Lumsden, 1972).

There is both epidemiological and analytical evidence linking MS with alterations in fatty acid (FA) metabolism. FAs form an important part of membrane phospholipids and relatively small changes in their concentrations may affect the regulation of membrane-bound enzymes and membrane fluidity. Whether one favors a viral, nutritional, metabolic or immunological theory of the aetiology of MS, the role of plasma membranes must fit into the argument at some stage.

There has been a great deal of speculation that MS may be related to a dietary insufficiency of polyunsaturated fatty acids (PUFA). This has largely stemmed from epidemiological studies which suggest MS to be more prevalent in areas which consume large amounts of animal (saturated) fats relative to oils high in PUFA (Smith and Thompson, 1977; Alter et al., 1974). Low levels of essential fatty acids (EFA) in the serum and formed blood elements of MS patients also suggest a need for dietary supplementation. Various animal studies have shown that changes in FA composition of the diet can result in an altered FA composition in myelin (Nowak and Munro, 1977). An altered FA composition may adversely affect the stability and fluidity of the myelin membrane and thus predispose to demyelinating processes. Therapeutic trials of PUFAs in the diet of MS patients have had some mildly encouraging, though controversial, results (Crawford and Stevens, 1981; Seidel, 1982).

There have been a number of CSF studies of lipids in MS but they have been somewhat limited by available analytical techniques (Thompson, 1977). Lumsden (1972) has reviewed the earlier work which has, in general, found increases in sphingomyelins, cephalins, cerebrosides and no significant changes in lecithin, phospholipids or cholesterol. These changes seemed also to be related to clinical activity of the disease and, it is suggested, may be the best index of active demyelination in MS. Seidel et al. (1980) suggest that CSF sphingomyelin and linoleic acid may have a primarily haematogenic, rather than CNS, origin. Their altered concentrations in MS then may be a reflection of BBB disturbances.

Neu (1984) looked at specific FAs in the CSF of MS and noted a marked deficiency of linoleic and arachidonic acids. This was most pronounced in the cholesterol ester fraction. He suggests that a deficiency of EFAs may aggravate immunopathological processes in MS, and that the membrane – sealing function of FAs on the myelin sheath may be impaired. Increased lipolysis through cAMP, by way of a lipotrophin – endorphin mechanism, or secondary to enzyme activation via a decrease in prostaglandin synthesis, are all possible causes of the impaired FA metabolism in MS (Neu, 1984).

Other CSF constituents in MS

Many other substances have been looked at in the CSF of MS patients. The reader is referred elsewhere for discussions of these constituents.

These include the following: other proteins and various amino acids (Lumsden, 1972); electrolytes, bromide, neuraminic acid (Tourtellotte, 1970); cAMP (Maida and Kristo Feritsch, 1981); complement (Delasnerie-Lanpretre *et al.*, 1982); Vitamin B12 and folate (Tourtellotte, 1970) and immune complexes (Salmi *et al.*, 1982).

Many enzymes have also been investigated in CSF, including glycolytic and respiratory enzymes (phosphohexose isomerase, lactic dehydrogenase, glutamic oxalcetic transaminase and isocitrate dehydrogenase) (Tourtellotte, 1970); hydrolytic enzymes (esterase, lysosomal hydrolases) (Rinne and Riekkinen, 1968; Kilpelainen *et al.*, 1982); proteinases (Rinne and Riekkinen, 1968; Richards and Cuzner, 1977); cholinesterase, pseudo-cholinesterase, phosphatases, and RNAase and DNAase (Lumsden, 1972), beta-glucuronidase (Kilpelainen *et al.*, 1980), and acid phosphatase (DeReuck *et al.*, 1984).

Parkinson's Disease (PD)

Parkinsonism is primarily due to a selective degeneration of dopaminergic neurons originating in the substantia nigra and ventral tegmental area. This has been demonstrated in both post-mortem studies as well as *in vivo* with positron emission tomography (Leenders *et al.*, 1986). There is also involvement of ascending NE, 5-HT, and cholinergic systems from lesions of the locus coeruleus, raphe nuclei and substantia innominata, respectively and abnormalities of GABA-ergic transmitter systems (Chase, 1980; Agid *et al.*, 1986) and various neuropeptides (see review of Uhl, 1988). CSF studies have played an important role in investigating these biochemical abnormalities in Parkinsonism.

The primary biochemical abnormality in Parkinson's disease (PD) seems to be an alteration in dopamine metabolism which is reflected in the CSF by the HVA and other DA metabolite concentrations. Decreased levels of HVA in the CSF have been reported by many investigators (Tabaddor *et al.*, 1978a; Chase, 1980; Sonninen *et al.*, 1982; Cunha *et al.*, 1983). Though HVA levels vary greatly, they have generally not been shown to correlate with clinical parameters of the disease or with response to therapy (Chase, 1980; Cunha *et al.*, 1983). Sonninen *et al.* (1982), however, found the CSF response to probenecid to correlate negatively with the degree of hypokinesia and rigidity, and with severity of the disease. They also suggested that, since normal CSF HVA levels are found in essential tremor and increased concentrations are found in patients with neuroleptic-induced extrapyramidal symptoms, the low CSF HVA of Parkinsonism may prove a valuable aid in the differential diagnosis of these disorders.

Studies by Vanderheyden *et al.* (1982) and by Cunha *et al.* (1983) suggest that the measurement of CSF-HVA levels before and after probenecid administration may be useful in predicting which patients will respond to L-DOPA therapy. Dopa-resistant patients tend to have higher HVA levels after probenecid administration than Dopa-sensitive patients. This was demonstrated in both prospective and retrospective studies. This may indicate two distinct subtypes of Parkinson's disease and may prove useful in the therapy of these patients. Nishi *et al.* (1989) found that CSF levels of HVA were clinically useful in differentiating L-DOPA non-responsive patients with striatonigral degeneration (SND) from patients with Parkinson's disease who responded to L-DOPA. Those patients with L-DOPA resistant SND had markedly lower levels of CSF HVA than those with PD. Patients with parkinsonian syndromes who have normal CSF HVA levels tend to have reduced CSF levels of somatostatin and/or metenkephalin suggesting that these also may be a particular subclass of PD patients (Lindvall and Olsson, 1990).

CSF levels of HVA and DA may also be useful in monitoring the effects of surgical transplants in PD with levels rising after surgery (Tyce *et al.*, 1989; Ahlskog *et al.*, 1990). CSF levels of neuropeptide Y, enkephalin, epinephrine, norepinephrine, and MHPG do not appear to be altered after autologous transplantation in PD (Tyce *et al.*, 1989; Yaksh *et al.*, 1990; Ahlskog *et al.*, 1990).

Since GABAergic neurons in the substantia nigra and globus pallidus are thought to be involved in the modulation of DAergic neurons, many investigators have looked at levels of GABA in the CSF of Parkinsonian patients. GABA is synthesised from glutamic acid by glutamic acid decarboxylase (GAD) which is decreased in activity in the striatal and substantia nigra tissue in these patients (Teychenne *et al.*, 1980; Chase, 1980; Manyam, 1982). This GAD activity will return to normal following long-term therapy with L-DOPA. Several investigators have found lower levels of GABA in the CSF of Parkinsonian patients (Hare *et al.*, 1980; Manyam, 1982; Kuroda *et al.*, 1982). Others, however, have not confirmed significantly lower levels than controls (Enna *et al.*, 1977b; Teychenne *et al.*, 1980). Various abnormalities in other amino acids in the CSF have also been noted in Parkinsonism (Gjessing *et al.*, 1974). Manyam *et al.* (1988) found GABA levels to be significantly decreased in the CSF of *de novo* patients with PD, as well as homocarnosine, phospho-ethanolamine, and threonine. These abnormalities tended to normalise with L-DOPA therapy.

Other CSF studies in PD have found reduced activity of hydroxylase cofactor (BH4) (Lorenberg *et al.*, 1979; Williams *et al.*, 1980; Fujishiro *et al.*, 1990), low neopterin levels (Fujishiro *et al.*, 1990), low somatostatin levels (Dupont *et al.*, 1982), low arginine vasopressin levels (Sundquist *et al.*, 1983), normal choline levels (Flentge *et al.*, 1984), variable 5-HIAA levels (Tabaddor *et al.*, 1978a; Chase, 1980), increased alpha-melanocyte-stimulating hormone (Rainero *et al.*, 1988a), the presence of antibody to substantia nigra and ventral tegmental area neurons (McRae-Degueurce *et al.*, 1988), and increased enkephalin and substance P (Pezzoli *et al.*, 1984). Sandyk (1988) suggests that the increased CSF enkephalin seen early in the disease could represent a hypothalamic compensatory mechanism to overcome striatal DA-deficiency. Williams *et al.* (1979) reported oligloclonal bands in the CSF of two patients with postencephalitic Parkinsonism. CSF levels of the NE metabolite, MHPG, are decreased in PD, whereas they are increased in MPTP toxicity-induced Parkinsonism (Kopin *et al.*, 1986). CSF studies of copper, iron, and ferritin have also produced mixed evidence of the oxidant theory of damage in PD, which have prompted recent trials of antioxidant therapy (Pall *et al.*, 1987; Halliwell, 1989; Pall *et al.*, 1990). CSF levels of levodopa have been shown to correlate with motor performance and dyskinesia in PD, suggesting that the wearing off of its therapeutic effects may be related to CNS drug concentrations (Olanow *et al.*, 1991). LeWitt *et al.* (1992) have recently described a method of simultaneous measurement of multiple DA metabolites in the CSF. They speculate that their detection of 3-O-methyldopa and levodopa in the CSF in early PD, could be an indication of DA synthesis and thus reflect compensatory processes among surviving DA neurons.

Huntington's Chorea

Huntington's disease (HD) is an autosomal dominant disorder characterised by choreiform movements and dementia. These symptoms usually occur between the ages of 35 and 50 years and progress slowly over many years. Postmortem analysis of the basal ganglia of these patients has shown abnormalities in various neurotransmitter systems. These include acetylcholine, serotonin, substance P, angiotensin converting enzyme (ACE), dopamine (DA), gamma aminobutyric acid (GABA), the enkephalins, vasoactive inhibitory polypeptide (VIP), and cholecystokinin (Beal and Bird, 1988).

CSF studies in Huntington's disease have indicated variable abnormalities in the concentrations of GABA, choline, 5-HIAA, and norepinephrine (Ziegler *et al.*, 1980; Butler *et al.*, 1980; Hayden, 1981). CSF levels of protein, glucose, polyamines, and cAMP as well as the cell count and electrophoretic pattern have all been found to be normal (Brooks *et al.*, 1980; Fishman, 1980; Kremzner *et al.*, 1979). HVA levels are generally normal, but somatostatin and met-enkephalin may be reduced (Lindvall and Olsson, 1990).

CSF analysis of GABA concentrations have received a lot of attention in Huntington's Chorea as they may prove useful for genetic counselling purposes, diagnosis, and monitoring response to drug treatment (Hare *et al.*, 1980). Both GABA and its primary synthetic enzyme, glutamic acid decarboxylase (GAD), are reduced in brain tissue of patients with Huntington's disease (Hare *et al.*, 1980; Hayden, 1981). Several investigators have reported low CSF levels of GABA both in patients with HD (Enna *et al.*, 1977b; Hare *et al.*, 1980; Hayden, 1981) and in patients at risk to develop the disease (Manyam *et al.*, 1978, 1979). Follow-up studies on these "patients at risk" are needed, however, before CSF GABA could be used for genetic counselling. A study by Perry *et al.*, (1982a), however, found both GABA and homocarnosine to be similar to their much lower control values. Their control values of GABA, using a modified ion exchange – fluorometric method, were less than half that of previously reported CSF GABA levels.

Alzheimer's Disease (AD)

The usual indices measured in CSF are generally normal in Alzheimer's disease except for occasional increases in protein content (Fishman, 1980). Postmortem studies of brain tissues in these patients have shown degeneration of 5-HT and GABA receptor cells, decreased NE levels, reduced frontal cortex glutamic acid decarboxylase (GAD) activity, and decreased choline acetyl transferase (CAT) activity (Bowen and Davison, 1980; Berger *et al.*, 1980). Central cholinergic pathways appear to be particularly vulnerable (Wood *et al.*, 1982; Bowen and Davison, 1980).

Several CSF studies have demonstrated reduced levels of HVA, 5-HIAA, and/or GABA in Alzheimer's disease (AD) (Enna *et al.*, 1977b; Bowen and Davison, 1980; Hare *et al.*, 1980; Soininen *et al.*, 1981a; Soininen *et al.*, 1982). Bareggi *et al.* (1982) studied CSF levels of HVA, 5-HIAA, and GABA in 15 patients with Alzheimer's disease. They found CSF HVA and GABA levels both decreased compared to control values while 5-HIAA concentrations did not differ significantly. They noted, however, that CSF HVA levels increased with age in their control group whereas GABA levels decreased. Thus, after accounting for these age-related changes, CSF HVA was found to be low but GABA and 5-HIAA did not differ from the age-matched controls. In contrast, Zimmer *et al.* (1984) found diminished CSF GABA levels in AD whereas HVA levels did not differ from controls. Low CSF HVA has been linked to various clinical subgroups of demented patients (Wester *et al.*, 1988; Wolfe *et al.*, 1990) but generally studies of the metabolites of NE, Serotonin, DA, and GABA have been conflicting and inconclusive in AD (see review of Cutler, 1987).

Several investigators have attempted to find a CSF cholinergic marker to parallel the reduced levels of cortical CAT and loss of cholinergic neurons detected in autopsy specimens. Both CSF choline and acetylcholinesterase (AChE) have been noted to be normal in Alzheimer's disease (Wood *et al.*, 1982). Soininen *et al.* (1981*b*), Gomez *et al.* (1986) and others have, however, detected low AChE in the CSF of patients with senile dementia of the Alzheimer type. They also studied CSF beta-glucoronidase in these patients as a potential glial marker but noted no differences from their control group. Butylcholinesterase and choline acetyltransferase have also been looked at in AD as potential cholinergic CSF markers. Despite the post-mortem and biopsy findings implicating ACh in AD, however, CSF studies of cholinergic markers have generally also been conflicting with both normal and decreased levels being found in several studies (Giacobini *et al.*, 1986; Rasmussen *et al.*, 1988; Kumar *et al.*, 1989; Wester *et al.*, 1988). Navaratnam *et al.* (1991) have recently, however, identified an anomalous molecular form of acetylcholinesterase in the CSF of patients with AD. They found this anomalous form of AChE in CSF obtained at necropsy in 19 of 23 patients with a histological diagnosis of AD and in none of their 19 non-demented patients, suggesting that this may prove a useful antemortem diagnostic test of AD.

Various neuropeptides have also been implicated in Alzheimer's disease. Wood *et al.* (1982) studied the CSF of patients with Alzheimer's disease, mixed dementias, and schizophrenics. They found CSF levels of somatostatin to be markedly reduced in their group of Alzheimer and mixed dementia patients. Only minor alterations were noted in CSF HVA, MHPG, and 5-HIAA and no change in AChE was observed.

Decreased somatostatin-like immunoreactivity has been found in most all CSF studies of AD (Bissette *et al.*, 1986*b*; Raskind *et al.*, 1986; Gomez *et al.*, 1986; Sunderland *et al.*, 1987; Davis *et al.*, 1988) as well as in cortical tissue in AD (Tamminga *et al.*, 1985; Beal *et al.*, 1985) and has proven to be one of the most reliable neurochemical changes seen in AD (see review of Vecsei and Widerlov, 1988). Soininen *et al.* (1988) have found CSF somatostatin to correlate with EEG changes seen in AD and with cognitive dysfunction.

Other neuropeptide findings in the CSF in AD include normal or decreased CRF (Pomara *et al.*, 1989; Bissette and Nemeroff, 1990), decreased neuropeptide Y (Alom *et al.*, 1990), decreased vasopressin and normal oxytocin and beta-endorphin (Raskind *et al.*, 1986), increased diazepam-binding inhibitor (Ferrarse *et al.*, 1990), decreased alpha-MSH (Rainero *et al.*, 1988*b*), and decreased thyrotrophin and gonadotrophin-releasing hormones (see review of Cutler, 1987).

Delaney (1979) noted decreased levels of aluminium in the CSF of ten patients with Alzheimer's disease. The significance of this observation is not clear. Hershey *et al.* (1983) did not find any relation between CSF concentrations of aluminium, arsenic, lead, or manganese with Alzheimer-type dementia, Alzheimer's disease or other dementia in their study of 19 trace elements in the CSF of 265 patients. They did note elevated CSF levels of silicon in 71% of their patients with AD and in 24% of those with Alzheimer-type dementia, suggesting silicon toxicity as a possible aetiology.

It is often important to differentiate AD from other types of dementia. Harrington *et al.* (1986) have isolated two abnormal proteins (designated "130" and "131") in the CSF of patients with Creutzfeldt-Jakob disease (CJD) which promise to be an important antemortem marker. Their detection uses a technique of gel electrophoresis in one direction and isoelectric focusing in the other. The origin of these proteins is not clear, but subsequent studies have shown a good correlation with biopsy and autopsy findings and their presence in the CSF of a patient with an appropriate clinical presentation strongly suggests the diagnosis of CJD (Block, 1992, personal communication).

Perhaps the most promising new finding in the study of CSF in AD and dementia is the development of a specific monoclonal antibody assay for amyloid β-protein precursor (APP) which may serve as a diagnostic test for AD. Van Nostrand *et al.*, (1992*a,b*) have found CSF APP levels to be 3.5 times lower in patients with AD than in either controls or in patients with dementia from other causes. It may also have prognostic value presymptomatically as those with the lowest values are those who become the most severely affected (Van Nostrand *et al.*, 1992*a,b*; Erickson, 1992; Farlow *et al.*, 1992; Wagner, 1992, personal communication).

Other CSF abnormalities noted in AD include increased albumin (Alafuzoff *et al.*, 1983), decreased glutamine (Procter *et al.*, 1988), decreased biopterin (Le Witt *et al.*, 1986) and decreased vitamin B12 levels (Van Tiggelen *et al.*, 1984; Nijst *et al.*, 1990).

Dystonia

Idiopathic torsion dystonia is a syndrome characterised by irregular, involuntary movements often occurring with abnormal postures. It may occur in autosomal recessive (among Jewish families) or autosomal dominant (in non-Jewish families) forms.

Many investigators have looked at the metabolites of dopamine and serotonin in dystonia since these neurotransmitter systems have been implicated in other movement disorders. Curzon (1973) reported slightly lower than normal concentrations of both 5-HIAA and HVA in lumbar samplings. Tabaddor *et al.* (1978*a,b*), in comparing adult and childhood onset forms of the disease, found significantly lower concentrations of HVA in the adult onset form in ventricular CSF samples. Concentrations of 5-HIAA were similar. Shaywitz *et al.* (1980) studied childhood-onset dystonia with probenecid loading and found both the 5-HIAA/probenecid and the HVA/probenecid ratios lower than in controls. The progressive form of dystonia is associated with markedly reduced LCSF HVA levels (Ouvrier, 1978). Thus both dopaminergic and serotonergic alterations may play a role in dystonia.

Because of reports of increased levels of plasma norepinephrine and dopamine-β-hydroxylase in dystonia (Waal-Manning, 1974; Ebstein *et al.*, 1974), Wolfson *et al.* (1983) recently measured ventricular CSF levels of the norepinephrine metabolite MHPG. Those with childhood-onset dystonia were found to have significantly lower levels of MHPG than subjects with other movement disorders or age-matched neurologic controls. Those with the adult-onset form, however, had levels similar to controls. Alterations in noradrenergic function may thus also play an important role in childhood dystonia.

Other CSF findings in childhood onset dystonia include increased butylcholinesterase and decreased somatostatin (Ruberg *et al.*, 1988; Wolfson *et al.*, 1988).

Benign Intracranial Hypertension

Benign intracranial hypertension (BIH) or pseudotumour cerebri (PTC) is a condition characterised by increased intracranial pressure (ICP) where known causes of this (e.g. tumour, infection, hypertensive encephalopathy) have been excluded. The ventricular system is of normal size and location and occasionally may be on the small side. This condition is not rare (estimated yearly incidence approximately 1:100 000) and is predominantly seen in women of childbearing years many of whom are obese and have menstrual irregularities.

The clinical symptoms of pseudotumour cerebri can relate only to those produced by increased intracranial pressure. This would include headache, transient visual obscurations or diplopia which may be attributable to 6th cranial nerve weakness from the ICP alone. Focal neurological signs and/or other posterior fossa signs such as ataxia would exclude the diagnosis of BIH. Alterations in mental function or cognition are not part of this syndrome. The diagnosis commonly is suspected when papilloedema is observed by an opthalmologist or neurologist in the course of fundoscopic evaluation in a young woman with headache or visual symptoms. As the list of associated disorders is long, the physician must take a careful history and inquire about recent weight gain, regularity of menses, pregnancy, symptoms consistent with endocrinopathies (hydroadrenalism, hypoparathyroidism), anaemia and medications, including phenothiazines, nalidixic acid, tetracycline, corticosteroids, excessive vitamin A intake and birth control pills (see review of Davson et al., 1987, pp. 778-80, and of Mann et al., 1983).

Once the diagnosis is suspected, the workup should include an image of the brain, either MRI or CT scan, to exclude the possibility of a mass lesion. Following this, a lumbar puncture may be performed, at which time the pressure will be between 200 and 600 mm of H_2O. The constituents of the spinal fluid are usually normal and no cells are found. The protein is normal or slightly on the low side and the glucose is also normal. Normal pulsations of CSF in the manometer are usually noted. The pressure should then be slowly lowered to approximately 50% of the opening pressure at which time headache may be relieved temporarily. It is also important to obtain binocular visual acuities and fields in this condition since impairement of visual fields and blindness are a possible consequence of this disorder when left untreated. The visual fields may demonstrate a large blind spot, nasal field defects or an acute arcuate scotoma (Wall and George, 1987). As there is no associated encephalopathy, the electroencephalogram is normal.

The pathogenesis of BIH is unknown. The clinical and physiologic aspects of the disorder indicate an increased amount of brain water which is not ventricular in location. Analysis of brain biopsy and the absence of encephalopathy suggest that the water content is extracellular (Sahs and Joynt, 1956). Spinal fluid infusion studies and cisternography have shown that there is a defect in CSF absorption in the arachnoid villi particularly in the superior sagittal sinus (Calabrese et al., 1978). However, if this were the only pathophysiological mechanism, the absence of hydrocephalus in this circumstance has never adequately been explained. BIH may be caused also by an increase in CSF formation, an increase in sagittal sinus pressure or an increase in extracellular brain oedema, possibly from metabolic or endocrine disturbance (Johnston et al., 1991).

The prognosis in BIH is generally good. Frequently the condition is self-limiting and serial fundoscopic evaluation with appropriate therapy may demonstrate resolution of papilloedema and symptoms associated with increased intracranial pressure. Nevertheless, because visual loss is an important and serious consequence of this disorder, serial visual fields are required perhaps at 6 week intervals making certain that the above mentioned abnormalities, if present, are not worsening.

The therapy of BIH includes medications to reduce the elaboration of cerbrospinal fluid and may include acetazolamide 250 mg three times a day or furosemide 40 mg daily. Acetazolamide appears to be a better choice but has side-effects that include nausea, vomiting and paraesthesias in the extemities. The weight reduction is an important part of therapy in obese individuals and reduction in body weight has been shown to correlate with improvement (Fishman, 1980). Repeated spinal taps are not recommended inasmuch as the rate of elaboration of CSF (0.38 cc per min) is such that the amelioration of symptoms would be transitory. Indeed patients find repeated spinal punctures so onerous that they may be lost to follow-up which, in a practical sense, may pose the biggest threat to their vision. When visual acuity is threatened as evidenced by loss of fields, surgical intervention may be necessary. This may take the form of lumboperitoneal shunt, subtemporal decompression or a neuropathalmological surgical procedure which would slit the optic sheath and allow spinal fluid to drain, thereby removing the immediate threat of excessive pressure upon the optic nerve (Keltner, 1988). Obviously, discontinuing offending medications, correcting endocrinopathies and parturition generally relieve the disorder. In general, a favourable outcome may be expected if the conservative measures outlined above are adhered to and visual fields are closely monitored.

Tumours of the CNS and Meninges

The procedure of lumbar puncture is extremely hazardous in patients with CNS tumours and increased intracranial pressure (ICP) because of the risk of herniation of cranial contents (Walker, 1982). Risk in patients with possible increased ICP may be minimised by the use of a small-calibre needle and slow withdrawal of fluid during the procedure. Pretreatment with steroids or mannitol may be indicated in some patients (Kornblith et al., 1982). Suspected CNS neoplasms should always be evaluated with CT or MR imaging when possible prior to consideration of lumbar puncture.

Pressure

Pressure may be normal or, more often, increased. The pressure is most elevated in those tumours of the posterior fossa and in rapidly growing tumours such as glioblastoma multiforme (De Jong, 1979). Obstruction of CSF pathways may occasionally cause reduced CSF pressure (Sayk, 1974).

Appearance

The fluid is usually clear in appearance. Yellow (xanthochromic) fluid suggests previous haemorrhaging, serum bilirubin transudation, or an elevated protein count (Kornblith et al., 1982). Spinal cord tumours may cause stasis of the CSF via obstruction of the subarachnoid space and this will yield a xanthochromic fluid with high protein content and an absence of RBCs (Levin et al., 1989). A marked pleocytosis such as in leptomeningeal carcinomatosis or any tumour encroaching the meninges or ventricles may occasionally cause clouding of the fluid (De Jong, 1979;

Wood, 1985). Melanocytic neoplasms may also produce melanin which may cloud the CSF (Sayk, 1974).

Glucose

The CSF glucose is usually normal but may be low in many neoplasms involving the meninges, particularly in leukaemic meningitis (Kornblith *et al.*, 1982). Alterations in the blood-CSF barrier, utilisation of glucose by neoplastic tissue or by leukocytes in the spinal fluid, and possibly other factors may play a role (Sayk, 1974; Bodansky, 1975). Extensive metastases of glioblastomas, leptomeningeal carcinomatoses, and sarcomatoses will often demonstrate values of 40 mg% or less (Sayk, 1974).

Protein

Elevation of CSF protein is a frequent finding. It is primarily due to an altered endothelial cell permeability. The electrophoretic pattern of these proteins generally reflects that of plasma proteins although increased immunoglobulins may be observed. Some specific proteins occurring in certain neoplasms (e.g. alpha-fetoprotein in dysgerminomas) have also been identified (Kornblith *et al.*, 1982; Sayk, 1974).

Cytology

CSF cytology is a good indicator of meningeal involvement in the diagnosis of CNS tumours and is also helpful in assessing the effectiveness of treatment (Glass and Wertlake, 1983). Malignant cells may be detected more easily in CSF than in other body fluids since there are fewer other cell types present. The yield of positive cytology runs about 15-30% for primary brain tumours and 20 to 50% in metastatic tumours, varying greatly depending on the type and grade of tumour (Balhuizen *et al.*, 1978; Sayk, 1974; Herndon and Brumback, 1989a). Rates of false negative results, even with meningeal involvement, may be high (up to 40%) but false positive results are rare (Glass and Wertlake, 1983). Tumours which seed early, e.g. medulloblastomas and, to a lesser extent, pineal tumours, supratentorial neuroblastomas, and primitive neuroectodermal tumours, are most amenable to cytological examination in the CSF (Edwards *et al.*, 1985).

CSF obtained postoperatively and ventricular samples tend to give higher rates of positive cytologies (Wood, 1985). Glass and Wertlake (1983) point out that a positive CSF cytology necessarily implies meningeal metastases and therefore a surgical cure is unlikely and therapy must be directed at the entire neuraxis. Oehmichen (1976), den Hartog Jager (1977), and Kolmel (1977) have all published excellent atlases of the cytology of CSF, and Bigner and Johnston (1981a), Glass and Wertlake (1983) and Herndon and Brumback (1989a) have also reviewed the CSF cytopathology seen in various neoplasms.

Biological tumour markers

The detection of polypeptides, hormone substances, enzymes and oncofetal antigens specific for certain neoplasms in various body fluids has been useful in the diagnosis and treatment of many systemic cancers. The role of measuring CSF biochemical tumour markers in CNS malignancy has not been as clear. Increased concentrations of substances released by neoplastic tissue may appear in the CSF from diffusion across an intact blood-CSF barrier with elevated serum levels, from alterations in the blood-CSF barrier, or from production within the CNS (Wasserstrom et al., 1981).

Biological tumour markers are of the most use in those tumours with leptomeningeal involvement or those in direct contact with or juxtaposed to the CSF pathways. Involvement of the leptomeninges by carcinoma may be detected early with the use of beta-glucoronidase, carcinoembryonic antigen (CEA), and lactate dehydrogenase (LDH). Measurement of their levels in the CSF appear to reflect the response to treatment (Schold and Bullard, 1980; Schold et al., 1980; Wasserstrom et al., 1981).

Interestingly, elevated CSF levels of CEA are often seen in tumours not necessarily associated with increased serum levels of CEA, e.g. lung cancer, breast cancer, malignant melanoma and bladder cancer (Bullard and Schold, 1985). Elevated CSF CEA is a frequent marker for metastatic tumours but seen far less frequently in primary CNS tumours (Edwards et al., 1985). CSF levels of α-fetoprotein (AFP) may be elevated in malignant germ cell tumours. It is a useful marker either alone or in combination with human chorionic gonadotrophin (hCG) for both diagnosis and as a measure of response to therapy (Bullard and Schold, 1985). Measurement of CSF hCG alone is not specific enough for the diagnosis of germ cell tumours without histologic confirmation.

The polyamines spermidine and spermine, as well as their precursor, putrescine, are produced during the growth phase of cells undergoing RNA synthesis. Meningiomas may be associated with an increase in spermidine and glioblastomas are frequently associated with increased CSF putrescine (Bullard and Schold, 1985). Polyamines are useful in the work up of gliomas adjacent to the ventricular system, but are not generally helpful in evaluating hemispheric gliomas (Fulton et al., 1983). The polyamines are also useful in the management of medulloblastoma, with elevation of both putrescine and spermidine found. Their levels may serve as an early indicator of recurrence in medulloblastomas and possibly other CNS tumours, and appear to correlate with the effectiveness of therapy (Marton *et al.*, 1981; Wassenstrom *et al.*, 1981; Fulton *et al.*, 1983; Leland *et al.*, 1983; Bullard and Schold, 1985).

Desmosterol, the immediate precursor of cholesterol, is another potentially useful tumour marker, being elevated in glioblastoma and oligodendroglioma but not in astrocytomas or in nonglial tumours (Butler *et al.,* 1982). Its detection in CSF, however, requires the use of triparanol which blocks the synthesis of cholesterol. The toxicity of this agent limits the routine clinical usefulness of desmosterol as a tumour marker (Bullard and Schold, 1985).

The CSF activity of various enzymes including aldolase, pyruvate kinase, enolase, adenylate kinase, LDH, creatine phosphokinase, glutamic oxaloacetic transaminase, glucose phosphate isomerase, leucine aminopeptidase, phosphohexose isomerase, lysozyme, acid phosphatase, and isocitrate dehydrogenase may also prove sensitive markers of neoplasia (Royds *et al.*, 1981*a*; Wasserstrom *et al.*, 1981; Timperley *et al.*, 1982; Hallgren *et al.*, 1982; Frithz *et al.*, 1982; Vivekanandan *et al.*, 1982). The various isoenzymes of enolase and of LDH may provide a reliable histologic marker for some tumours and may be a very early and sensitive index of cerebral pathology (Gu *et al.*, 1981; Parsons *et al.*, 1981; Tapia *et al.*, 1981; Timperley *et al.*, 1982; Vivekanandan *et al.*, 1982). Other CSF tumour markers of potential use include ectopic hormones, beta-2-microglobulin, immuno-chemically defined markers (e.g. S-100 protein and glial fibrillary acidic protein), myelin basic protein, creatine kinase BB, somatostatin, various adenohypophyseal hormones, endorphins, eosinophil cationic protein (ECP), cyclic nucleotides, various lipids, and glial-derived proteins (Schold and Bullard, 1980; Wasserstrom *et al.*, 1981; Cramer and Schindler, 1982; Cutler and Spertell, 1982; Coombs *et al.*, 1982; Hallgren *et al.*, 1983; Mattias-Guiu *et al.*, 1986). The interested reader is referred to the reviews of Wasserstrom *et al.* (1981), Sayk (1974), Edwards *et al.* (1985) and Bullard and Schold (1985).

CSF markers in paraneoplastic syndromes

CNS paraneoplastic syndromes are thought to be a result of an immune reaction directed against antigens shared by the underlying neoplasm and certain neurons. Two specific autoantibodies – anti-Yo, associated with paraneoplastic cerebellar degeneration, and anti-Hu, associated with paraneoplastic sensory neuronopathy – encephalomyelitis – have recently been identified in the CSF and appear to be useful diagnostic markers (Furneaux *et al.*, 1990; Peter, 1993 pp. 268-285).

Bacterial Meningitis

The CSF in bacterial meningitis is classically characterised by increased pressure, white cell count, protein, and decreased glucose levels. The pressure is elevated to about 190 mm H_2O in 85% of cases (Hayward et al., 1987) and above 500 mm in 15% (Merritt and Fremont-Smith, 1938). Horwitz et al. (1980) reported a 6% incidence of cerebral herniation and a 1% death rate from herniation in their series of 302 infants and children with acute bacterial meningitis. Although suspicion of meningitis is an important indication for lumbar puncture, the procedure should be postponed in patients with signs of increased intracranial pressure until the pressure can be reduced with hyperosmolar agents. Prompt treatment with antibiotics and further evaluation with CT scanning is indicated (Greenlee, 1990).

As discussed in Chapter 5, the cloudiness of the fluid may give a quick estimate of the cell count in helping to distinguish between the various types of meningitis. The increased protein in bacterial meningitis frequently results in xanthochromia.

The leukocyte count is usually greater than 1000 WBC/mm^3 in 85% of patients (Merritt and Fremont-Smith, 1938) with a predominance of polymorphonuclear (PMN) cells. Cell counts may reach up to 10,000 cells/mm^3. The cell count must be determined promptly as delay will artificially reduce the count due to cell lysis and adhesion. PMNs are more susceptible than lymphocytes to disintegration and this decrease is thus not proportional. A reduction of 50% of the total WBC count may be caused by the sample remaining at room temperature for 1/2 hour (Meena et al., 1989).

The cell count is generally a sensitive indicator of a bacterial aetiology in meningitis, with a sensitivity approaching 1.0 (Marton and Gean, 1986). It is important to note, however, that early in the course of meningitis there may be a lack of significant cellular response. In the very young, the very old, immunocompromised patients, and in overwhelming *Streptococcus pneumoniae* infection, there may also be an absence of pleocytosis (Moore and Ross, 1973; Wood and Anderson, 1988). One-third of patients with a total WBC count less than 1000/mm^3 may demonstrate a lymphocytosis (Powers, 1985). The leucocyte count in the CSF also has prognostic as well as diagnostic significance, with counts below 1000/mm^3 associated with a poorer prognosis. The pleocytosis may commonly persist after adequate treatment and is not an indication for prolonging therapy (Fishman, 1980).

Since the CSF glucose concentration is directly dependent on the blood glucose level, simultaneous blood glucose determination should always be obtained. It takes approximately one to two hours for plasma glucose changes to be reflected in the CSF and four hours to reach equilibrium. The normal CSF/serum glucose ratio is about 0.6 for adults. In neonates CSF glucose levels are approximately 75-80% of serum levels (Sarff *et al.*, 1976). Levels in neonates may on occasion be more than 100% of the serum value (Wood and Anderson, 1988). Glucose levels must be measured promptly after LP, as it may be factitiously reduced unless fluoride is added to stop glycolysis (Fishman, 1980).

Values below 50% of serum levels in adults and below 60% in infants are suggestive of meningitis. The sensitivity of CSF glucose in the diagnosis of bacterial meningitis is about 0.58 (Marton and Gean, 1986). A low CSF glucose is also seen in tuberculous, fungal, carcinomatous, amoebic, chemical, and rheumatoid meningitis, and in haemorrhagic leuko-encephalitis, Behcet's syndrome, and other illnesses (Swartz, 1980; Fishman, 1980). The CSF/serum glucose ratio is also affected by elevation of blood glucose levels; a ratio of less than 0.3 has been suggested to be abnormal in diabetic patients (Greenlee, 1990).

The CSF protein may be elevated in all CNS infections, but is generally highest in purulent meningitis. Most determinations of CSF protein in meningitis of bacterial aetiology range from 100-500 mg/100 ml (Adams and Petersdorf, 1980). It is elevated above 45 mg/100 ml in 86% of cases (Hayward *et al.*, 1987). CSF protein levels may remain abnormal for several months, returning to normal much more slowly than glucose levels or cell counts. Although nonspecific, a CSF protein level over 100 mg/100 ml, associated with a PMN pleocytosis, is highly suggestive of a bacterial aetiology.

Although a low glucose associated with a polymorphonuclear pleocytosis, and usually an increased CSF protein, is classically seen in purulent bacterial meningitis, it is important to note that these may also be seen in the early stages of viral meningitis, in 15-20% of patients with subarachnoid haemorrhage, and in a variety of other conditions (Swartz, 1980; Hayward *et al.*, 1987).

CSF lactate levels are generally independent of serum levels and thus directly reflect CNS production (Fishman, 1980). High levels are indicative of tissue acidosis and increased anaerobic glycolysis. Both CSF lactate and its enzyme (lactate dehydrogenase) are elevated in bacterial meningitis and have been suggested to be sensitive aids to its early diagnosis (Knight *et al.*, 1981). CSF lactate is significantly higher in pyogenic meningitis than in tuberculous meningitis. In both types of meningitis, levels are markedly increased over lactate concentrations found in encephalitis, aseptic meningitis, partially treated bacterial meningitis and controls (Controni *et al.*, 1977; Brook *et al.*, 1978; Berg *et al.*, 1982). CSF lactate levels may be valuable in following the response to therapy of meningitis, as they tend to return to normal after treatment (Controni *et al.*, 1977; Murata and Vemura, 1981). It should be noted that although CSF lactate is consistently elevated in bacterial meningitis, there is considerable overlap in the values obtained for individual patients with various meningitides. Berg *et al.* (1982) have shown lactate to be equal to, but not better than, standard biochemical methods in the diagnosis of meningitis. Lactate concentrations above 6 mmol/l are highly suggestive of bacterial meningitis and concentrations less than 3 mmol/l of a viral aetiology (Bailey *et al.*, 1990). CSF lactate may be measured with commercially available kits in about 15 minutes. Although it is not a specific test for bacterial meningitis, it may be a valuable adjunct in the diagnosis and therapy of bacterial meningitis. It must, however, be interpreted along with the other CSF parameters and the clinical situation.

Gram staining and culture are the most valuable and specific CSF measures in bacterial meningitis. Sixty to ninety per cent of patients with bacterial meningitis may have the causal organism detected on gram staining and this has a specificity approaching 100%. False positives occasionally occur as a result of contamination (Marton and Gean, 1986). Gram stain will detect 90% of cases of pneumococcal or staphylococcal meningitis, but may pick up only half the cases of gram negative meningitis and less than half due to listeria monocytogenes or anaerobes (Greenlee, 1990). The sensitivity of gram stain decreases to 60% in patients who have received antibiotic therapy. Acridine orange staining (AOS) may be a more sensitive staining method, particularly in partially treated patients (Benson *et al.,* 1988). Cultures approach 100% specificity but may be positive in only about 80% of patients thought to have bacterial meningitis (Marton and Gean, 1986).

Because of the importance of instituting prompt antibiotic therapy, a number of rapid diagnostic tests have been developed for detection of bacterial meningitis. These include immunological methods for detection of antigens, e.g. counterimmunoelectrophoresis (CIE), enzyme-linked immunosorbent assays, and latex particle agglutination. In addition, a number of non-immunologic methods show promise, including gas liquid chromatography (GLC), the limulus lysate test and polymerase chain reactions (PCR).

CIE has the advantage of being a rapid test of antigen detection. Results are available within one to two hours and it does not require viable organism. CIE is currently used for detection of bacterial, fungal, and protozoal antigens. It is rapid and specific but false negative results are common (Thadepalli *et al.*, 1982; Rytel, 1975). Occasional false positive results have also been reported. For meningococcal meningitis, the sensitivity of CIE is between 50 and 90% and for pneumococcal meningitis 60-100%. It is most sensitive in detecting haemophilus meningitis, picking up 80-90% of cases (Wood and Anderson, 1988).

Latex agglutination involves the absorption of antigens or antibodies to latex particles. It is more sensitive than CIE in meningitis due to *H. influenzae* and group B streptococci, with a detection rate of greater than 90% (Wood and Anderson, 1988). Coagglutination is another agglutination test which has also been shown to be more sensitive than CIE for meningitis due to meningococcus and *H. influenzae* type B. The use of antigen detection techniques is overall somewhat less sensitive than cultures but the major bacterial causes of meningitis may be detected in 75-80% of cases. These have been reviewed by Kaplan (1983).

The main nonimmunologic methods used for bacterial meningitis are GLC and the limulus lysate test. GLC may be performed in less than four hours and is an expensive technique, but it is particularly reliable in detecting antigens of anaerobic bacteria. It may also detect bacteroides, *H. influenzae*, *S. pneumoniae* and a variety of other bacteria as well as fungi. It may be difficult to discriminate if there is more than one pathogen in the sample. French *et al.* (1990) have used GLC with mass spectrometry and selected ion monitoring, finding this to be a more rapid and more sensitive test than microscopy and culture. They found it to be a useful marker for the common organisms causing bacterial meningitis, with a sensitivity of 88% and a specificity of 98%. The limulus lysate test is extremely valuable for the rapid diagnosis of gram negative bacterial meningitis. It may be performed in under one hour. Its major drawback is that it is nonspecific and does not discriminate between various types of gram negative organisus present. These nonimmunologic methods have been reviewed by Martin (1983).

A number of other tests have also been used for the rapid diagnosis of bacterial meningitis. The Quellung test is useful in the diagnosis of pneumococcal meningitis. It involves mixing antisera against serotypes of the organism with CSF. There are 83 serotypes of *S. pneumoniae,* 14 of which may cause infections in humans (Graves, 1989). The nitroblue tetrazolium dye test (NBT) is an assay for the presence of superoxide free radicals generated by granulocytes in CSF as an index of purulent meningitis. Its sensitivity and specificity are not yet clear. C-reactive protein and α-2 macroglobulin have also been found useful in differentiating bacterial meningitis from aseptic meningitis (Abramson *et al.*, 1985; Virji *et al.*, 1985). Several investigators have detected marked increases in total amino acid concentrations in patients with purulent meningitis (Corston *et al.*, 1981b; San Joaquin *et al.*, 1982; Briem *et al.*, 1982). This may be due to increased permeability of the blood-brain-CSF barriers, inhibition of amino acid transport across the choroid plexus, and/or altered CNS metabolism (Fishman, 1980). Briem *et al.* (1982) found the total concentrations of amino acids in patients with purulent meningitis to be higher than in patients with aseptic meningitis. A high concentration in those with bacterial meningitis seemed to indicate a poor prognosis. Olson and Arnoldi (1982) have found the CSF anion gap to be significantly elevated in bacterial meningitis compared to aseptic meningitis and to other systemic and localised bacterial or viral infections. There was, however, considerable overlap in these values.

The interested reader is referred to the reviews of Benson *et al.* (1988), Wood and Anderson (1988), and Greenlee (1990).

Viral Meningitis

Viral meningitis is usually diagnosed by the clinical features and by the exclusion of other possible causes. Characteristically there is a predominantly monocytic CSF pleocytosis with cell counts ranging from 10-1000 cells/mm^3. The protein is often mildly elevated in the 50-100 mg/dl range and the glucose levels are usually normal. The CSF glucose may occasionally be decreased. A PMN pleocytosis is often seen early in the illness and this may be confused with bacterial meningitis. Repeat lumbar puncture may be necessary to demonstrate the progression of the CSF abnormalities to a lymphocytic pleocytosis after 24-36 hours (Greenlee, 1990). The sensitivity of repeat lumbar punctures in these instances approaches 1.0. The CSF is usually clear in viral meningitis. Mumps and lymphocytic choriomeningitis virus (LCM) infection may present with a decreased glucose and increased protein (less than 200 mg/dl) (Graves, 1989).

Viral cultures may be useful in isolating enterovirus, LCM, or mumps within two to three days (Jackson and Johnson, 1989). Viral cultures of CSF generally show a sensitivity of 0.40, but the sensitivity is much higher with enteroviral infections (Health and Public Policy Committee, ACP, 1986). The use of viral cultures is rarely necessary clinically but may be useful for epidemiological purposes. Rapid means of viral detection include electron and immuno-fluorescent microscopy, specific antiviral antibody assays, and viral antigen and nucleic acid assays. The use of the polymerase chain reaction (PCR) also holds promise in the rapid identification of viruses. (See review of Eisenstein, 1990). The various methods of virus detection have been reviewed by Daumgarten (1987) and by Salmi (1989). CSF interferon levels have also been suggested as a rapid diagnostic test in viral infections and this appears to have a high specificity for virus infections, but is not a particularly sensitive indicator and does not appear to relate to the clinical status of the patients (Flowers and Scott, 1985). Organism-specific antibody indices are also available for meningoencephalomyelitis due to CMV, HSV, arbovirus, influenza A and B, mumps, varicella-zoster, echovirus, coxsackie A and B, LCM, and adenovirus infection (Peter, 1993).

Fungal Meningitis

The CSF findings in fungal meningitis are similar to those in tuberculous meningitis. The pleocytosis is predominantly lymphocytic. The glucose level is usually decreased and protein levels increased. It is almost always associated with an increased WBC count in the CSF. The CSF glucose levels may be lower than that of tuberculous meningitis. Patients who are immunocompromised may sometimes lack the characteristic pleocytosis.

Candida albicans, Cryptococcus neoformans, Blastomyces dermatidis and *Coccidioides immitis* may all very occasionally be detected with gram or silver staining of the CSF sediment, but this is usually unproductive (Greenlee, 1990). Cryptococcus may be detected with the India Ink smear with a sensitivity of approximately 0.26. Latex agglutination is somewhat more sensitive in identifying cryptococcus, with a sensitivity between 0.58-0.90 (Health and Public Policy Committee, ACP, 1986). Repeated lumbar punctures may be needed to detect the organism. Cryptococcus may be recovered from CSF cultures in 60-70% of cases with the first lumbar puncture but this may require large quantities of CSF (5-10 ml) and cisternal puncture may occasionally be needed (Berger and Paz, 1976). The complement fixation test for cryptococcal antigen is extremely specific, but not a very sensitive test, with about one-third of cases being detected. The latex agglutination test detecting cryptococcal antigen is the most useful test for the diagnosis, requiring only 25-60 ng of cryptococcal antigen, and may detect over 90% of cases even when cultures and India Ink preparations are negative (Sabetta and Andriole, 1985). Rheumatoid factor may cause false positive reactions.

Besides cryptococcus, the only common fungus that is easily isolated from CSF is *Candida albicans*. Large volumes of CSF are often needed for culture. Yeasts, aspergillus and zygomycetes may produce positive cultures in 1-3 days, but culture of Histoplasma capsulation may require six weeks, and the rate of successful culture is low (Graves, 1989). An ELISA assay is available for Histoplasma capsulation for serum and urine (Wheat *et al.*, 1986). *Coccidioides immitis* may be detected in 76% of patients by complement fixation antibody testing. Gas liquid chromatography with or without mass spectrometry shows promise in detection of fungal meningitis (Craven *et al.*, 1977). McGinnis (1983) has reviewed the various available methods for detection of fungi in CSF. Intra-BBB synthesis of organism-specific IgG may be detected for coccidioides and cryptococcus using the organism-specific antibody index (Peter, 1993).

Tuberculous Meningitis

Introduction

In tuberculous meningitis (TBM) the basis of the pathological process is thought to be a caseating tubercle (Rich's focus), which has ruptured into the subarachnoid space (Rich and McCordock, 1933; Parsons, 1988). The following release of mycobacteria provokes a Mantoux reaction with inflammatory changes in the cerebrospinal fluid (CSF). Spreading out from the ruptured tubercle, basal meningitis develops which is responsible for the characteristic neurological complications such as cranial nerve palsies, infarctions due to occlusion of arteries and veins, hydrocephalus and spinal block. In tuberculomas, major inflammatory responses may be absent in the CSF, depending on their proximity to the subarachnoid space (De Angelis, 1981).

The CSF changes reviewed below will be subjected into two groups. First, general parameters will be described, such as cell count, protein, and glucose. As in all infectious diseases of the nervous system, alterations of these parameters are nonspecific. Even the association of increased protein and lymphocyte response with a fall of CSF glucose does not prove the diagnosis of TBM, as a similar pattern can be found in partially treated pyogenic meningitis, meningeosis carcinomatosa, sarcoidosis and fungal infections (Parsons, 1988). Secondly, the use of more specific tests in the CSF will be discussed. These tests are addressed to establish a rapid and sensitive diagnosis of TBM by the detection of mycobacteria and their compounds and of a specific host response directed against the bacilli.

General changes

The CSF in TBM is usually a clear or slightly opalescent fluid, and may form a clot if it is allowed to stand. The opening pressure is elevated with a mean of 190 mm H_2O (range 80 to 540, Ogawa et al., 1987). The white cell count is increased, most commonly in the hundreds and seldom above 1000 cells/ul (Kasik, 1988). When tubercle bacilli and their cellular compounds are first released into the CSF, polymorphonuclear cells may be observed initially. These are replaced by lymphocytes within a few days, which represent the main white cell population during the course of the disease (Kasik, 1988). Beside these, neutrophils and eosinophils can be found in up to 25% and 10% respectively. During the course of TBM, a transient increase of polymorphonuclear cells up to 80% of white cells, has been reported in anti-tuberculous treated patients. This was not accompanied by a change of their clinical condition and disappeared even without antibiotic treatment (Teoh et al., 1986; Parsons, 1988). The authors considered that an exacerbation of meningeal inflammation due to compounds of dead mycobacteria was responsible for the increase. It is important to realise that such changes do not necessarily indicate a superinfection complicating the course of TBM.

Considerable variation of CSF protein values has been observed, which is usually elevated in the range of 100 to 500 mg/dl. However, values below 100 mg/dl have been reported in 25% of TBM patients (Kennedy and Fallon, 1979). Parsons (1988) noted a rough correlation between total protein and the white cell count. The blood-CSF barrier permeability is increased. Autochthonous production of IgG and oligoclonal IgG banding can be found in the majority of patients, whereas production of IgA and IgM occurs less frequently. In advanced stages of the disease, protein levels of 1000 to 1500 mg/dl can lead to a spinal block, which correlates with a poor prognosis (Molavi and Le Frock, 1985).

In most patients with TBM, the CSF glucose levels are moderately low in the range of 40-50 mg/dl (Molavi and Le Frock, 1985). Some patients will show a CSF glucose within the normal range. Moreover, in diabetics the usually high CSF glucose levels fall to "normal" during TBM (Parsons, 1988). Thus the blood:CSF ratio of glucose must also be considered. The presence of hyperglycaemia, glucose infusion or insulin administration can influence this ratio by causing rapid changes in blood glucose levels, and changes in the CSF lag some hours behind those in blood.

Specific tests

The search for mycobacteria is the crucial stage of the CSF analysis. Acid fast bacilli staining (Ziehl-Neelson) has a low sensitivity, detecting only 10-40% of proven cases of TBM (Molavi and Le Frock, 1985), as large numbers of organisms ($> 10^4$) must be present to be reliably detected. Culture of the organisms is a much more sensitive test but may require 4-8 weeks. Decisions about treatment of suspected TBM can often not be delayed until the results of culture are able to confirm the diagnosis. To overcome these difficulties in establishing the diagnosis of TBM, several more rapid and sensitive tests have recently been developed to aid in the diagnosis of TBM. These include direct tests for the mycobacterium and mycobacterial antigens and indirect tests detecting antibody to the organism.

Direct tests screen for mycobacteria and their compounds. They are thus independent of the extent of the patient's inflammatory response, which is advantageous in immunocompromised patients. A radiometric detection method ($BACTEC^R$) is available using ^{14}C palmitic acid, which is incorporated into mycobacteria and is evolved as $^{14}CO_2$ during growth and respiration (Roberts, 1988). Its sensitivity has been considered to be equivalent to conventional culturing, but its clinical utility is limited, as the mean recovery time for M. tuberculosis is 14 days (range 2 to 43).

The detection of mycobacterial antigen in the CSF is both a sensitive and a specific test for the diagnosis of TBM. Krambovitis et al. (1984), using a latex-agglutination immunoassay, looked at the initial CSF samples of TBM patients, and demonstrated a sensitivity of 94% and a specificity of 99%. The single false positive result was obtained in a patient with Haemophilus influenzae meningitis. In contrast, Chandramuki et al. (1985) were able to demonstrate a specificity of only 79%, with antigen being detected in four out of 19 patients with pyogenic meningitis. These false positive results were considered to be due to antigen sharing of mycobacteria with other microorganisms (Daniel, 1987). The use of more specific antigens in the preparation of assays should yield tests of greater specificity.

Tuberculostearic acid (TBSA) is a fatty acid compound of the mycobacteria cell wall and does not exist in human tissues. It was introduced for the rapid diagnosis of TBM by Mardh et al. (1983) using the combined gas chromatography/mass spectroscopy (GC/MS) method. Larger series using GC/MS (French et al., 1987) have confirmed the high sensitivity of this method (95%). In the study of French et al. (1987) a single false positive result was obtained in a patient who underwent intrathecal treatment with amikacine, which is a derivative of actinomyces. In addition, TBSA was found in the CSF eight months after the initiation of anti-tuberculous treatment, suggesting that this method is useful to confirm the diagnosis retrospectively (French et al., 1987).

The polymerase chain reaction (PCR) offers the opportunity of detecting minimal amounts of mycobacterial genome by amplification of specific DNA sequences. PCR is able to distinguish even closely related species in samples containing less than 10 organisms (Böddinghaus et al., 1990). PCR is a more sensitive technique than either ELISA or conventional culturing (Shankar et al., 1991). It has to be mentioned that due to the high sensitivity of PCR, cross-contamination of 12% of samples from patients not suffering from TBM was observed in this study. However, nucleic acid technology provides an interesting diagnostic approach and may initiate a new era in clinical microbiology.

Indirect tests usually measure the products of the host response to the infection. Hernandez et al. (1984) demonstrated IgM or IgG antibody to mycobacterial antigen in the CSF of 20/20 patients with TBM and in 0/70 control subjects suffering from other infections of the nervous system and from non-infectious diseases. Chandramuki et al. (1985), however, found a high rate of false positives in patients with pyogenic meningitis (73%) and controls living in an area with a high prevalence of tuberculosis. Coovadia et al. (1986) also detected antibodies to mycobacterial antigen in the CSF of 8% of South African children with pyogenic meningitis. In areas with a low prevalence of tuberculosis, however, detection of measurable amounts of antibodies in the CSF is uncommon (Chandramuki *et al.*, 1985). It would appear then that CSF antibody titres may result from contact with environmental mycobacteria, limiting the usefulness of this method in areas with a high rate of tuberculosis.

Adenosine deaminase (ADA) is an enzyme produced by T-lymphocytes. Elevated CSF levels have been found in 63 to 100% in TBM (Daniel, 1987). Segura *et al.* (1989) found a specificity of 95% measuring CSF ADA. However, ADA release of stimulated lymphocytes is not a specific response to mycobacteria. Elevated levels of ADA may also be seen in viral meningitis. Furthermore, as CSF ADA levels correlate with alterations of the blood-CSF barrier (Donald *et al.*, 1987), one must consider that levels may also reflect a general lymphocyte response in the blood.

In summary, most of the direct and indirect tests provide considerable sensitivity and can be performed rapidly. The better specificity seems to be obtained by direct tests as discussed above. However, to date, the main drawback of many of these techniques is the need for complex and expensive analytical equipment, which is often available in Western countries but not usually in developing countries where TBM is common.

Acquired Immunodeficiency Syndrome (AIDS)

The neurological manifestations of AIDS may occur during any phase of the illness and affect 31-65% of adults and 50-90% of children infected with human immunodeficiency virus (HIV-1) (American Academy of Neurology AIDS Task Force, 1989). Up to 10% may present initially with neurological symptoms (Levy *et al.*, 1985). The neurological complications include HIV meningitis, peripheral neuropathy, myelopathy, encephalopathy, cerebrovascular disease, lymphomas, and various opportunistic infections. These have been reviewed by McArthur (1987) and by Harrison and McAllister (1991). Perry (1990) has recently reviewed the psychiatric complications of AIDS.

HIV appears to be a neurotropic virus and may invade the CNS at an early stage. Patients with seroconversion illness may develop a mild meningitic illness shortly after seroconversion. They frequently develop CSF abnormalities even when asymptomatic, including a mild pleocytosis and increased CSF protein. McArthur *et al.* (1988) isolated the HIV virus in two of seven patients who were asymptomatic but had seroconverted within six to 24 months. Eight of eleven such patients also had an increased IgG index and two were found to have a pleocytosis or increased CSF protein. Hollander and Levy (1987) also isolated the virus in the CSF in five of eight patients with normal neurologic examinations. Thus, although HIV has been isolated from the CSF more often in patients with neurological and neuropsychiatric findings (Ho *et al.*, 1985; Levy *et al.*, 1985; McArthur *et al.*, 1988), occult infection of the nervous system may occur early on in the illness. Specific antibodies to HIV, increased cell counts, protein and immunoglobulins, and cytological abnormalities have also been detected in the CSF of asymptomatic seropositive individuals (Lobenthal *et al.*, 1983; Resnick *et al.*, 1985; Goudsmit *et al.*, 1986; Appleman *et al.*, 1988; Bukasa *et al.*, 1988; McArthur *et al.*, 1988; Portegies *et al.*, 1989).

HIV meningitis may occur at any point in the illness from seroconversion to full-blown AIDS. It is often associated with cranial nerve palsies and long tract signs and is usually self-limiting. A mononuclear pleocytosis is usually present (mean 41 WBC/mm³; range 5-176 WBC/mm³), and may persist for six to 12 months after infection (McArthur, 1987). While other types of viral meningoencephalitis cause a selective recruitment of T-helper/inducer (CD4) cells into the CSF in preference to T-suppressor/cytotoxic (CD8) cells, HIV meningitis is characterised by increased proportions of CD8 cells and a reduction of CD4 cells in the CSF (McArthur, 1987). Total protein (mean 65 mg/dl, range 20-186 mg/dl) and IgG are also frequently elevated, oligoclonal bands may be detectable, and HIV may be isolated from the CSF in about 50% of patients with HIV meningitis (McArthur, 1987).

In AIDS-related peripheral neuropathies the CSF protein is usually elevated. Patients presenting with Guillain-Barré syndrome or chronic inflammatory demyelinating polyneuropathy have atypical CSF findings with a pleocytosis (mean 23 WBC/m³) in addition to the increased CSF protein, which is markedly elevated (mean 178 mg/dl) (McArthur, 1987; Harrison and McAllister, 1991). The CSF in mononeuritis multiplex associated with AIDS is also often cellular (Harrison and McAllister, 1991).

CSF abnormalities are common in AIDS-related dementia (ARD) but there is no specific test yet available to confirm the diagnosis. The CSF in ARD is usually hypocellular and the glucose is usually normal (Katz *et al.*, 1989). A predominantly mononuclear pleocytosis (range 4-51 cells/mm³) is seen in about 20% of cases and the increased CSF protein (range 42-189 mg/dl) rises progressively during the clinical course (Navia *et al.* 1986). CSF IgG is also usually elevated and oligoclonal IgG banding may be seen (McArthur, 1987; Navia *et al.*, 1986). As with other AIDS-related neurological conditions, the CSF composition of mononuclear cells parallels that of the blood with inverted CD4:CD8 ratios and there appears to be a relationship between the blood and CSF CD4 lymphocyte proportions and the severity of dementia (McArthur *et al.*, 1989). The detection of HIV p 24 antigen in the CSF correlates with dementia in adults and with progressive encephalopathy in children, but is not useful in predicting neurological deterioration. It is detected uncommonly in asymptomatic individuals (Epstein *et al.*, 1987; McArthur, 1987; Portegies *et al.*, 1989).

Intrathecal synthesis of HIV specific antibody has been demonstrated in AIDS-related dementia and HIV has been isolated from the CSF in these patients, but these CSF abnormalities have also been frequently demonstrated in neurologically asymptomatic patients as well (Resnick *et al.*, 1985; Bukasa *et al.*, 1988; McArthur, 1987).

A number of other substances in the CSF have also been looked at as potential markers of CNS involvement, including neopterin (Brew *et al.*, 1990; Griffin *et al.*, 1991), alpha-tumour necrosis factor (Grimaldi *et al.*, 1991), and β-2-microglobulin (Elovaara *et al.*, 1989; Brew *et al.*, 1989).

McArthur *et al.* (1992) have found β-2-microglobulin to be a useful marker for HIV dementia with elevations (>3.8mg/l) showing a sensitivity of 44%, specificity of 90%, and a positive predictive value of 88%.

Heyes *et al.* (1989, 1990*a,b*) have demonstrated increased quinolinic acid in the CSF of humans and rhesus macaques with AIDS, suggesting a possible role for excitotoxicity in the pathogenesis of CNS involvement with AIDS.

The most important indication for CSF analysis in AIDS is in the diagnosis of opportunistic infection, particularly fungal and mycobacterial meningitis. One must be aware that the CSF formula is highly variable in AIDS and the typical cellular and protein changes in meningitis may not always be present (Britton *et al.*, 1989). The VDRL may also be initially negative in the CSF in neurosyphilis (Feraru *et al.*, 1990). In cryptococcal meningitis the cell count is often normal, but the India Ink preparation may be positive in over 80% and the sensitivity of cryptococcal antigen detection approaches 100% in these patients (McArthur, 1987; Greenlee, 1990).

Neurosyphilis

CNS involvement of *Treponema pallidum* usually occurs with dissemination of syphilis but may occur early in the disease even with no symptoms evident. A CSF pleocytosis may be present in 9-35% of patients with primary or secondary syphilis (Merritt and Fremont-Smith, 1938). Lukehart *et al.* (1988) isolated *T. pallidum* in the CSF of 12 (30%) of 40 patients with untreated primary and secondary syphilis. An additional four of their patients had a reactive Venereal Disease Research Laboratory (VDRL) test indicating that 16 of their 40 patients had evidence of CNS involvement, even at this early stage of the illness.

The CSF changes seen in syphilis vary with the stage of the illness and with the type of CNS involvement. About 20% of patients with primary syphilis will develop persistent CSF abnormalities (and thus by definition asymptomatic neurosyphilis) and of these approximately one-fifth will become symptomatic with neurosyphilis. Prior to the advent of antibiotics, approximately two-thirds of patients with asymptomatic neurosyphilis would develop meningeal (6%), vascular (10%), tabetic (30%), or paretic

(12%) neurosyphilis (Graves, 1989). In primary and secondary syphilis, the CSF pleocytosis is usually lymphocytic with cell counts up to 100/mm^3. The protein content may be slightly raised and the pressure is usually normal. The pleocytosis may be evident before the appearance of a secondary rash (Merritt and Fremont-Smith, 1938; Wood and Anderson, 1988). During the latent stage of the illness the CSF may continue to show a variable lymphocytic pleocytosis (Merritt and Fremont Smith, 1938; Herndon and Brumback, 1989). The CSF may also continue to show a positive serology at this time.

In general paresis the cell count is usually between 25 and 75 cells/mm^3, but a mononuclear pleocytosis as high as 175/mm^3 may be seen. The pressure is usually normal or slightly increased. The protein is usually between 50 and 100 mg/dl. There is usually increased gamma-globulin and a positive Wassermann reaction (Fishman, 1992).

In acute syphilitic meningitis there is a markedly increased pressure usually greater than 200 mm (range 80 to 600 mm), a lymphocytic pleocytosis between 2 and 21 000 (mean 450) cells/mm^3, and a decreased glucose. The protein may be elevated up to 380 mg/dl with an average of 110 mg/dl (Merritt and Fremont-Smith, 1938). The pleocytosis seen in menigovascular syphilis is predominantly mononuclear between 11 and 100 cells/mm^3 and the protein is usually elevated between 45 and 260 mg/dl in about two-thirds of patients (Merritt et al., 1946).

The findings in tabes dorsalis are extremely variable depending on the activity of the disease. The cell count may vary between 0 and 200 cells (mean 38 cells) per mm^3 and approximately one-third have a normal cell count. The protein content may vary between 17-320 mg/dl (mean 61 mg/dl) and the pressure is usually normal but occasionally moderately increased (Merritt and Fremont-Smith, 1938).

T. pallidum cannot be grown in routine cultures but may be identified in the CSF using dark field microscopy, immunofluorescence, silver stained sections of artificially cultured CSF, or rabbit infectivity tests. The inoculation of rabbits for the identification of T. pallidum is a more cumbersome procedure but is less likely to be compromised by artefacts and has a sensitivity of approximately ten organisms (Lukehart et al., 1988).

Serological tests for syphilis

The colloidal gold test has been used in the past as a reflection of qualitative changes in the CSF proteins with the three patterns – paretic, tabetic, and meningitic curves – thought to be associated with general paresis, tabes dorsalis, and non-syphilitic meningitis respectively. As a variety of serological tests and other more specific tests for proteins are now available, the colloidal gold test is no longer used.

There is considerable debate about when to do a lumbar puncture in syphilis and the usefulness of the various serological tests available. Dans *et al.* (1986) have pointed out that the CSF-VDRL is often inappropriately ordered to exclude neurosyphilis, finding only three of 2,536 CSF-VDRL tests ordered at Johns Hopkins Hospital to be positive. They recommend that it be used either in seropositive patients with neuropsychiatric signs or in seronegative patients with neuropsychiatric signs suggestive of syphilis, and, due to its low sensitivity, that it not be used to rule out neurosyphilis but rather to "rule it in" when clinically indicated. Wiesel and colleagues (1985) compared treatment strategies of performing a lumbar puncture to test for asymptomatic neurosyphilis or empirical treatment with penicillin G benzathine without lumbar puncture. They found both strategies to give a similar cure rate of 99.7% and recommended that lumbar puncture offers little additional benefit in patients with asymptomatic late syphilis. Their recommendations have been criticised, however, (Simon and Fishman, 1986) for not taking into account the treatment failures that may occur with intramuscular penincillin G. benzathine. This, along with the fact that such treatment does not result in detectable levels of penicillin in the spinal fluid, has prompted the World Health Organisation to recommend that penicillin G. benzathine not be used in the treatment of neurosyphilis and that patients with syphilis of more than two year's duration have a lumbar puncture to exclude asymptomatic neurosyphilis (Simon and Fishman, 1986). The Centre for Disease Control (CDC) has also recommended that lumbar puncture be done to check CSF VDRL in asymptomatic patients with untreated syphilis of greater than one year's duration. In the past, patients with neurosyphilis would receive the same amount of penicillin as other patients with syphilis without evidence of neurological involvement of over one year's duration. The evidence that this may occasionally have been insufficient to cure CNS disease led the CDC in 1985 to recommend that neurosyphilis be treated with larger doses of penicillin for a longer period of time. The use of CSF serological tests for syphilis to exclude CNS involvement is thus essential in the management of patients with syphilis.

Both specific treponemal and nontreponemal serological assays are available for syphilis. The CSF VDRL is a nontreponemal test which is the most specific for neurosyphilis with a specificity of approximately 1.0, but with a sensitivity of only 0.40-0.60 (Health and Public Policy Committee, ACP, 1986). Elevation of CSF gamma-globulin, or of the WBC count, are suggestive of neurosyphilis, being seen in 70-80% of patients, but both measures are relatively nonspecific. Because of its high specificity the CSF VDRL is the serological test of choice in the diagnosis of neurosyphilis, but its low sensitivity does present some limitations and it must be considered that a negative CSF-VDRL does not rule out neurosyphilis. A false positive serum VDRL test occurs in a variety of diseases but false positives rarely occur with the CSF test. A false positive may occur in a patient with a positive serum VDRL in the event of a traumatic lumbar puncture. A positive CSF VDRL does not differentiate between active or inactive forms of neurosyphilis.

There are a number of specific treponemal antibody tests which are more sensitive than the VDRL but considerably less specific. The fluorescent treponemal antibody absorption test (FTA-ABS) is a sensitive test for neurosyphilis, but its use has been controversial as it is felt that it may overdiagnose CNS involvement in syphilis. False negative tests are rare except in immunocompromised individuals and false positive tests may occur when the antibody leaks into the CSF either through contamination with a traumatic lumbar puncture or through breakdown of the blood-brain-CSF barriers. The CSF FTA-ABS does not differentiate between active asymptomatic and treated neurosyphilis and a positive test may persist for years, even with treatment. Davis and Schmitt (1989) have reviewed the samples of 1665 CSF FTA-ABS tests used as a screening procedure and found, of these, 48 samples were reactive. Those samples which tested positive for FTA-ABS also underwent a CSF VDRL test and they found that although the specificity of the CSF VDRL was 100%, the sensitivity was only 27%. They stressed the importance of clinical judgment in the diagnosis of active neurosyphilis and considered 15 of their 48 patients with reactive FTA-ABS to have active neurosyphilis with a reactive CSF FTA-ABS, neurological signs consistent with the diagnosis, no other recognised cause for neurological illness, and either a pleocytosis or elevated protein. It is of note that only four of these 15 patients had a reactive CSF VDRL.

Concomitant measures to correct for protein leakage across the blood-brain barrier may help to correct for false positive treponemal tests which may be caused by antibody leakage from the serum. The TPHA index and TPHA-IgG index measure local CNS production of antibody to *T. pallidum* and can thus help establish the diagnosis of neurosyphilis (Tramont, 1991). Specific treponemal IgM (FTA-IgM) may also aid in establishing the diagnosis, as serum IgM does not cross the blood-brain barrier (Tramont, 1991). Wolters and colleagues (1988) in a study of 203 syphilitic patients, found that the TPHA may be accurately interpreted by measurement of IgG and IgM indices. They found that either a positive CSF VDRL or a combination of raised IgG and/or IgM index with an elevated CSF cell count, were both useful criteria in establishing the diagnosis of asymptomatic neurosyphilis.

Other immunoglobulin findings in neurosyphilis include the presence of oligoclonal bands and the presence of *T. pallidum*-specific IgA, which has been postulated to inhibit the antitreponemal activity of IgG and thus to play a part in the pathogenesis of neurosyphilis (Gschnait *et al.*, 1981).

In summary, neurosyphilis is often accompanied by increased CSF protein, decreased CSF glucose and an increased WBC count. These findings are nonspecific but are useful when considered with the clinical state and with the CSF serology testing. The CSF VDRL is a nontreponemal test which is the serological test of choice, because of its specificity. Its major disadvantage, however, is its low sensitivity. Treponemal antibodies may be demonstrated by a number of different tests including treponemal haemaglutination and indirect fluorescent antibody testing, as well as by ELISA testing. These tests are much more sensitive than the VDRL but their major drawback is their tendency to overdiagnose neurosyphilis. This is largely due to antibody from serum crossing the blood-brain-CSF barriers accounting for false positive tests. This may be corrected for, however, by considering the clinical state of the patient, evidence of pleocytosis or increased CSF protein, and with measurement of albumin in the serum and CSF to correct for BBB leakage as a measure of CNS antibody production to *T. pallidum* (Luger *et al.*, 1981; Wolters *et al.*, 1988; Davis and Schmitt, 1989; Tramont, 1991). Isolation of *T. pallidum* is still largely restricted to research laboratories.

Lyme's Disease

Borrelia burgdorferi (B.b.) was identified as being the causative agent of Lyme's disease in 1982 (Burgdorfer *et al.*). Ixodid ticks have been shown to be the most important vector of the spirochaete. Lyme's disease is a multisystem disease mainly affecting the skin, musculoskeletal, cardiovascular and nervous systems and is divided into three stages according to clinical features and incubation time (Steere *et al.*, 1986).

Stage 1 is characterised by *erythema chronicum migrans* (ECM), *lymphadenosis cutis benigna* and nonspecific influenza-like symptoms. Incubation time is up to one month. Recent reports suggest that up to 25% of patients with stage 1 disease have asymptomatic CNS-involvement (Schmidli and Meyer, 1990).

Stage 2 occurs weeks to months after inoculation and classically presents with meningopolyradiculitis (MPR), otherwise known as the Garin-Bujadoux-Bannwarth-Syndrome. Less common are "aseptic" meningitis and cardiovascular involvement. There are marked differences in the incidence of stage 2 in North America and Europe. These variances in frequency of clinical expression are thought to be related to heterogeneity of antigens in *B.b.* (Barbour *et al.*, 1985).

Stage 3, seven months to twelve years after initial infection, is typified by progressive encephalomyelitis, cranial nerve palsies, arthritis, and mononeuritis multiplex. Other rare syndromes have also been described (Ackermann *et al.*, 1988; Kohlhepp *et al.*, 1989).

CSF laboratory tests

Diagnosis of Lyme's disease is based on clinical symptoms and signs. However, as more and more "idiopathic" syndromes are being investigated or suspected of being caused by the *B.b.* spirochaete, increasing emphasis is being placed on confirmatory laboratory tests. Most important among these are the examination of the cerebrospinal fluid (CSF) and serological tests. The identification of intrathecally synthesised IgG antibodies against *B.b.* is currently the most specific test available for Lyme neuroborrelioses (Steere *et al.*, 1990). Detection rate and level of antibodies to *B.b.* show considerable variation between laboratories, as there has been little interlaboratory standardisation and comparability of tests (Hedberg and Osterholm, 1990).   Compounding this is the marked *Borrelia burgdorferi* strain heterogeneity caused by plasmid encoded DNA (Have *et al.*, 1986). This has led to widely differing results on the presence of antibodies to *B.b.* in Lyme's disease (Hedberg and Osterholm, 1990). Although international standards are slowly being introduced, it is at this stage still prudent not to rely on results of antibody testing as sole criterion for the diagnosis or abscence of Lyme disease (Hedberg and Osterholm, 1990).

The diagnostic usefulness of lymphocyte stimulation tests (LST) is still controversial. Some groups have found a good positive correlation between antibody levels and LST. In contrast other researchers found up to 50% of LST positive in otherwise seronegative Lyme disease, and the highest positive rates were in healthy technicians working with *B.b.* (Schmidli and Meyer, 1990). At this stage the use of LST in Lyme's disease is still in the experimental stage.

Halperin and Heyes (1992) have recently found CSF levels of quinolinic acid to be substantially elevated in neuroborreliosis. As quinolinic acid is an excitotoxin and N-methyl-D-aspartate (NMDA) agonist, this suggests that some of the neurological deficits in Lyme's disease may be due to excitotoxicity.

The polymerase chain reaction (PCR) will undoubtedly become more and more established and enable earlier and more definite diagnosis of Lyme's disease than other laboratory tests currently available. Keller *et al.* (1992) demonstrated PCR's high specifity and sensitivity in detecting *Borrelia burgdorferi* oligonucleotides. They point out that, in addition, PCR may have a role in predicting clinical outcome after antimicrobial therapy.

B.b. can be cultured from CSF and other body fluids and tissues, but the low yield and high costs are prohibitive for routine use.

Humoral immune response

In the CSF, antigen detection precedes the specific immune reaction
(Garcia-Monco *et al.*, 1990). The intrathecal humoral immune response
involves the production of polyclonal IgG, IgM and IgA. As presented in
Tables 6-2 and 6-3, CSF oligoclonal IgG production is nearly always
elevated in Lyme neuroborreliosis. Not all of the oligoclonal IgG, as tested
by immunoblotting, is directed towards *B.b.* specific antigens (Hansen *et
al.*, 1990). One of the major immunogens in the CSF humoral response is
the 41-kDa-flagellar *B.b.* antigen, which shows a marked reactivity with
CSF oligoclonal bands (Wilske *et al.*, 1986). The specificity of non-reactive
IgG is as yet unknown (Hansen *et al.*, 1990). The temporal profile of CSF
oligoclonal *B.b.* specific IgG antibodies early on in MPR was studied by
Hansen *et al.*, (1990). Two and six weeks after onset of symptoms 42% and
100% of patients respectively had identifiable specific intrathecal antibody
production, making it clear that the diagnostic sensitivity of this and other
techniques depends largely on the disease duration. This is confirmed by
the reports of 100% antibody detection rate in stage 3 patients (Ackermann
et al., 1988). In stage 2, quantitative IgA and IgM levels are reported to
be elevated in 0-30% and 86-100% of patients respectively (Henriksson and
Link, 1985, Pohl *et al.*, 1986). Both early and late Lyme neuroborreliosis
have a specific and non-specific IgA and IgM response (Steere *et al.*, 1990).
There is as yet no clear picture of the extent and distribution of the
non-specific and specific IgA and IgM response. In the largest study of stage
3 neuroborreliosis (44 patients), nearly all were shown to have all three
immunoglobulin fractions raised and intrathecal IgG antibody synthesis was
positive in 100% (Ackermann *et al.*, 1988).

Cellular immune response

Cellular immune mechanisms precede the development of a measurable
humoral response and are described by Dattwyler *et al.* (1986). Measurements of cellular immune responses are currently being investigated for
their use in the diagnosis and evaluation of Lyme's disease.

CSF changes in relation to clinical syndromes

Stage 1:
Although *B.b.* is thought to spread to the CNS within several days of
inoculation (Barthold *et al.*, 1988), the CSF generally shows no detectable
changes in stage 1 (Steere *et al.*, 1983). Garcia-Monco *et al.* (1990)
demonstrated CSF *B.b.* antigens in three out of five patients with early
evidence of neurological involvement (headache, meningism). Monoclonal

antibodies directed against two specific outer surface proteins of *B.b.* were utilised for this purpose. Serum or CSF antibodies could not be detected. The dormant nature of the *B.b* spirochaete is well demonstrated by a report of the isolation of *B.b.* from the otherwise normal CSF of an asymptomatic patient (Pfister *et al.*, 1989).

Stage 2:
(a) Spontaneous course   Recent studies have confirmed the original finding of Bannwarth (1941), that most MPR follows a benign self-remitting course. CSF changes parallel the clinical course, usually normalising over a period of several months. Antibody titres both in serum and CSF may remain detectable for years after clinical recovery. Highly specific and sensitive assays are able to detect oligoclonal IgG and intrathecal *B.b.* IgG antibody production in otherwise normal CSF for years after clinical evidence of disease (Hansen *et al.*, 1990; Kruger *et al.*, 1989). This is likely to be similar to persistent treponemal IgG antibody synthesis reported years after adequate treatment of neurosyphilis and can be regarded as an "immunological scar" (Kruger *et al.*, 1989).

(b) Course after treatment   Antibiotics are the treatment of choice as they induce rapid clinical response and combat the (albeit small) possibility of chronic progressive disease. CSF changes normalise more rapidly than without treatment. As mentioned above, without specific therapy, in-trathecally produced *B.b.* IgG antibody and oligoclonal IgG levels may occasionally persist for years in an otherwise healthy patient (Kruger *et al.*, 1989; Hansen *et al.*, 1990). However, levels should be decreasing or at a generally stable low concentration. If assays reveal rising or high stable levels of intrathecal *B.b.* antibody, continuing pathogen activity must be considered and clinical follow-up is indicated. Table 6.2 summarises the CSF findings of stage 2 neuroborreliosis.

TABLE 6.2. *Typical CSF findings of stage 2 neuroborreliosis.*

Cells per mm^3	100-1000 (range 50-2000)
Cytology	50-80% small lymphocytes
	10-35% large lymphocytes
	1-10% plasma cells,
	occasional atypical plasma cells or polynuclear cells
Total protein content (mg/dl)	50-150 (range 30-300)
*IgG *B.b.* antibody titre	detected in 40-100%
CSF/Serum glucose index	< 0.6 in 50%
Oligoclonal IgG bands	detected in 80-100%

(*Antibody titres done 2-6 weeks after onset of neurological symptoms. The longer symptoms are present the higher the antibody detection rate. Antibody titres may vary widely between different laboratories)

Stage 3:

Though there are increasing numbers of reports of chronic progressive neurological disease, the overall number is still small. The course of tertiary disease without treatment is not known as the disease entity has only been recognised for the past half decade and all cases have been treated vigorously. Even then the majority of patients only partially respond, as irreparable damage to the nervous system has already taken place (Ackermann *et al.*, 1988). Half a year after specific therapy, the cell count should be back in the normal range. Likewise, after one year, protein levels should be decreasing or stable at a low level. As in stage 2 disease, with normalisation of inflammatory CSF changes, oligoclonal *B.b.* specific IgG antibodies can persist, and this may be regarded as a harmless residual finding. Mononeuritis multiplex presents with normal CSF findings (including absent CSF antibodies), but with highly elevated serum IgG antibodies (Steere *et al.*, 1990).

Regardless of the clinical stage, unabated intrathecal synthesis of *B.b.* antibodies is currently the best laboratory index of pathogen activity. In patients who have responded to treatment but continue to show significant intrathecal synthesis of *B.b.* antibodies, however, the need for further treatment ultimately rests on clinical acumen (Ackermann *et al.*, 1988). Table 6.3 summarises the CSF findings in stage 3 neuroborreliosis.

TABLE 6.3. *Typical CSF findings of stage 3 neuroborreliosis.*

Cells per mm^3	5-500 (range 5- 1000)
Cytology:	mostly lymphocytes and plasma cells, rarely polymorphs
Total protein content (mg/dl)	50-300 (range 50-1200)
Intrathecal IgG *B.b.* antibody production	40-100%
CSF/Serum glucose index	< 0.6 in 50%
Oligoclonal IgG bands	80-100%

Sarcoidosis

The neurological manifestations of sarcoidosis are protean and estimated to occur in 5% of patients with sarcoidosis (Stern *et al.*, 1985; Delaney, 1977). Clinical syndromes include cranial and peripheral neuropathy, hydrocephalus, aseptic meningitis, hypothalamic dysfunction and intracranial mass lesions.

CSF changes in neurosarcoidosis are reported in 53 to 70% (Delaney, 1977; Stern *et al.*, 1985; Chapelon *et al.*, 1990). Mononuclear pleocytosis (< 200/mm^3) is common, occurring in 43-72% of patients with CSF alterations. The only study on CSF lymphocyte subpopulations to date showed an increased T4/T8 cell ratio in three of eight patients (Stern *et al.*,

1987). Exceptionally, eosinophilia may be present (Scott, 1988).

Total protein is elevated in approximately 70% and may be as high as 350 mg/dl. Hypoglycorrhachia (CSF glucose level/blood glucose level <0.6, or CSF glucose level <40 mg/dl) is present in 10-20%, may be as low as 15 mg/dl, and is associated with diffuse meningeal sarcoidosis (Gaines et al., 1970; Stern et al., 1985).

Increased CSF IgG levels have recently been detected in four of five patients studied (Borucki et al., 1989), and there have been isolated reports of the presence of oligoclonal IgG bands (Kinnman and Link, 1984; Scott et al., 1989).

Serum angiotensin converting enzyme (ACE) levels are a good index of systemic disease activity (Gronhagen-Riska and Selroos, 1979). Similarly, CSF ACE levels appear to correlate well with the clinical course of neurosarcoidosis (Oksanen et al., 1985a). Oksanen et al. (1985b) have published the largest cohort to date and established the following ranges in CSF ACE activity: normal adult (0.78 ± 0.27 u/ml), sarcoidosis without neurological involvement (0.88 ± 0.34), active neurosarcoidosis (1.42 ± 0.27). Many patients with neurosarcoidosis, however, may still have normal CSF ACE levels.

It must be kept in mind that raised levels of ACE are not unique to neurosarcoidosis, and can also be found in bacterial meningitis and malignant CNS tumours.

With the exception of CSF ACE levels, cerebrospinal fluid findings have not been found to reliably correlate with the subsequent disease course (Stern et al., 1985). Kveim-specific IgG has been detected in the CSF in neurosarcoidosis, but further work needs to be done to establish its role as a diagnostic tool.

Peripheral Neuropathies

The CSF protein levels are increased in a wide variety of neuropathies (Table 6-4). The raised level of CSF protein can be looked upon, most simply, as a reflection of generalised root disease. Some neuropathies in which nerve roots are involved extensively, e.g. Guillain-Barré syndrome, chronic inflammatory demyelinating neuropathy, diabetic neuropathy, and Refsum's disease, show gross increases of CSF protein. However, in most neuropathies an increased CSF protein is mild, usually below 200 mg/100 ml. It should be emphasised that the CSF may be normal in these neuropathies.

Guillain-Barré syndrome

Guillain-Barré syndrome (acute idiopathic inflammatory poly-radiculoneuropathy) is the most common acute areflexic quadriparesis and its diagnostic criteria has been recently reviewed (Arnason, 1984; Asbury and Cornblath, 1990). The disease, characterised by a lymphocytic cellular infiltration of peripheral nerve and destruction of myelin, is inflammatory in nature, possibly an autoimmune disorder of delayed hypersensitivity.

It is well known that Guillain-Barré syndrome is accompanied by an increase in the CSF protein without pleocytosis, the "albumino-cytologic dissociation". In most cases, during the first days or week of illness, protein levels in the CSF are normal. After several days of illness, the protein value begins to rise steadily. Later, even while the clinical condition is becoming stabilised, the CSF protein value continues to rise. Peak protein values occur approximately two to six weeks after onset of clinical symptoms (Wiederholt and Mulder, 1965; McLeod *et al.*, 1976), and may reach levels as high as 2 g/100 ml. Extreme elevation of the protein level has been suggested as correlating with raised intracranial pressure and with papilloedema. However, papilloedema can also be seen in conjunction with only modest increases in CSF protein. No correlation has been established between increased CSF protein levels and severity and/or duration of disease. The CSF protein may remain elevated for several months, even after recovery is underway. In contrast, CSF protein may be normal throughout the illness, suggesting minimal root involvement.

Cells in the CSF are not prominent in Guillain-Barré syndrome and the absence of cells is supportive, although not necessary, for its diagnosis. Mononuclear cells, usually less than $10/mm^3$, are present in up to one-half of the cases. The maximal cellular responses were noted between 10 and 20 days after the onset of symptoms. Exceptionally, they may number up to above 50 cells per mm^3 (McLeod *et al.*, 1976). The CSF pleocytosis is of no value as a prognostic sign. In human immunodeficiency virus seropositive patients with demyelinating neuropathy, CSF pleocytosis is commonly seen (see section 6-12).

The origin of increased CSF proteins in Guillain-Barré syndrome is unclear, although it may be caused by leakage from serum through a damaged blood-CSF barrier or by intrathecal immunoglobulin synthesis. The fact that cisternal CSF protein levels may be only slightly increased despite marked elevations of LCSF protein suggests that the protein may derive from the capillary endothelial cells of the spinal roots traversing the subarachnoid space (Fishman, 1992, p.333). Vedeler and colleagues (1986) examined CSF from 80 patients with Guillain-Barré syndrome, and found an increased CSF concentration of IgG, correlating with increased CSF total protein, in more than 90% of patients. Serum IgM and IgA were increased in approximately 25% of patients, while serum IgG was at normal levels in all patients. Different results have been reported on the frequency of oligoclonal bands in the CSF with Guillain-Barré syndrome. Oligoclonal IgG, if positive, is usually transient and disappears when neurological signs subside (Dalakas *et al.*, 1980; Segurado *et al.*, 1986). Antineural antibodies to nerve root and brain may be found not only in serum but also in CSF.

Chronic Inflammatory Demyelinating Polyradiculoneuropathy (CIDP)

CIDP may be the peripheral nervous system counterpart of multiple sclerosis, being a recrudescent or chronic inflammatory and demyelinating process possibly due to an autoimmune process, although not proved. CIDP has been distinguished from Guillain-Barré syndrome only in recent years; other names for CIDP include chronic Guillain-Barré syndrome and chronic relapsing polyradiculoneuropathy. The criteria for the diagnosis of CIDP have been recently outlined by Cornblath *et al.* (1991).

CSF protein is often elevated in this disease and especially so during relapses (Austin, 1958; Thomas *et al.*, 1969), although an elevated protein level is not essential for the diagnosis. In general, the severity of neuropathies appears to be related to the protein level (Dyck and Arnasan, 1984). Dyck and colleagues analysed the CSF in 44 patients with CIDP, and CSF protein values of between 23 and 600 mg per 100 ml (mean 137.6 mg per 100 ml) were recorded. The CSF gamma globulin was elevated in a few cases. A pleocytosis of more than five lymphocytes and polymorphonuclear cells per cubic millimeter is not uncommon (Dyck and Arnason, 1984).

Whereas transient CSF IgG banding may be found in Guillain-Barré syndrome, CIDP patients may show a stable IgG band in the CSF. Monoclonal IgG banding in CSF is not affected by immunosuppressive therapy and does not correlate with the severity or chronicity of the disease (Dalakas *et al.*, 1980; Segurado *et al.*, 1986).

Diabetic neuropathy

The typical finding in the CSF of diabetic neuropathy is a moderate increase of the protein content (Ives, 1957; Thomas and Eliasson, 1984). Bischoff (1963) found an elevated CSF protein in 66% of 318 cases, with an average value of 60 mg per 100 ml. Rundles (1945) reported protein levels of over 250 mg per 100 ml in very severe diabetic polyneuropathy. Increased globulin values in the CSF were also found in the majority cases of diabetic neuropathy (Gribbels and Schliep, 1970; Kutt *et al.*, 1961). There was no correlation with vascular complications, nor was there any with the severity and duration of the diabetes or with the age of the patient. The cell count is normal in diabetic neuropathy. The CSF sugar content is strictly related to the blood sugar level and therefore of no specific diagnostic value (see section 5-6). An increased sorbitol concentration associated with a reduced myoinositol in the CSF has been reported in patients with diabetic polyneuropathy (Servo *et al.*, 1977).

TABLE 6.4. *Peripheral neuropathies with an increased CSF protein.*

Guillain-Barré syndrome
Chronic inflammatory demylinating polyradiculoneuropathy
Diabetic neuropathy
Hereditary neuropathy

> Hereditary motor and sensory neuropathy Type III (Déjerine-Sottas disease)
> Heredopathia atactica polyneuritiformis (Refsum disease)
> Hereditary motor and sensory neuropathy Type I (Charcot-Marie-Tooth disease) (Serratric and Roux, 1979; Hagberg and Lyon, 1981)
> Porphyric neuropathy (Ridley, 1984)

Neuropathy associated with systemic disease

> Uraemic neuropathy (Asbury, 1984)
> Hypothroid neuropathy (Bastron, 1984)
> Paraproteinemia (multiple myeloma, macroglobulinemia, monoclonal gammopathy, cryoglobulinemia) (McLeod, 1984; Smith *et al.*, 1983; Dalakas and Engel, 1981; Bady, 1988; Kelly *et al.*, 1983)
> Amyloid neuropathy (Cohen and Rubinow, 1984)
> Herpes varicella-zoster neuropathy (Baringer and Townsend, 1984)
> Human immunodeficiency virus infection (Dalakas and Pezeshpout, 1988; Leoport *et al.*, 1987; Parry, 1988)
> Diphtheritic neuropathy (McDonald and Kohn, 1984)
> Sarcoid neuropathy (Matthews, 1984)
> Systemic lupus erythaematosus (Conn and Dyck, 1984)
> Serum sickness (Iqbel and Arnason, 1984)
> Carcinomatous neuropathy (McLeod, 1984; Vincent *et al.*, 1986)
> Lymphoma neuropathy (McLeod, 1984)
> Leukaemia (McLeod, 1984)
> Polycythaemia vera (McLeod, 1984)
> Plasma cell neoplasia (Delauche *et al.*, 1981; Read and Warlow, 1978)
> Ulcerative colitis (Chad *et al.*, 1986; Konagaya *et al.*, 1989)

Toxic neuropathies

> Triorthocresyl phosphate (TOCP) (Schaumburg and Spencer, 1984)
> Arsenic intoxication (Windebank *et al.*, 1984)
> Lead intoxication (Windebank *et al.*, 1984)
> Drugs (gold, perhexiline, thalidomide) (Le Quesne, 1984; Windebank, *et al.*, 1984)

Hereditary neuropathy

Hereditary motor and sensory neuropathy, Type III (HMSN III; Dejerine-Sottas disease)

Elevated CSF protein has been found in 75% of patients of HMSNIII (Hagberg and Lyon, 1981). Dyck reported that the CSF protein level ranged from 76 to 180 mg/100 ml in five cases; the lowest value was found for the patient with the least involvement (Dyck and Arnason, 1984).

Refsum's disease (Heredopathia atactica polyneuritiformis)

The CSF protein is increased in almost all cases, while the cell count is normal. This was originally considered one of the cardinal features of this disease (Refsum, 1946). Protein levels are usually in the range of 100 to 700 mg/100 ml, but may be higher in some cases. A correlation between the severity of the clinical picture and the CSF protein concentration has been observed (Campbell and Williams, 1967).

Migraine

There have been few studies looking at the CSF changes in migraine. The CSF is generally normal between migraine attacks. Severe attacks, especially with focal neurological signs, may be associated with a pleocytosis and a slightly increased CSF protein (Fishman, 1980). This may relate to a transient meningeal inflammation in migraine (Kremenitzer and Golden, 1974), but also raises the question of whether such migrainous episodes may be symptomatic of an underlying inflammatory disorder (Bartleson et al., 1981).

Various neurotransmitter substances have also been looked at in migraine. Barrie and Jowett (1967) found no significant differences between migraine patients and controls looking at CSF levels of serotonin, acetylcholine, adrenaline, bradykinin and kinin-forming enzyme. They did note two of their migraine patients with severe continuous migraine had an unidentified smooth-muscle contracting substance present in the CSF. Welch et al. (1976a,b) noted increased GABA and cyclic AMP in the CSF of patients during or shortly after a migraine attack. Kovacs et al. (1989) measured CSF obtained by suboccipital puncture in 52 migraine patients, examining 18 of them during a migraine attack. They noted significantly lower total CSF protein content with no changes noted in the CSF protein fractions in their migraine patients, as well as increased levels of 5-hydroxyindoleacetic acid (5-HIAA) which did not appear to relate to the occurrence of a migraine attack. CSF levels of homovanillic acid (HVA) did not differ between migraine patients and controls. The increased CSF 5-HIAA may indicate a defect of serotonin metabolism in migraine which appears to be independent of paroxysms.

Stroke and Transient Ischaemic Attacks (TIAs)

CSF examination may be useful in both the differential diagnosis and in the assessment of the prognosis of strokes and TIAs. The main indication for lumbar puncture in the evaluation of strokes is in the diagnosis of subarachnoid haemorrhage, where lumbar puncture is more sensitive than either CT or MRI scanning. CT and MRI scanning, however, are both superior to LP examination in the diagnosis of intracerebral haemorrhage and of cerebral infarction. Lumbar puncture, however, is indicated in the evaluation of stroke where a CNS vasculitis is suspected (with a pleocytosis and increased IgG), when tuberculous meningitis is suspected (with a low CSF glucose) or other CNS infection needs to be excluded, in young patients with unexplained strokes, and in patients with AIDS or with positive serum syphilis serology (Fishman, 1992, p. 347).

Ruff and Dougherty (1981) did a retrospective study of 512 patients admitted with transient ischaemic attacks (TIAs) or stroke-in-evolution (SIE). Of their 37 cases of intracerebral haemorrhage, all were picked up on CT scanning, but only nine were detected by lumbar puncture. However, of their 17 cases of subarachnoid haemorrhage, LP detected eight cases which were not seen on CT. They noted a 6.7% incidence of major complications (severe back pain or/paraparesis) in their 342 patients who were given anticoagulants after LP. This risk of major complications was greatly increased if the patient had a traumatic LP (76.29% vs 2.2%) or if anticoagulants were started within one hour of the LP (17.4% vs 1.5%). All of their major LP-related complications occurred in anticoagulated patients, and they recommend that if an LP is performed in the evaluation of patients with TIAs or SIEs, anticoagulation not be started in these patients for at least one hour to minimise the risk of spinal haematoma.

Subarachnoid haemorrhage (SAH)

As mentioned above, lumbar puncture is more accurate than CT or MRI scanning in the diagnosis of SAH. A CT scan will pick up most cases of SAH, but an LP is indicated if SAH is suspected on clinical grounds and the CT is negative. Repeat LPs may be necessary in some cases, as 10% of patients with SAH will demonstrate clear CSF examination up to 12 hours after the bleed (Nadis and Klawans, 1989).

The differentiation between subarachnoid haemorrhage and a traumatic LP is often difficult. The most important aspects in the differentiation between SAH and traumatic LP are: (1) noting the appearance and cell count in at least three separate tubes, collected serially at the time of LP, and (2) examination of the supernatant. In subarachnoid haemorrhage there will be equal blood in all the tubes collected and the supernatant will be xanthochromic due to pigments released from the lysis of RBCs. A supernatant may, however, remain clear for two to four hours after the onset of SAH. In a traumatic LP the supernatant will be clear and either the first or last tube collected will contain more blood than the others (Fishman, 1980).

Analysis of the specific pigments may also be helpful in the diagnosis of SAH. Oxyhaemoglobin and bilirubin are characteristically detectable in SAH, but are not seen in traumatic taps. Oxyhaemoglobin may be detectable in a traumatic LP initially, but will clear in the analysis of serial tubes. In subarachnoid haemorrhage, oxyhaemoglobin will appear within two hours, peak in one to three days, and clear in seven to nine days. Bilirubin will be detectable between ten hours and three days following SAH, peak at one week, and clear at two to four weeks (Nadis and Klawans, 1989). Methaemoglobin, a reduction product of haemoglobin usually associated with old encapsulated haemorrhages, may also contribute to xanthochromia and may be measured, but is not generally seen in SAH or in traumatic LP (Brumback, 1989b). The detection of these pigments and assessment of the cell counts is discussed further in Chapter 5.

Cerebral haemorrhage

In cerebral haemorrhage, the CSF may show (1) an increased pressure in more than half of the cases, (2) varying degrees of pigmentation in some 80% of cases, (3) a WBC count initially proportional to the RBC count but progressively increasing as a reflection of the blood-induced meningeal reaction, and (4) an increased protein content again initially proportional to the RBC count and progressively increasing disproportionately as a reflection of the influx of serum proteins across the blood-brain barrier (Merritt and Fremont-Smith, 1938). Occasionally, the CSF may contain 500 to 4000 white cells/mm^3 in cases of intracerebral haemorrhage with few or no RBC's present. This may be due to an aseptic meningeal reaction from haemorrhagic necrosis of the ventricular wall.

Lee et al. (1975) noted that 25% of their cases with intracerebral haemorrhage had a clear CSF. Sornas et al. (1972) noted a polymorphonuclear neutrophilic leukocyte (PNL) reaction in 70% of their patients with haemorrhagic infarction and lobar haematoma. This was most prominent in those patients with lobar haematoma and peaked in three to four days after onset. Thirteen of their 16 patients with intracerebral lobar haematoma demonstrated an increased total WBC count, whereas 90% of those with presumed bland infarcts had normal total WBC counts. They also noted a correlation between the PNL reaction and the CSF oxyhaemoglobin concentration in their patients with haematoma.

Britton *et al.* (1983) evaluated 231 stroke patients with CT and/or autopsy to assess the accuracy of lumbar puncture in the diagnosis of stroke. They also noted an increased WBC count in 75% of their cases with cerebral haemorrhage compared to 35% of those with haemorrhagic cerebral infarction, and 12% of those with ischaemic infarction. They found the mean protein level in the CSF to be highest in those with stroke associated with haemorrhage. Using a protein value of greater than 1 g/l as being characteristic of haemorrhage, they found LP to have a sensitivity of 89% and specificity of 92% in diagnosing stroke associated with haemorrhage. With spectrophotometry they found CSF examination to have a sensitivity of 72% and specificity of 94% in the diagnosis of haemorrhage. They also noted a high consistency between visible xanthochromia and spectro-photometric analysis of 93%. They suggest that in centres where CT or MRI scanning are not readily available, that simple CSF analysis may have a high diagnostic utility in the evaluation of stroke, particularly analysis of protein and xanthochromia to differentiate haemorrhagic from non-haemorrhagic stroke when one is considering anticoagulants or platelet inhibitors.

Hayakawa *et al.* (1979) have found that astroprotein (immunologically identical to glial fibrillary acidic protein, GFAP) may also be useful clinically in differentiating intracerebral haemorrhage from SAH and cerebral infarction. They found CSF concentrations of astroprotein were markedly elevated in intracerebral haemorrhage, reflecting the size of the lesion and also the likely clinical outcome. Slight to moderate elevations were also seen in SAH and in cerebral infarctions, but these did not relate to prognosis in these cases.

In patients with multiple lobar haemorrhages, where cerebral amyloid angiopathy [CAA] is suspected, measurement of cystatin C in the CSF may be a useful diagnostic marker. Shimode *et al.* (1991) have found low levels of this proteinase in the CSF of 15 patients with CAA, related to its deposition in the cerebral microvasculature. Van Nostrand *et al.* (1992*b*) have also found decreased amyloid β-protein in the CSF of patients with hereditary cerebral haemorrhage with amyloidosis, Dutch type, similar to their Alzheimer's patients.

Cerebral thrombosis and embolism

In non-haemorrhagic cerebral infarction due to thrombosis or to nonseptic embolism, the CSF pressure is usually normal or only slightly elevated and the cell count is normal in 85-90% of patients. Occasionally increased CSF pressure may occur with extensive cerebral infarction and ooedema and a mild leukocytic response may also occasionally be seen in the first few days (Merritt and Fremont-Smith, 1938; Sornas *et al.*, 1972; Fishman, 1980).

The usual CSF indices may be helpful in differentiating septic from nonseptic embolic stroke. Pruitt *et al.* (1978) reviewed the neurological complications of bacterial endocarditis in 218 patients, including 42 patients with cerebral embolism. The CSF was found to be purulent, with a PMN leukocytic pleocytosis and decreased glucose in seven patients, aseptic with a lymphocytic reaction and normal glucose in 13 patients, and haemorrhagic in three patients, with the remainder having normal CSF cell counts. In their total of 69 patients with neurological complications who underwent lumbar puncture, CSF cultures were positive in 11 of these. Powers (1986) has advocated that although the diagnostic yield may be small, CSF analysis should be a routine evaluation in patients with cerebral embolism suspected to be of cardiac origin. Cell counts are usually normal in cases of aseptic embolism, but when the embolus is from a septic focus, the pleocytosis maybe up to 4000 cells/mm^3, relating often to an aseptic meningeal reaction.

A number of investigators have looked at a variety of CSF enzymes and other proteins as markers of prognosis in cerebral ischaemia. Wolintz *et al.* (1969) measured creatinine phosphokinase (CPK), aldolase and lactate dehydrogenase (LDH) and found these to be elevated in patients with both haemorrhagic and non-haemorrhagic stroke. There was no clear correlation between enzyme rise and clinical course, but marked elevations were associated with a poor prognosis. They suggest that CPK, being a brain specific enzyme, may be the most appropriate enzyme indicator of cerebral damage, particularly in blood stained fluid. Bohmer *et al.* (1983) have found that creatinine kinase may have prognostic value in global cerebral hypoxia associated with cardiac arrest. Donnan *et al.* (1983) have also suggested that creatine kinase, LDH, and glutamate oxaloacetate transaminase (GOT) may be helpful in differentiating cortical from lacunar strokes, being elevated in 80% of the cases of cortical stroke and showing minimal or no elevation in lacunar stroke.

Strand *et al.* (1984) noted both myelin-basic protein (MBP), indicative of damage to myelin, and tau-fraction to be elevated in haemorrhagic and non-haemorrhagic strokes. They noted the level of CSF MBP correlated to visibility of the lesion on CT and also to prognosis in their patients. Hay *et al.* (1984) looked at CSF levels of enolase in cerebral infarction and noted a positive correlation between CSF enolase and the volume of the infarct. High levels tended to be related to poor prognosis. Other possible CSF markers of prognosis in stroke include adenylate kinase (Terent and Ronquist, 1980), cyclic AMP (Papageorgiou *et al.*, 1983) neuron-specific enolase and S-100 protein (Persson *et al.*, 1987), and CSF lactate (Busse and Hoffman, 1983). The interested reader is referred to the recent review of Nadis and Klawans (1989).

Narcolepsy and Hypersomnia

Narcolepsy is an illness characterised by excessive daytime sleepiness and cataplectic attacks occuring with a sudden loss of muscle tone often brought on by startling stimuli. Sleep paralysis, hypnagogic hallucinations, automatic behaviour and nocturnal sleep disruptions are also common in narcolepsy (Parkes, 1985). Narcoleptic sleep is distinguished from other abnormal sleep patterns by the occurence of a rapid eye movement (REM) period within several minutes of sleep onset (Hishikawa, 1976). In idiopathic hypersomnia patients complain of excessive daytime sleepiness without cataplexy. Sleep apnoea and various neurological, psychiatric and endocrine diseases may also result in hypersomnia.

The use of methylphenidate, amphetamines and tricyclic antidepressants in the therapy of narcolepsy has suggested investigating central catecholamine and serotonin metabolism since these drugs are known to affect these neurotransmitter systems. Parkes *et al.* (1974) first investigated CSF biogenic amine metabolites and amino acids in 20 patients with narcolepsy. They noted CSF HVA and aspartate levels to be significantly depressed in these patients while concentrations of CSF phenylalanine, tyrosine, serotonin, tryptophan, 5-HIAA and several other amino acids studied were normal. Their data may, however, represent in part a drug effect in these patients, as medications were discontinued only eight hours prior to lumbar sampling. Mouret *et al.* (1976) measured CSF HVA and 5-HIAA levels in narcoleptics, mixed hypersomniacs, and hypersomniacs with excessive REM sleep patterns. They found no significant difference in either HVA or 5-HIAA before or after probenecid loading in their narcoleptic or mixed hypersomniac patients. After probenecid, CSF HVA was significantly increased in the hypersomniacs with excessive REM sleep. They concluded that the pathological defect in narcolepsy probably involves neurotransmitter systems other than dopaminergic or serotonergic ones. The usual CSF indices of protein, pressure, cell count, and glucose are normal in narcolepsy and hypersomnia.

Epilepsy

The CSF levels of protein, glucose, pressure, and cell count are generally normal in idiopathic epilepsy (Fishman, 1980; DeJong, 1979). Transient elevations of pressure, protein, lactate and acidosis may, however, occur following a seizure episode (DeJong, 1979; Brooks and Adams, 1975). During seizures there may be an acute increase in pressure due to increased cerebral blood flow and cerebral metabolism (Merritt and Fremont-Smith, 1938; Fishman, 1980). A pleocytosis (up to 80 cells/mm^3) may also occur after seizures, but attributing such a pleocytosis to the seizure should always be a diagnosis of exclusion, as CNS infections may often present with seizures (Fishman, 1992).

Thompson and Salinsky (1988) reviewed the records of 95 patients who underwent LP for evaluation of partial epilepsy. Although 24 of their patients had CSF abnormalities, it provided additional diagnostic information only for four patients with clinically suspected subarachnoid haemorrhage. They concluded that routine LPs are not indicated in the evaluation of epilepsy provided that CT scanning is performed.

The CSF electrolytes also are not greatly altered in seizures. CSF concentrations of potassium, sodium, and chloride, as well as those of calcium and phosphate are generally normal. Brooks (1980) and Heipertz *et al.* (1979) demonstrated CSF levels of magnesium to be elevated following seizure activity. They considered this to originate primarily from release by cells in the CNS since it did not seem to depend on alterations in the blood-brain-barriers or on the CSF cell count. Brooks and Adams (1975) did not, however, find any change in CSF magnesium level for 1-6 hours following a seizure. Brooks (1980) has also reviewed the changes in acid-base status and CSF metabolites seen in seizures.

Various studies have indicated that GABA levels in lumbar CSF samplings are lower in subjects with seizure disorders (Enna *et al.*, 1977b; Hare *et al.*, 1980; Wood *et al.*, 1979). The association of reduced levels of CSF GABA with seizure disorders suggests that seizures could result from the loss of neural inhibition, since GABA acts as an inhibitory neurotransmitter. This is probably, however, an oversimplification. The dependency of glutamic acid decarboxylase (GAD) (the primary enzyme in GABA synthesis) on vitamin B_6 and the association of B_6 deficiency with seizures supports this idea. Many convulsant drugs actually interfere with B_6 metabolism. The anticonvulsants phenytoin, sodium valproate, and phenobarbital are all thought to enhance GABAergic systems in the CNS (Wood and Brooks, 1980; Eadie and Tyrer, 1983). Mao *et al.* (1974) showed GABA to be inversely related to cyclic guanosine monophosphate (cGMP) levels in the cerebellum of rats treated with various drugs affecting GABA metabolism. The work of Gross *et al.* (1979) has also implicated cGMP in epilepsy.

There have been a number of conflicting results looking at the various neurotransmitters, metabolites, and amino acids in epilepsy. Pitkanen *et al.* (1989) looked at CSF levels of inhibitory and excitory amino acids in treated drug-refractory epileptics. They noted decreased aspartate and increased levels of glutamine and homocarnosine compared to controls, and normal levels of glutamate, asparagine, total GABA, taurine, and glycine. Many investigators have also found alterations in CSF concentrations of dopamine, norepinephrine, HVA, 5-HIAA, and cyclic nucleotides (Myllyla *et al.*, 1977; Meldrum, 1978; Wood and Brooks, 1980; Shaywitz *et al*., 1980; Chadwick, 1981; Reynolds, 1981; Smidt and Loscher, 1981;

Hiramatsu *et al.*, 1982; Airaksinen and Leino, 1982; Loscher, 1982; Mohan *et al.*, 1982).

As somatostatin appears to have epileptogenic activity in various animal models of epilepsy and as levels have been found increased in human epileptic foci (Schacker *et al.*, 1987), this neuropeptide has recently received a lot of attention in epilepsy. Pitkanen *et al.* (1988) found CSF levels of somatostatin-like immunoreactivity (SLI) to be decreased in 60 patients with complex partial seizures who were medicated. An earlier study by the same group (Pitkanen *et al.*, 1987) noted that somatostatin levels do not appear to be altered by the acute effect of seizures, although beta-endorphin was found to be increased in patients with tonic-clonic seizures post-ictally. Pitkanen *et al.* (1989) also measured SLI and beta-endorphin in the CSF of unmedicated newly diagnosed epileptics and in chronic medicated epileptics. They found lower SLI levels in patients with chronic epilepsy on anticonvulsants compared to both newly diagnosed epileptics and patients with panic disorder. Unmedicated, newly-diagnosed epileptics did not differ from controls. It is difficult to be certain whether the decreased somatostatin activity observed by Pitkanen *et al.* is due to the effects of chronic epilepsy or, more likely, due to medication effects. Rubinow *et al.* (1985) and Steardo *et al.* (1986) have both reported carbamazepine to have a lowering effect on CSF SLI activity and this appears to be related to its anticonvulsant activity.

Tourette Syndrome

Gilles de la Tourette syndrome (GTS) or Tourette syndrome is a neuropsychiatric condition of childhood onset, characterised by multiple motor and vocal tics, and associated with a variety of psychiatric features, including attention deficit disorder, learning disorders, hyperactivity, obsessive compulsive features, and conduct disorder. The clinical, genetic, and biochemical features have recently been reviewed by Robertson (1989), Leckman *et al.* (1987), and by Comings (1990*b*).

A number of neurotransmitter systems acting alone or in combination have been suggested to be of aetiological significance in GTS. The role of dopamine has received particular attention, based largely on the pharmacological studies and observed treatment responses in patients to agents which block dopamine receptors (e.g. haloperidol, pimozide) and from the observation that dopamine agonists (e.g. stimulants) will exacerbate the symptoms of GTS. Johansson and Roos (1974) first reported a single patient with very low levels of the dopamine metabolite homovanillic acid (HVA) in the CSF, and subsequently van Woert *et al.* (1976) reported an elevated probenecid-induced accumulation of HVA in the CSF. However, Van Woert *et al.* did not control for activity level, which may influence HVA in the CSF and the increased motor activity in GTS may possibly have contributed to their HVA levels. Subsequently, Shapiro et al. (1978) studied post-probenecid HVA levels in eight GTS patients and found these levels to be similar to previously published reports of normal values for CSF HVA levels. They did not, however, have a control group with which to compare, and did not control for probenecid concentrations. Most other studies of CSF HVA have found decreased levels in Tourette syndrome.

Cohen et al. (1978) investigated the serotonin metabolite 5-HIAA, as well as HVA, in the CSF of six children and one adult with Tourette syndrome and found their levels of HVA and 5-HIAA to be significantly lower both pre- and post- probenecid compared to the control group of 27 other paediatric patients. In the adult patient with GTS, dextroamphetamine produced a dramatic decrease in the CSF HVA level, an increase in the 5-HIAA level, and an exacerbation of symptoms. There was an apparent association between the severity of the tic syndrome and the ratio of CSF 5-HIAA to HVA, patients with the least severe disorder having the highest accumulation of 5-HIAA relative to HVA. They postulated that the relatively lower dopamine turnover was related to a receptor super-sensitivity. They also highlighted the importance of the interaction between the serotonin and dopamine systems, with reduced functioning of inhibitory serotonergic mechanisms, and thus a functional dopaminergic overactivity. Butler et al. (1979) also investigated CSF HVA and 5-HIAA in nine children with GTS, finding decreased pre- and post-probenecid levels of both metabolites, compared to age matched controls.

Cohen et al. (1979) followed up on their previous study and reported decreased HVA and 5-HIAA in ten children with GTS compared to 51 children with a variety of neuropsychiatric and medical illnesses. Inter-estingly, Cohen et al. also found one patient with GTS who demonstrated increased CSF MHPG, the major norepinephrine (NE) metabolite, relative to both the other neuropsychiatric and other GTS patients. This suggested, at least in this patient, that there may be a role for noradrenergic overactivity in addition to any serotonergic or dopaminergic contributions. This prompted them to give this patient a trial of clonidine, a centrally active imidazoline which reduces central turnover of norepinephrine, presumably by its action on presynaptic neurons leading to the inhibition of the locus coeruleus. This trial yielded sustained improvement of this patient's GTS symptoms as well as being beneficial in two other cases. Clonidine has since become a standard therapy in GTS, in addition to neuroleptics, because of its low incidence of side-effects (Comings, 1990b). This provides a good example of how the investigation of CSF metabolites may lead to rational treatment strategies. The fact that haloperidol responsiveness in GTS appears to predict a therapeutic benefit from clonidine could indicate a link between the dopaminergic and noradrenergic systems in GTS (Caine, 1985).

Koslow and Cross (1982) have reviewed the CSF and pharmacological studies in GTS and the methodological problems with each. They point out several methodological problems with the studies of both Cohen *et al.* and Butler *et al.* They suggest that the indirect evidence for dopaminergic involvement in GTS with the findings of low levels of HVA and the effectiveness of haloperidol in reducing the symptoms may indicate that hypersensitive dopamine receptors represent the principal malfunction in GTS, with other neurotransmitter alterations secondary to this. They point out, however, that the fact that this hypersensitivity develops during childhood rather than being present at birth suggests that there may be a more primary dysfunction in GTS, postulating the presence of a "dopaminergic supersensitivity-producing factor (SSPF)" which they state could possibly be prolactin or another neuropeptide. This they base on the finding that hypophysectomy of rats prior to haloperidol or estrogen treatment will block the increase in the number of dopamine receptors in the striatum that one would expect to see with chronic estrogen or haloperidol treatment in rats. Haloperidol will also produce increased prolactin release as a result of dopaminergic blockage, as does estrogen, and hypophysectomy will eliminate prolactin release. Furthermore, chronic prolactin infusion in hypophysectomised rats will cause supersensitivity of dopamine receptors. The fact that higher levels of estrogen may serve to counteract the effect of increased release of prolactin in humans, they speculate, could account for the three-to-one male to female sex ratio observed in GTS.

The evidence for dopaminergic dysfunction in Tourette syndrome has been confirmed by subsequent CSF studies. Singer *et al.* (1982 *a,b*) demonstrated low CSF HVA levels in patients with GTS, with clinical improvement associated with increased CSF HVA levels after haloperidol treatment, providing further evidence for a dopaminergic supersensitivity mechanism in Tourettes. In contrast to the findings of Cohen *et al.*, who noted the severity of tics to be inversely related to the ratio of 5-HIAA to HVA, they were unable to confirm this correlation and found 5-HIAA reduced in less than 25% of their patients. They point out the fact that GTS patients improve with remarkably low oral doses and low serum levels of haloperidol and that this may indicate that the response to haloperidol acts by different mechanisms in Tourette patients than in schizophrenics who will usually require higher oral doses and serum levels. Haloperidol treatment produced little change in 5-HIAA, and the response of CSF MHPG was variably altered on treatment.

Singer *et al.* (1984) have also looked at CSF cholinesterase activity in GTS based on the postulated abnormality of acetylcholine metabolism in GTS. This follows some pharmacological reports of effects with administration of cholinergic and anticholinergic agents and reports of increased RBC choline content and reduced choline uptake into fibroblasts. They found no significant differences between CSF acetylcholinesterase (ACHE) activity between untreated or haloperidol treated patients and controls, which thus does not appear to support the postulated involvement of the cholinergic system in the pathophysiology of GTS.

There has been a remarkable paucity of post mortem studies in GTS which might be helpful in interpreting these biochemical abnormalities. Haber *et al.* (1986) performed immunocytochemical studies of enkephalin-like (ELI), dynorphin-like (DLI), and substance P-like (SPLI) immunoreactivity in the brain of a patient with GTS. They reported ELI and SPLI positive "woolly fibres" densely stained and of normal distribution, with DLI staining considerably less dense and the most striking finding being a total absence of DLI-positive woolly fibres in the dorsal part of the external segment of the globus pallidus with the ventral pallidum showing very faint staining. Theirs is the first study to show a distinct neurochemical pathological change in Tourette syndrome. Dynorphin is an opioid peptide first isolated from the pituitary. Its name comes from the Greek "*dynamis*", meaning power, as it appears to be some 700 times more potent than leu-enkephalin (which comprises the first five amino acids of its chain of 13 amino acids). There is pharmacological evidence from case reports to support a role for either increased or decreased endorphins in GTS (Comings, 1990*b*). Sandyk (1989*a*,*b*) have discussed the neuroendocrine functions of dynorphin in the hypothalamic pituitary axis as they relate to Tourette syndrome, and the evidence that opioids appear to have a direct modulation of striatal dopaminergic neurons. Sandyk has postulated a protective function of beta endorphin in movement disorders and discussed the possible pathophysiology behind a dynorphin deficiency in Tourette syndrome.

Leckman *et al.* (1988), following up on Haber's neuropathological findings, examined CSF dynorphin A in seven GTS patients. They noted CSF levels of dynorphin A to be on average 32% higher than for the normal controls. They found lower mean CSF HVA and 5-HIAA concentrations among the GTS patients and no significant differences in CSF tyrosine, MHPG, tryptophan, neurotensin, somatostatin, or corticotrophin releasing factor. They also noted (Leckman and Chittenden, 1990) that the level of dynorphin A correlated with the severity of obsessive-compulsive symptoms in GTS. They suggest that, in view of Haber's findings, the observed increase in CSF dynorphin A concentrations may not be an indicator of the levels found in the basal ganglia. Comings (1990*b*) has pointed out that the assay in Leckman *et al.*'s CSF study was for dynorphin (1-8), and not dynorphin (1-13) which was observed to be absent in the globus pallidus by Haber *et al.* He states these may be regulated independently. Robertson (1989) also points out that many of the clinical features of Haber's patient were atypical for GTS. Alternative explanations of the apparent discrepancy between the CSF and neuropathological findings might include a down-regulation of the opioid receptors which dynorphin binds to, or an alteration of the enkephalinase which breaks down dynorphin.

In summary, CSF studies in Tourette syndrome have generally substantiated the pharmacological studies demonstrating the involvement of dopaminergic, serotonergic, and noradrenergic mechanisms in GTS. Dynorphin, and possibly other neuropeptides, also appear important. Comings (1990b) has hypothesised that the primary defect in GTS involves the tryptophan oxygenase gene on the long arm of chromosome 4 at band q 31, causing a decrease in serotonin with secondary involvement of the other neurotransmitter systems and a syndrome of disinhibition of the frontal lobes and limbic systems. His views on GTS, however, are highly controversial and await confirmation (see review of Robertson, 1989). As the genetics and neurochemistry of Tourette syndrome are beginning to unfold, further CSF studies will need to be correlated with neuropathological and positron emmission tomography (PET) studies to further define the roles of DA, NE, 5-HT and dynorphins in this disorder.

7. CSF in Psychiatric Illness

Schizophrenia

Investigations into the mechanisms of action of antipsychotic medications and the psychotogenic effects of various stimulant drugs have implicated various biogenic amines in the aetiology and pathogenesis of the schizophrenias. These studies have largely focused on catecholamine and indoleamine systems, though altered metabolism of other neurotransmitter substances has also been postulated.

Dopaminergic processes

Evidence for the "dopamine hypothesis" of schizophrenia stems primarily from observations on the similarity of amphetamine psychosis to acute paranoid schizophrenia, from the fact that dopamine (DA) agonists will exacerbate schizophrenic symptoms, and from studies on the DA antagonist effects of neuroleptics (Crow and Johnstone, 1978). This theory regards schizophrenia as a state of excessive activity of dopaminergic neurons in certain areas of the brain. Amphetamine psychosis is believed to be due primarily to an increased central release of catecholamines. CSF studies suggest that doses of amphetamine sufficient to produce psychotic symptomatology do increase central DA turnover (Angrist *et al.*, 1974; Crow and Johnstone, 1978). Chlorpromazine, haloperidol and other antipsychotics have also been shown to increase DA turnover, however, as demonstrated by increased CSF levels of the DA metabolite homovanillic acid (HVA) after treatment with these drugs (Sedvall *et al.*, 1975). This has been interpreted as representing a compensatory feedback response of presynaptic neurons to the postsynaptic blockade of DA receptors by the neuroleptics (Crow and Johnstone, 1978; Sedvall *et al.*, 1975).

If the DA hypothesis of schizophrenia is correct, one might expect this to be reflected in elevated concentrations of HVA in the CSF of these patients, indicating a state of increased DA turnover. Such an increase has not, however, been demonstrated. There is even some evidence that decreased levels may be associated with increased severity of some symptoms in schizophrenia (Bowers, 1974b; Post *et al.*, 1975). Some have argued that, since the HVA detected in CSF is thought to originate largely from the corpus striatum, caudate nucleus and the nigrostriatal DA system bordering the lateral ventricles, CSF-HVA levels may not reflect changes in DA metabolism in the mesolimbic and/or mesocortical DA systems classically thought to be involved in schizophrenia. There still exists, however, considerable controversy over the anatomical origin of CSF HVA as well as over the anatomy of schizophrenia.

Normal or decreased DA turnover, as has been seen in the majority of CSF-HVA studies, could coexist with a state of functional DA overactivity in schizophrenia as postulated by the DA hypothesis of schizophrenia. This could occur if there were either a decreased activity of an inhibitory transmitter acting on dopaminergic systems or, alternatively, if mesolimbic receptors were supersensitive to the effects of DA (Crow and Johnstone, 1978).

Relationship of CSF DA metabolites to symptoms and CT findings

Although several studies have noted a positive correlation between CSF HVA levels and acute psychotic symptoms in schizophrenic patients, others studies have shown a negative correlation with ratings of psychosis and positive symptoms. Rimon et al. (1971) reported a positive correlation of CSF HVA levels with paranoia. Lindstrom (1985) noted lower levels of CSF HVA in 40 drug-free schizophrenic patients compared to 21 healthy controls, and found levels to correlate positively with social interest and total positive scores on the Nurses' Observation Scale for Inpatient Evaluation and negatively with lassitude and slowness of movements. Lindstrom found no relation between CSF HVA and family history of schizophrenia. This contrasts with Sedvall et al. (1980a,b) who found an increase in CSF HVA levels in healthy subjects and schizophrenics with a family history of schizophrenia.

Lindstrom's findings of low HVA being associated with lassitude, psychomotor retardation and social withdrawal would be consistent with the findings of several other studies associating low HVA with negative symptoms in schizophrenia. Low HVA levels have also been related to poor prognosis and may reflect a dopamine receptor supersensitivity (Bowers, 1974b, 1978b). Several other studies have also shown low CSF HVA levels to be related to negative symptoms and to have a significant negative correlation with cortical atrophy or enlarged ventricles on CT scans (Nyback et al., 1983; Houston et al., 1986; Van Kammen et al., 1986b; Doran et al., 1987; Heritch 1990). These results suggest there may be a loss of dopaminergic neurons and/or decreased dopaminergic turnover related, perhaps in part, to cerebral atrophy and to the development of negative symptoms in schizophrenia. These CSF and CT studies may link decreased dopaminergic activity with Crow's (1980, 1987) postulated type 2 schizophrenic syndrome, characterised by frequently unremitting negative symptoms, and may help to distinguish it from the type 1 syndrome characterised by more reversible positive psychotic symptoms.

It is tempting here to assume that a reduction in cortical dopaminergic activity brought about by cerebral atrophy may occur in schizophrenia and may represent a distinct subgroup of patients. Reynolds (1989) has suggested that these findings might not be due to a decrease in dopaminergic neurons or activity, but rather to the increase in ventricular volume causing an increase in the amount of CSF, effectively decreasing the overall concentration of CSF HVA, as well as other brain metabolites. It is also not clear whether these patients demonstrating negative symptoms, decreased CSF HVA, and apparent increased cerebral atrophy represent a distinct clinical subgroup or whether this is the severe end of a continuous spectrum of illness in schizophrenia. Interestingly, van Kammen *et al.* (1986*b*) have also found a significant decrease in the DA metabolite, DOPAC, in the CSF of schizophrenic patients associated with brain atrophy on CT scans and a non significantly increased dopamine in the CSF of patients with brain atrophy. They calculated that intraneuronal, extra-neuronal and total dopamine utilisation were all significantly decreased in the group with brain atrophy.

Van Kammen *et al.* (1984*b*) noted cerebral atrophy in schizophrenics to be associated with low levels of CSF 5-hydroxyindoleacetic acetic acid (5-HIAA), 3,4-hydroxyphenyl-acetic acid (DOPAC), NE and dopamine-β-hydroxylase (DBH) as well as of HVA. They suggest that this is representative of a global monoamine disturbance in this schizophrenic subgroup, with the monoamine systems interacting with each other. They argue against this being a dilution effect by pointing out that measurements of other CSF constituents were not reduced in these patients.

Relationship of CSF DA metabolites to treatment

CSF HVA and other dopamine metabolites have also been widely studied during treatment with antipsychotic drugs. Many of these studies have suggested that increased CSF HVA levels may predict treatment response to neuroleptics. Although there have been some discrepancies between studies, HVA levels have generally been found to rise during treatment with neuroleptics (see van Kammen *et al.* 1986*a* for review). Tolerance to this effect is usually observed with time. Bowers (1984) noted that a subgroup of his schizophrenics, characterised by a positive family history, more extrapyramidal side-effects and more residual symptoms, did not develop this tolerance reflected in CSF HVA levels after one month of neuroleptic treatment. The CSF HVA tolerence effect may thus be an indication of treatment responsiveness and may relate to a subgroup with a genetic predisposition. Van Praag and Korf (1975) reported higher treatment HVA levels after probenicid were related to improvement during the first week of neuroleptic treatment. Lower HVA levels prior to treatment were related to more parkinsonian side-effects. Van Kammen (1986*b*) also found post-probenecid CSF HVA levels increased in pimozide-responsive patients. Alfredsson *et al.* (1984) found in their chlorpromazine treated patients that improvement of psychotic morbidity and HVA elevation tended to be positively correlated to drug concentrations in serum and CSF.

Frecska *et al.* (1985) measured dopamine, DOPAC, and HVA in the CSF of 14 schizophrenic inpatients before and two weeks after withdrawal of long term neuroleptic medication. They found dopamine and its metabolites significantly reduced after neuroleptic discontinuation and this decrease was correlated with positive symptoms of post-withdrawal deterioration. Low pre-withdrawal DOPAC levels predicted severe relapse. Bagdy *et al.* (1985) also found a decrease in dopamine, DOPAC, and HVA two weeks after discontinuation of neuroleptics correlating with the decrease in neuroleptic activity. They also suggest (Bagdy *et al.*, 1984) that the persistence of elevated levels of CSF catecholamine metabolite levels after withdrawal may have a predictive value for poor response and/or development of tardive dyskinesia.

Cooper *et al.* (1988) looked at the effects of electroconvulsive therapy (ECT) on the CSF amine metabolites in schizophrenic patients and noted a significant increase in the concentration of CSF HVA observed after the first ECT treatment, but not after the final treatment. They suggest that, with ECT, the increase in dopamine turnover might reflect a decrease in receptor density, resulting in the clinical improvement. A concomitant decrease in density of pre-synaptic dopamine receptors would initially decrease negative feedback and increase dopamine turnover, with biochemical tolerance developing, as with neuroleptic drugs, to this effect.

Relevance of plasma and PET studies to CSF studies

Investigations of the plasma concentrations of the dopamine metabolite homovanillic acid have shown some interesting findings relative to the CSF studies. Concentrations of plasma homovanillic acid before treatment, as well as after treatment, have been found to correlate highly with global severity of illness in schizophrenia (Davis *et al.*, 1984). Pickar *et al.* (1984) found both the absolute concentrations and the neuroleptic-induced reductions in plasma HVA to correlate with ratings of psychosis and an improvement in psychosis respectively. They also found neuroleptic treatment to be associated with a significant time-dependent decrease in plasma HVA. Bowers and Swigar (1987) noted increased plasma HVA levels before treatment in schizophrenic patients, decreasing with neuroleptic treatment with a high pre-treatment value correlating with a favourable early response to neuroleptics. Bowers (1991) has suggested that high plasma HVA levels may be a useful prognostic indicator of early neuroleptic response. Pickar *et al.* (1986*b*) also found neuroleptic treatment to be associated with time-dependent decreases in plasma HVA and neuroleptic withdrawal with increases in levels of HVA, in a double-blind placebo-controlled study. The changes in individual mean levels of plasma HVA they found to be predictive of treatment response.

These apparent discrepancies between the plasma and CSF studies of HVA, reviewed above, have been further examined by Pickar *et al.* (1990). They measured CSF and plasma monoamine metabolites in 22 drug-free schizophrenic patients and found the CSF levels did not differ significantly from normal controls, but correlated negatively with ratings of psychosis and with positive symptoms. Consistent with previous studies, they also found plasma HVA to correlate positively with psychosis and positive symptom ratings. They have postulated a "bidirectional" model of psychosis to explain the apparent discrepancies between the various plasma and CSF studies in schizophrenia. They suggest that CSF HVA levels may well relate to frontal cortical dopaminergic activity. This is supported by the studies reviewed above of lower levels of CSF HVA correlating with cortical or prefrontal cortical atrophy on CT scans, and the post-mortem study of Stanley *et al.* (1985) correlating CSF HVA levels with HVA levels in the frontal cortex but not with HVA levels in the caudate. Plasma HVA, on the other hand, originates principally from activity of the peripheral sympathetic nervous system. That plasma HVA levels correlate well with the clinical state, however, suggests that plasma HVA levels may also reflect brain stem and hypothalamic centres influencing the control of the peripheral sympathetic system. They suggest that the finding that plasma HVA correlates positively with psychosis, while CSF HVA correlates negatively, may relate to CSF HVA originating from both cortical and subcortical sources. Plasma HVA, largely derived from peripheral metabolism, may reflect activity of monoaminergic subcortical neurons modulating peripheral nervous system activity. Based on this evidence, they postulate that decreased frontal cortical release and/or metabolism of dopamine could be coupled with increased subcortical activity resulting in the psychotic symptoms of schizophrenia. This "bidirectional" model could then be one possible explanation of the apparent discrepancies between the plasma and CSF studies in schizophrenia.

Future studies correlating CSF dopamine metabolites with post mortem and with positron emission tomography (PET) studies are likely to be fruitful in helping to clarify some of these issues. Post mortem studies to date have been somewhat conflicting and have been confounded by the use of neuroleptic drugs affecting dopamine receptor studies. Although there was some initial enthusiasm over the PET study by Wong *et al.* (1986) showing increased D2 dopamine receptor densities in the caudate nucleus in schizophrenics compared to normal volunteers, subsequent studies have shown some conflicting results (Farde *et al.*, 1987, 1990; Martinot *et al.*, 1991; see discussions of Swart and Korf, 1987, Waddington, 1989; Seeman and Seeman, 1988; and Zeeberg *et al.*, 1988). In addition, the cloning and expression of a rat D2 dopamine receptor cDNA has been recently reported and promises to shed further light on the genetic expression of dopamine receptor subtypes in various regions of the CNS (Bunzow *et al.*, 1988). Sedvall (1990) has recently reviewed the biochemical, post mortem, and PET studies related to the monoamine hypotheses of schizophrenia.

Summary of CSF DA studies
CSF studies of dopamine and its metabolites have proven to be highly variable and have shown no consistent differences between drug-free schizophrenics and controls. There have, however, been several studies indicating dopamine turnover to correlate positively with some schizophrenic symptoms, particularly paranoia. It has generally correlated negatively with indicators of severe and/or chronic illness, particularly when these findings are related to the findings of cerebral atrophy on CT scans. These may indicate that CSF dopamine turnover is reduced in a subgroup of schizophrenic patients with cerebral atrophy, characterised as having more negative symptoms and being more chronic and treatment refractory, consistent with Crow's type 2 schizophrenia. Heritch (1990) suggests that reduced turnover is primarily due to a deficiency in dopamine release and that dysregulation of dopamine may result from disruption of feedback mechanisms. He further speculates that acute psychosis may be associated with a relative increase in the release of dopamine impinging on super-sensitive post-synaptic receptors made so by chronic synaptic depletion. These findings must, however, be treated with caution at this stage; further correlation of clinical data with MRI and PET scanning should help elucidate the role of dopaminergic mechanisms in schizophrenia. The dopaminergic hypothesis of schizophrenia has undergone significant changes in recent years (see Reynolds, 1989; Meltzer, 1987, and Crayton, 1990 for reviews), and CSF studies of dopamine metabolites appear promising in helping to clarify the role of dopamine, as well as to assist in the prognosis and prediction of treatment response.

Dopamine-beta-hydroxylase (DBH)

Some investigators have proposed that the primary defect in schizophrenia may be a low activity of the enzyme dopamine-beta-hydroxylase, which converts DA to NE (Hartman, 1976). This would cause a relative deficit of NE while producing an excess of DA. While no such consistent deficit of DBH in the CSF of schizophrenics compared to controls has been found (Major *et al.*, 1983, 1984), Sternberg *et al.* (1978) did find a lower CSF-DBH activity in patients with "reactive" schizophrenia relative to patients with "process" schizophrenia. Major *et al.* (1983) suggest that decreased CSF-DBH may be associated with an increased vulnerability to psychopathology in general, rather than to schizophrenia or a specific illness type. A study by Sternberg *et al.* (1983*b*) found CSF-DBH activity significantly lower in schizophrenic patients who improved with neuroleptic treatment than in those patients who remained psychotic after treatment. Van Kammen *et al.* (1983) have also found decreased CSF-DBH (in addition to HVA) in schizophrenics with cerebral atrophy. CSF-DBH levels may thus be useful in delineating certain subgroups of schizophrenics.

Norepinephrine (NE)

Investigations of NE metabolites in CSF have also yielded conflicting data. Subrahmanyam (1975) found lower levels of the NE metabolite methoxy hydroxy-phenyl glycol (MHPG) in both acute and chronic schizophrenics. Other investigators have not, however, succeeded in detecting significant differences in the CSF concentrations of either MHPG or VMA in schizophrenics compared to controls (Post *et al.*, 1975; Matthysse, 1978; van Kammen and Sternberg, 1980). Lake *et al.* (1980*b*) measured CSF NE concentrations in schizophrenics and found them to be increased over control values. They noted particularly high levels in a subgroup of some paranoid patients.

Relationship of CSF NE and metabolites to treatment response and relapse
Sedvall *et al.* (1977) noted that a reduction in the MHPG level (as well as an increase in HVA level) correlated with clinical improvement during treatment with chlorpromazine in psychotic patients. They also found the HVA/MHPG ratio useful in following improvement with several anti-psychotics, correlating positively with recovery. This suggests that anti-psychotics act by affecting both dopaminergic and noradrenergic systems.

Many antipsychotics are also potent α-2 adrenergic blockers, but this effect does not seem to correlate with antipsychotic activity (Meltzer, 1987). Although beta-blockers have been reported to demonstrate some anti-psychotic effects, α-2 adrenergic blockers do not appear to have marked antipsychotic activity. Hornykiewcz (1982, 1986) has reviewed the evidence implicating norepinephrine in schizophrenia, and argues that hyper-arousal in schizophrenia could be mediated by increased NE activity and that this may act by its effect on dopaminergic transmission.

Van Kammen *et al.* (1989*c*) found four of 13 drug-free relapsed schizophrenic patients improving with double-blind clonidine (an α-2 adrenergic agent) treatment and suggested that patients with normal or high α-2 receptor activity and normal CSF norepinephrine were likely to respond to clonidine treatment. Those with either high or low CSF NE levels were non-responders. Clonidine treatment in these patients acted to decrease both CSF NE and MHPG. Van Kammen *et al.* (1985*a*) also argued that norepinephrine may be associated with a hyper-aroused state as indicated by loss of sleep. They noted higher CSF NE levels found in patients who slept four hours or less the night prior to lumbar puncture. Their group of responders to clonidine also demonstrated a higher growth hormone response to clonidine challenge, which could indicate increased α-2 receptor function.

Van Kammen *et al.* (1989*b*) have also reported elevated CSF norepinephrine in drug-free relapsed schizophrenic patients correlating significantly with the psychosis ratings, and with hours of sleep the night prior to the lumbar puncture. They suggest that elevated CSF norepinephrine levels during neuroleptic treatment may be a predictor of relapse after discontinuing haloperidol. They postulate that elevated norepinephrine levels may be from cells which escape a haloperidol-induced nonresponsive state, analogous to the depolarisation block in the dopamine neuronal system in animals treated with chronic haloperidol, making these patients perhaps more vulnerable to relapse. Kemali *et al.* (1985) also found the elevated CSF norepinephrine levels correlated significantly with computerised EEG indicators of arousal, and did not clearly relate to ratings of psychosis.

Relationship of CSF NE to symptoms

Van Kammen *et al.* (1990) have also recently published further data on their group of schizophrenics, looking at their negative symptoms and relapse. Drug-free CSF NE and MHPG levels correlated significantly with the severity of negative symptoms and psychosis ratings. When the patients were divided into relapsers and non-relapsers, a significant positive correlation between negative symptoms and CSF NE and MHPG was observed only in the patients who relapsed. They suggest that these CSF noradrenergic indices indicate not only that negative symptoms may be aggravated by increased noradrenergic activity, but that similar significant relationships with positive symptoms occur.

CSF NE and tardive dyskinesia

Noradrenergic hyperactivity may also be related to the development of tardive dyskinesia in schizophrenic patients. Jeste *et al.* (1984) measured CSF noradrenaline in 28 patients, eight with tardive dyskinesia, five with spontaneous dyskinesia and 15 without dyskinesia. They found significantly elevated norepinephrine levels in those with tardive dyskinesia compared to the other groups, but no significant difference in MHPG. They suggest that tardive dyskinesia may be a result of noradrenergic hyperactivity rather than post-synaptic dopamine receptor supersensitivity.

Summary of CSF NE studies
Increased CSF noradrenergic activity appears then to be associated with both positive and negative symptomatology in schizophrenia as well as with tardive dyskinesia. It may also be a useful indicator for risk of relapse of schizophrenic illness when discontinuing neuroleptic treatment. Whether these findings are specific for schizophrenia or whether they represent non-specific hyperarousal or stress-response in schizophrenia, it would appear that further studies should be done to replicate these findings and to further investigate the possible therapeutic role of alpha- and beta-adrenergic related treatments (Hornykiewicz, 1986; Meltzer, 1987). Lake *et al.* (1987) have reviewed the plasma, CSF, urine and post-mortem studies of NE and its metabolites and have discussed the methodological difficulties with these studies.

Serotonin (5-HT)

The implication of serotonergic systems in the pathophysiology of schizophrenia has largely stemmed from studies of the psychotomimetic effects of the hallucinogen D-lysergic acid diethylamide (LSD), and from structural similarities observed between brain amines and other hallucinogens (Curzon, 1972). LSD is believed to produce its effects via inhibition of serotonergic neurons. LSD, as well as several other hallucinogens (psilocybin, bufotenine, harmine, and DMT), all contain the same indole ring structure as the endogenous indoles tryptamine and serotonin (5-hydroxytryptamine, 5-HT). These observations have led to the "transmethylation hypothesis" of schizophrenia which implicates abnormal methylation of indolealkylamines in the aetiology of schizophrenia. This theory also suggests that catecholamines could also undergo a similar process since they contain the same phenethylamine structure as the hallucinogens mescaline and 3,4-dimethoxyphenethylamine (DMPEA). Thus, some of the symptoms of schizophrenia could be explained by the formation of methylated amines which function as endogenous psychotogens (Curzon, 1972). Mehl *et al.* (1977) have described a substance detected in human CSF which can displace LSD from its receptor sites. This "LSD-displacing factor" was detected in higher concentrations in the CSF of psychotic patients. Brown *et al.* (1983) have detected the presence of the endogenous hallucinogen dimethyltryptamine in the CSF of schizophrenics, but noted no association between its presence or concentrations and schizophrenic illness relative to controls. There have been a large number of CSF, blood, and urine studies of various endogenous hallucinogens over the years, but no consistent repeatable findings have emerged from these (see DeLisi and Wyatt, 1987 for review).

Bowers (1978a,b) measured the serotonin metabolite 5-HIAA in acute and chronic schizophrenic patients. He noted relatively decreased levels in acute schizophrenics, and an inverse relationship between 5-HIAA and psychomotor agitation in these patients. Bowers (1978a,b) postulated that many of the symptoms of schizophrenia may be due to a loss of the inhibitory effects of serotonergic neuronal activity on behaviour, or, alternatively, to a circulating psychotomimetic substance acting on 5-HT receptors. CSF 5-HIAA has also been found to be negatively correlated with the presence of Schneiderian First Rank Symptoms (Post et al., 1975), favorable prognostic signs, motor movements (Kirstein et al., 1976), with ventricular size in schizophrenic patients (Potkin et al., 1983), and with phasic eye movement activity (Benson et al., 1983). Csernansky et al. (1990) have also found a positive correlation between 5-HIAA and negative symptoms in schizophrenia. The study of Benson et al. found serotonin turnover to correlate inversely with REM sleep eye-movement activity. This may then be a non-invasive indicator of central serotonin activity, and be a simpler and safer measure than lumbar puncture.

High CSF 5-HIAA has been reported in a group of chronic, drug-free schizophrenics (Gerner et al., 1984a) and has been associated with a family history of schizophrenia (Sedvall et al., 1980, 1984), indicating this as a possible marker for a familial predisposition to schizophrenia.

There have been a large number of studies looking at the role of serotonin as a marker for suicide risk in schizophrenics, with most of these (van Praag, 1982; van Praag and Einstein, 1983; Ninan et al., 1984; Banki et al., 1985) but not all (Roy et al., 1985; Lemus et al., 1990) demonstrating low CSF 5-HIAA as a biological marker of suicide risk. Banki et al. (1985) found the low CSF 5-HIAA to correlate with Mg^{++} levels in psychiatric patients, suggesting that Mg^{++} may be a factor maintaining normal serotonergic activity. As low CSF 5-HIAA levels have been found to be a biological marker for suicide and aggression in a variety of diagnostic groups, this probably indicates a more general involvement of serotonin in the biology of aggression towards self or others, rather than a specific finding in schizophrenia (see section 7-2). The role of serotonin in schizophrenia has been reviewed by Stahl and Wets (1987).

Amino acids

Gamma-amino butyric acid (GABA)

CSF studies of GABA in schizophrenia have produced conflicting results. Lichtshtein et al. (1978) found that CSF GABA levels were not significantly different in untreated schizophrenics when compared with controls. GABA concentrations did decline significantly in schizophrenics following neuroleptic treatment. Their use of an enzymatic procedure to measure

GABA has, however, been criticised by some (Hare *et al.*, 1980). Another study using an ion/exchange fluorometric method did find significantly lower levels of CSF-GABA in drug-free schizophrenics (van Kammen and Sternberg, 1980). Van Kammen *et al.* (1982) detected lower levels of GABA in young female schizophrenics (< 30 years) compared to age and sex matched controls. They noted the GABA activity to increase with duration of illness, number of hospitalisations, months of hospitalisation, and with age. Gattaz *et al.* (1986a), however, used a radio-receptor assay to measure CSF GABA in 19 paranoid schizophrenics before and after three weeks on haloperidol treatment and found no relation of GABA levels to treatment or to symptoms rated by the Brief Psychiatric Rating scale.

GABA may also be important in the development of tardive dyskinesia, (TD) as CSF levels are significantly decreased in schizophrenics with TD compared to non- dyskinetic controls. Treatment with GABA agonists may also ameliorate TD in some patients and will increase CSF GABA accordingly (Thaker *et al.*, 1987).

Glutamate and other amino acids

Since phencyclidine (PCP) can induce schizophreniform symptoms in concentrations where it blocks N-methyl-d-aspartate (NMDA) channels, and since schizophrenic patients are particularly sensitive to the schizophreniform effects of PCP, it has been suggested that NMDA receptor mediated neurotransmission may be implicated in schizophrenia (Javitt and Zukin, 1990). Decreased NMDA receptor activation results in increased DA release and this hypothesis could thus still be consistent with the dopamine hypothesis of schizophrenia. Attention has turned to CSF levels of glutamate, an endogenous NMDA agonist, looking for evidence for the "glutamate hypothesis" of schizophrenia. Decreased concentrations of glutamate have been reported in neuroleptic treated subjects with schizophrenia relative to non-psychiatric controls (Kim *et al.*, 1980). This might suggest impaired functioning of glutamatergic neurons in schizophrenia. These results, however, have not been replicated.

Gattaz *et al.* (1982) measured CSF glutamate levels in paranoid schizophrenics and found higher concentrations in patients treated with neuroleptic drugs. No difference was noted in schizophrenics not taking neuroleptics when compared with controls. Similarly, Perry (1982) measured glutamate in both CSF and brain tissue of schizophrenics and found no difference from control levels.

The requirement of glycine for NMDA receptor activation, the fact that glycine may act as a neuromodulator of dopamine release, and the observation that some schizophrenics may benefit from large doses of glycine therapy (Waziri, 1988; Javitt and Zukin, 1990) indicate a possible role for disturbances of glycine metabolism in schizophrenia. Korpi *et al.* (1987), however, found no difference in the concentrations of glycine, glutamate or several other amino acids in 17 chronic schizophrenic patients compared to neurological controls.

In contrast, Reveley *et al.* (1987), did find increased glycine as well as several other amino acids in schizophrenic patients compared to healthy controls. In their study, they found significantly higher levels of CSF alanine, glycine, leucine, and phenylalanine in 12 patients with schizophrenia compared to nine orthopaedic controls undergoing myelogram. Bjerkenstedt *et al.* (1985) also found increased CSF concentrations of isoleucine, leucine, and histidine as well as increased plasma concentrations of taurine, methionine, valine, isoleucine, leucine, phenylalanine and lysine. The plasma levels of the amino acids competing with tyrosine and tryptophan for transport into the brain were all negatively correlated to the CSF concentrations of the DA metabolite HVA and the 5-HT metabolite 5-HIAA. They suggested that the raised plasma levels of competing amino acids which share the L-transport system of neutral amino acids, may limit the brain uptake of tyrosine. This could lead to a diminished dopamine turnover and result in a compensatory development of supersensitive dopamine receptors. Similarly, competition for tryptophan across the blood-brain-barrier may affect indoleamine metabolism in schizophrenia.

Although CSF studies of amino acids in schizophrenia have not given any consistent support for the glutamate hypothesis of schizophrenia, or for a clear role of excitatory amino acids in schizophrenia, their study has helped to understand the alterations in transport systems across the blood-brain-barrier occurring in schizophrenia.

Proteins

Increased total protein concentration in the cerebrospinal fluid of schizophrenics has been reported by a large number of studies. This probably relates to increased permeability of the blood-CSF-barrier in these patients. A number of studies have shown subgroups of schizophrenic patients with increased permeability of the blood-CSF barrier, looking at the CSF/serum albumin ratio and other measures (Kirch *et al.*, 1985; Bauer and Kornhuber, 1987). Bauer and Kornhuber (1987) found evidence of increased blood-CSF barrier permeability in eight of 15 newly diagnosed male schizophrenic patients. They noted a high correlation between CSF total protein and the CSF/serum albumin ratio, with no evidence of intrathecal IgG synthesis detected. Other studies have also demonstrated an increase in abnormal gamma globulin fractions in the CSF of schizophrenic patients (Dencker and Malm, 1978; Hunter *et al.*, 1969; Kirch *et al.*, 1985), and one study has shown decreased CSF IgG (De Lisi *et al.*, 1981). Harrington *et al.* (1985), have demonstrated the presence of some abnormal protein constituents in the CSF of a subgroup of schizophrenics that were not present in the CSF of normal volunteers, suggesting that these are disease associated proteins, but the significance of these findings awaits further study.

Cyclic nucleotides

The cyclic nucleotides, adenosine-3',5'-cyclic monophosphate (cAMP), and guanosine-3',5'-cyclic monophosphate (cGMP) are thought to be important as "second messengers" for neurotransmitters and hormones in the CNS (Brooks *et al.*, 1980). Catecholamines, 5-HT, and various peptides will stimulate cAMP in neural tissue, while cGMP is stimulated primarily by cholinergic activity (van Kammen and Sternberg, 1980; Gattaz *et al.*, 1983*a,b*).

Smith *et al.* (1976) found no difference in either baseline or neuroleptic induced levels of cAMP in the CSF of schizophrenics. Zohar *et al.* (1978) noted that increased levels of cAMP related to several factors suggesting a poor prognosis in schizophrenics, including early onset, lack of hallucinations, slow first remission, diagnosis of simple type schizophrenia, and poor intermorbid adjustment. Several other CSF studies have yielded variable results (van Kammen and Sternberg, 1980).

Ebstein *et al.* (1976) and Smith *et al.* (1976) both noted a trend towards somewhat lower concentrations of cGMP in schizophrenics, with chronic neuroleptic treatment seeming to increase cGMP levels. However, these differences were not significant. Gattaz *et al.* (1983*a,b*, 1984) also found decreased levels of CSF cGMP in drug-free schizophrenics and increased cGMP in neuroleptic treated patients. Since DA and HVA concentrations were not altered in their study, they suggest that the proposed cholinergic-DA imbalance in schizophrenia is due to a reduction of cholinergic activity with only a relative dominance in dopaminergic systems.

CSF studies of cGMP may thus shed further insight on the "cholinergic hypothesis" of schizophrenia. CSF studies of cholinergic systems have been difficult, generally due to the rapid enzymatic destruction of acetylcholine. CSF acetylcholinesterase has also been looked at in various studies in schizophrenia but has not been found to differ significantly (Davis *et al.*, 1979; Deutsch *et al.*, 1983). Tandon and Greden (1989) have reviewed the role of cholinergic mechanisms in the pathogenesis of schizophrenia.

Prostaglandins

Horrobin *et al.* (1978) postulated that the psychotic symptoms of schizophrenia may be associated with a lack of prostaglandins (PGs), while catatonic symptoms are due to an excess of PGs. Diminished PGE1 activity is associated with an increase in dopamine release (Crayton, 1990). Mathé *et al.* (1980) noted an increase in PGE in the CSF of drug-free schizophrenic males. Linnoila *et al.* (1982) measured CSF concentrations of PGE2, PGF2α, and 6-keto-PGFlα of 11 schizophrenic patients. They found no evidence of elevated prostaglandins in these patients. Gerner and Merrill (1983) also found no difference in CSF PGE in their population of 18 schizophrenics compared to depressed and manic patients or to normal controls. Van Kammen *et al.* (1988) and Brody *et al.* (1987) have reviewed the role of fatty acids and prostaglandins in schizophrenia.

Peptides

Opioid peptides
Because of the marked effect of opiate alkaloids on human behaviour, many investigators have looked at the role of peptides with opioid activity in various mental disorders. Evidence for a link between endorphins and schizophrenia comes from observations that CSF endorphins (especially fraction I) are frequently elevated in drug-free patients with schizophrenia and tend to decline on treatment with neuroleptics and propranolol (Lindstrom *et al.*, 1978; Verhoeven and van Praag, 1982). Patients with puerperal psychosis also demonstrate elevated CSF endorphin levels (Lindstrom *et al.*, 1978). Indirect evidence of the "endorphin theory" of schizophrenia comes from studies showing some positive results reported in schizophrenics with administration of the opiate antagonist naloxone (Watson *et al.*, 1978). Several other studies with naloxone have, however, yielded conflicting results (Volavka *et al.*, 1977; Lindstrom *et al.*, 1982). Both an opioid deficiency state and excess state have been postulated to play a role in the pathogenesis of schizophrenia (Frecska and Davis, 1991).

Lindstrom *et al.* (1982) looked at CSF endorphin fractions I and II in 53 schizophrenics and 19 healthy controls. They detected elevated levels of either fraction I or II in at least one CSF sample in 72% of their schizophrenic population. Those patients with a hebephrenic type of schizophrenia had elevated levels of fraction I more often than the undifferentiated group of schizophrenics.

Beta-endorphin has also been detected in increased concentrations in the CSF of schizophrenics. Domschke *et al.* (1979) noted a ten-fold increase in five patients with acute schizophrenia. They found beta-endorphin levels to be normal or slightly decreased in those with a chronic course. In contrast,

Hollt *et al.* (1982) found only a slight increase in beta-endorphin-like immunoreactivity in the CSF on 15 schizophrenics. Their subject group, however, consisted of both acute and chronic cases.

Pickar *et al.* (1982*a,b*) demonstrated a nearly two-fold decrease in CSF opioid activity in male schizophrenics compared to male controls. Female schizophrenics had levels similar to their controls. CSF beta-endorphin immunoreactivity levels, however, were similar for all groups.

There have since been several different fractions of opioid activity investigated in the CSF in schizophrenia (Wen *et al.*, 1983; Naber and Pickar, 1983; Rimon *et al.*, 1983; Lindstrom *et al.*, 1986; Berger *et al.*, 1986; Bissette *et al.*, 1986*a*; Nemeroff and Bissette, 1988). There seems, however, to be no clear trend at this time as to the role of opioid peptides in the pathogenesis of schizophrenia, and similarly, treatment with opioid agonists and antagonists in schizophrenia have met with mixed reports of efficacy. Bissette and Nemeroff (1988) have recently reviewed the post mortem, CSF, and treatment studies, and Naber and Pickar (1983) have discussed the methodological problems in the measurement of endorphins in body fluids.

Neurotensin (NT)
There has been a lot of attention recently looking at the interplay between NT and DA. It has been reported to co-localise with DA in several areas of the CNS. Atypical antipsychotics have been found to increase NT in the nucleus accumbens only, whereas the more standard antipsychotics, which pose a larger problem with extrapyramidal effects, will increase NT in the nucleus accumbens and striatum (Nemeroff *et al.*, 1989).

Several investigators (Nemeroff *et al.*, 1983; Manberg *et al.*, 1985; Garver *et al.*, 1991) have noted decreased levels of neurotensin in subgroups of untreated schizophrenic patients, with normalisation of neurotensin levels after neuroleptic treatment. This is particularly notable in view of the findings of increased neurotensin in the accumbens and caudate nucleus of rats after dopamine antagonist treatment (Levant *et al.*, 1991). Nemeroff *et al.* (1989) found a subgroup of schizophrenics, nonparanoid type, with reduced NT levels to increase following treatment with neuroleptics. Conversely, centrally administered neurotensin will increase dopamine turnover and produces a number of pharmacological effects similar to antipsychotics (Levant *et al.*, 1991). This putative endogenous antipsychotic thus appears to hold great promise in the study of schizophrenia, and neurotensin receptor agonists may prove a potentially novel class of antipsychotics (Garver *et al.*, 1991).

Vasopressin, oxytocin and neurophysins
Because of their effects on the processes of learning and memory, vasopressin and oxytocin have been investigated in the CSF of schizo-

phrenics. Moreover, oxytocin selectively increases post-synaptic DA receptor sensitivity in the mesolimbic system but decreases presynaptic DA receptor sensitivity in the nigrostriatal system (Pedersen, 1991). Vasopressin has also been shown to increase DA turnover in the nigrostriatum and tuberoinfundibular DA systems (Pedersen, 1991). Although van Kammen *et al.* (1981) reported vasopressin to be reduced by some 40% in the CSF of male schizophrenics, Beckmann *et al.* (1985) noted no difference in either their untreated schizophrenic patients or in those treated with halperidol, compared to controls.

Beckmann *et al.* (1985) also looked at oxytocin, noting CSF concentrations of oxytocin to be increased in their schizophrenic group and higher in those receiving neuroleptic treatment. Oxytocin has been reported to have opposite effects to vasopressin in inhibiting dopamine and norepinephrine in some areas. Beckmann *et al.* suggest that the increased oxytocin concentrations may be of significance in the clinically observed amnestic syndromes in neuroleptic treated schizophrenics.

As neurophysins are the carriers of vasopressin and oxytocin in the hypothalamus, Linkowski *et al.* (1984) looked at the levels of neurophysin 1, associated with vasopressin, and neurophysin 2, associated with oxytocin, in affective illness and in schizophrenia. They felt these might reflect long term oxytocinergic and vasopressinergic function being more stable than the active peptides in the CSF and being released simultaneously at the synaptic level. They found lower levels of neurophysin 1 and higher levels of neurophysin 2 in schizophrenics compared to controls. Vasopressin was first used to treat schizophrenia by Foriz in 1952 with one-third of his patients showing improvement, and subsequent studies have shown variable therapeutic effects (Nemeroff and Bisette, 1988; McDonald and Krishnan, 1991).

Somatostatin
Somatostatin has been shown to exert a number of behavioural actions including alterations in sleep, locomotion, memory, learning, and eating behaviours. It also appears to stimulate the release of dopamine from the striatum in animals and is reduced in the brain by neuroleptic treatment. Dopamine may, conversely, stimulate the release of somatostatin in several brain areas. There have been a number of studies with variable results looking at CSF somatostatin in schizophrenia. Rubinow (1986), Doran *et al.* (1986), Wood *et al.* (1982), and Gerner *et al.* (1985) have all found normal or elevated CSF somatostatin in schizophrenia. However, Bissette *et al.* (1986*b*) noted reduced levels in schizophrenics. Gattaz *et al.* (1986*b*) found somatostatin-like immunoreactivity in the CSF of schizophrenic patients to increase after haloperidol treatment, whereas Doran *et al.* (1989) noted CSF somatostatin to be significantly reduced and CSF HVA significantly

elevated during fluphenazine treatment. Doran *et al.* (1986) looked at the effect of the dexamethasone suppression test in schizophrenic and depressed patients on CSF somatostatin. They found lower levels of CSF somatostatin in dexamethasone non-suppressors regardless of diagnosis. The reason for the disparity between these studies is not clear at this time.

Cholecystokinin (CCK)

Because cholecystokinin immunoreactivity (CCK-IR) co-localises with dopamine in some neurons in the ventral tegmental area, many investigators have looked at CCK peptides as possibly modulating dopamine function and thus being relevant to the pathogenesis of schizophrenia. Although Gerner and Yamada (1982) found no significant difference in CSF CCK-IR concentrations in schizophrenics compared to controls, several other studies (Verbanck *et al.*, 1984; Lotstra *et al.*, 1985) have noted decreased levels of CCK immunoreactivity in schizophrenics. These results, along with the findings of post mortem studies, have prompted therapeutic trials of CCK peptides in schizophrenia, many of which have been shown to have at least some therapeutic effect. Nair *et al.* (1986) has reviewed the role of CCK in schizophrenia and the results of these therapeutic trials. Adequate trials of CCK have not yet been done, however, as all studies have been with systemically administered CCK which penetrates the blood-brain and blood-CSF barriers poorly (Tanimoto *et al.*, 1991).

Neuropeptides Y and YY

Widerlov *et al.* (1988a) recently looked at neuropeptide Y and peptide YY in the CSF of patients with major depression and schizophrenia compared to healthy volunteers. Neuropeptide Y was significantly lower in the CSF patients with depression, whereas neuropeptide YY was significantly reduced in drug-free schizophrenic patients, but not in the depressed patients. Treatment with neuroleptics did not affect the level of either neuropeptide Y or YY. They suggest that the reduced concentrations of neuropeptide Y or YY may be used as trait markers for depression and schizophrenia respectively.

Other neuropeptides

Other neuropeptides that have been looked at in schizophrenia include increased corticotrophin releasing factor (Banki *et al.*, 1987), decreased levels of delta sleep inducing peptide (Lindstrom *et al.*, 1985), decreased bombesin levels (Gerner and Yamada, 1982; Gerner *et al.*, 1985), and prolactin levels increasing with neuroleptic treatment (Rimon *et al.*, 1985). Bissette and Nemeroff (1988) have reviewed the CSF and post-mortem studies of neuropeptides in schizophrenia as well as the clinical trials of CCK, thyrotrophin-releasing-hormone (TRH), vasopressin, and opioid agonists and antagonists in schizophrenia.

Calcium

Various studies of CSF calcium in schizophrenia have shown no difference from control levels (Jimersen *et al.*, 1979, 1980). Jimersen *et al.* (1979) did, however, find increased CSF levels of calcium in eight of nine schizophrenics who were restudied in a drug-free period. Gattaz *et al.* (1983*b*) also noted increased CSF Ca^{++} as well as CSF Mg^{++} levels in drug-free schizophrenics. Both electrolytes correlated negatively with CSF cGMP levels. They suggested that neuroleptics may act by restoring Mg^{++} and Ca^{++} levels to normal, thus correcting the relative cholinergic-dopaminergic imbalance.

Immunological and viral studies

There has been a considerable amount of speculation about a possible viral and/or autoimmune aetiology in schizophrenia (van Kammen and De Lisi, 1984; De Lisi, 1984). As mentioned earlier, a number of studies have shown signficantly increased IgA, IgM and IgG in schizophrenics, indicating possible recent or past infection.

De Lisi *et al.* (1981), however, noted a generalised reduction in IgA, IgG and IgM, suggesting that there may be a diminished immunological competence in schizophrenia, perhaps related to the use of longterm neuroleptics, or perhaps related to the illness itself.

There have also been a number of studies demonstrating specific anti-viral antibodies in the CSF of schizophrenics, particularly to cytomegalovirus (CMV) (Albrecht *et al.*, 1980; Torrey *et al.*, 1982; De Lisi, 1984), although others have not found any association with CMV antibodies (Shrikhande *et al.*, 1985). Van Kammen *et al.* (1984) looked at CMV antibodies in relation to brain atrophy and CSF monoamine metabolites, but found them to be unrelated.

There have also been many studies looking at the cytotoxic effects of CSF in schizophrenics *in vitro* and *in vivo* and either relating these to possible toxic or autoimmune effects, or to virus-like bodies in the CSF causing these effects. Mikheyeva (1963) has reviewed the extensive Russian and Eastern European work done in this field since the 1920s. Polini (1954) found that intravenous injection of 10-20 ml of CSF from schizophrenics caused a decrease in frequency and voltage of the EEG, when injected into normal subjects. The ethics of many of these earlier studies obviously casts doubt on them. More recent studies have shown a cytopathic effect (CPE) from CSF derived from schizophrenics (Tyrrell *et al.*, 1979, 1983; Taylor *et al.*, 1982, 1985*a,b*; Vilkov *et al.*, 1986, 1987; Crow *et al.*, 1979), but it is not clear whether this cytopathic effect has been related to a virus-like agent, a toxin, or "anti-brain antibodies". Crow *et al.* (1979) reported a virus-like agent

(VLA) with a cytopathic effect on cultured cells in 18 of 47 patients with schizophrenia. They subsequently reported, however, that this cytopathic effect was more probably related to a toxic factor than to a virus (Taylor *et al.*, 1982, 1985*a,b*). The CSF in these patients produced an unusual degenerative change in human fibroblast tissue culture lines (Tyrrell, 1983) but was not specific to schizophrenic patients, occurring also in a similar proportion of patients with progressive neurological illnesses. The CPE effect has not been found to be prevented by either nucleic acid or protein synthesis inhibition, appears to be resistant to ultraviolet radiation and is associated with increased CSF enolase levels. This group initially reported that marmosets injected intracerebrally with CPE-positive CSF from schizophrenics became behaviourally less active over time compared to marmosets injected with CPE-negative CSF from control patients. In a recent reinvestigation of this phenomenon, however, they failed to replicate their findings, concluding that the original findings were due to factors unconnected with the nature of the CSF (Baker *et al.*, 1989).

Conclusion

CSF studies in schizophrenia have been hampered by lack of control for the heterogeneity of patients, different stages of the disease studied, diurnal and seasonal variations of neurotransmitter metabolites, different assays used and other sources of variance such as age, sex, and activity levels, which may all affect CSF metabolite levels. These have led to a number of conflicting results in these studies. There are, however, several promising trends and recent results which may have potential clinical value. These include the distinction of some biological subgroups of schizophrenics by HVA and 5-HIAA, the possible use of HVA and NE as predictors of treatment response and relapse, and the use of 5-HIAA in the prediction of aggression and suicide risk, and perhaps of familial predisposition.

The study of proteins and amino acids have led to a better understanding of the blood-brain-CSF barriers in schizophrenia and the study of neuropeptides and other neurotransmitters has shed light on the various neurochemical theories of schizophrenia and paved the way for the development of trials of neuropeptide treatment in schizophrenia. The CSF studies of CCK, and of neurotensin in particular, appear very promising in leading to new treatment strategies in schizophrenia.

Affective Illness

The usual CSF indices of pressure, cell count, and glucose are usually normal in both mania and depression (Fishman, 1980). Pharmacological studies of the effects of tricyclic antidepressants (TCAs), monoamine oxidase inhibitors (MAOIs) and other centrally acting drugs have implicated various neurotransmitter systems in the pathophysiology of unipolar and bipolar affective illness. We will focus here on the CSF studies of the neurotransmitters and their metabolites and discuss also the CSF abnormalities of neuropeptides, prostaglandins, enzymes, calcium and protein in affective illness.

Catecholamines

There have been many indirect pharmacological data suggesting that central catecholamine activity, norepinephrine (NE) in particular, is diminished in major depression and elevated in manic states. Drugs known to increase NE activity via various mechanisms, e.g. MAOIs, TCAs, have proved useful in the treatment of depression, while drugs which decrease NE activity, e.g. reserpine, propranolol, methyldopa will produce depression as a side-effect (van Praag, 1980b; Post et al., 1978a).

CSF studies of NE, its metabolites MHPG and VMA, and the enzyme DBH (which converts DA to NE) have all been used as indices of central noradrenergic activity in affective illness, yielding a variety of conflicting results (Subrahmanyam, 1975; Vestergaard et al., 1978; Lerner et al., 1978; van Praag, 1980b; Post et al., 1978a, 1980b). In general, these studies have tended to show normal levels of VMA, normal to elevated MHPG, elevated NE and decreased DBH activity in mania (Post et al., 1980b). Studies relating these parameters to depression have tended to find concentrations of VMA low, low to normal levels of MHPG, normal to elevated NE and normal DBH activity in the CSF (Post et al., 1980b).

Subrahmanyam (1975) reported lower levels of MHPG in depressed patients which improved slightly with treatment. Other studies have reported MHPG to be normal in depression but elevated in mania or in certain subpopulations of depressed patients (Vestergaard et al., 1978; Post et al., 1980b). In looking at CSF levels of NE, Post et al. (1978a) found higher than normal levels of NE in the CSF of manic patients and normal levels in their depressed population. Those depressed patients with high levels of anxiety, however, demonstrated higher NE concentrations compared with those with lower anxiety levels. A study by Lerner et al. (1978) showed that manic patients tended to have lower DBH activity in CSF, whereas it was noted to be higher in their bipolar depressed patients.

Studies over the last decade have tended to use the more sensitive methods of gas chromatography-mass spectrometry (GC-MS) or high pressure liquid chromatography with electrochemical detection (HPLC-EC) for measurement of amine metabolites and radioenzymatic or isotope derivative techniques for measurement of the amines themselves. These studies have, however, also been very inconsistent and have generally shown normal levels of norepinephrine and normal-low levels of its metabolites in the CSF in depression, and variable results in mania (see reviews of Post *et al.*, 1984*a*; Gjerris, 1988*a,b*). Two studies have looked at epinephrine in depression, with both finding decreased levels in the CSF compared to controls (Christiensen *et al.*, 1980; Gjerris *et al.*, 1987*a*).

The observations that amphetamines, which potentiate central catecholamines, produce a euphoric state and that Parkinson's disease, a DA-deficient state, is frequently associated with depression have caused many investigators to look at the role of DA metabolism in affective illness (van Praag, 1980*b*). Investigations of the DA metabolite HVA in the CSF of manic-depressive patients have also been highly variable. They have generally demonstrated normal to increased levels in mania and normal to decreased concentrations in depression (Post *et al.*, 1980*b*; van Praag, 1980*b*; Asberg *et al.*, 1984*a,b*). Niklasson *et al.* (1983) found CSF HVA as well as 5-HIAA to correlate positively with CSF levels of xanthine and hypoxanthine in depressed patients, indicating parallel purinergic and monoaminergic activation. CSF HVA levels may have therapeutic implications in that low levels tend to indicate an increased tendency toward bipolarity of affective illness and to respond to L-DOPA and piribedil (Bowers, 1974*a*; Post *et al.*, 1978*b*, 1980*b*).

More recent studies of dopamine metabolites have continued to show variable results but have generally shown normal (Gerner *et al.*, 1984; Gjerris *et al.*, 1987*c*) or decreased (Asberg *et al.*, 1984*a,b*; Roy *et al.*, 1985*b*) levels of HVA in the CSF of depressed patients. Gerner *et al.* (1984*a*) noted a significant interaction of CSF HVA with age in their depressed patients, which they feel may in part explain some of the high variability between studies. They noted HVA levels to be lower in younger depressed patients and higher in older depressed patients compared to normal subjects. They noted no relationship between mania ratings and CSF HVA level, although their manic group tended to have moderately higher HVA levels than their normal controls. Gjerris *et al.* (1987*c*) noted higher CSF concentrations of total CSF dopamine and normal CSF HVA, NE, and MHPG, compared with controls. The increased CSF dopamine levels tended to occur in patients with delusional symptoms when compared to patients without delusions. This finding is interesting in view of the suggestion by Schatzberg *et al.* (1985) that psychotic depression may relate to increased activity of central dopamine. They suggest that their findings would be consistent with a hypothesis of an imbalance between central neurotransmitter systems, rather than solely diminished dopaminergic function.

CSF studies have thus provided inconsistent results in support of the catecholamine hypothesis of affective disorder generated by the pharmacological studies. One possible contribution to these apparent discrepancies may be related to the controversy over the origin of norepinephrine, dopamine and their metabolites in the lumbar CSF and whether they do indeed measure central catecholamine function. Although it is felt that these measures do most likely originate from CNS metabolism, there is still some debate about their origin in lumbar CSF. If manic-depressive illness is related to catecholamine dysfunction in specific areas of the brain, it is possible that lumbar CSF (LCSF) measurements may not be indicative of changes in these areas. Alternatively, if affective illness is related to catecholamine dysfunction throughout the brain, studies of these metabolites in LCSF will be relevant only if they are indicative of general CNS catecholamine metabolism. These issues have been discussed in detail in Chapter 3.

Another possible contribution to the inconsistencies in the catecholamine studies of the CSF in affective illness may be the lack of standardisation in the different methods used in these studies. Gjerris (1988*a,b*) has recently reviewed the methodologies in these various studies in some depth and has pointed out the difficulties in comparing studies using different analytical methods of CSF measurements. She also discusses the lack of control in many of these studies, particularly the earlier studies, for adequate drug washout period, and for the CSF sampling procedure, taking into account the gradients of the metabolites, age, height, sex and activity levels. She also points out that many of the studies using probenecid to block the acid transport system in measuring the metabolites have not adequately controlled for probenecid concentrations. These discrepancies between studies have lessened in recent years, but nonetheless make it difficult to be certain in comparing the results of given investigations. There is also the ever present problem in CSF studies of comparing one's data to an adequate control group and the problems with some of the earlier studies using patients with neurological disorders as controls. Although the studies in recent years have generally used healthy volunteers, there has been significant variation between age, sex and height in the control groups in various studies and monoamine metabolites may even vary significantly between inpatient and outpatient healthy volunteers (Guthrey *et al.*, 1985).

Gjerris (1988*a,b*) also points out the problem of the heterogeneity of patients with depression in the various studies. Particularly in the earlier studies there were no standardised assessment systems for diagnostic classification. Studies within the last decade, however, have used more standardised assessment, notably the International Classification of Diseases (ICD9), the Diagnostic and Statistical Manual of Mental Disorders (DSM-III and DSM-III-R) and Newcastle rating scales. The use of these more standardised assessments in the last decade has tended to decrease the frequency of studies reporting low levels of the CSF amine metabolites in depression.

There have been a number of recent studies which have attempted to take into account the heterogeneity of affective illness, looking for abnormalities of the amine metabolites in various subgroups of patients. Banki *etal.* (1981) has noted CSF HVA levels to correlate positively with sleep disturbances, anxiety and agitation on the Hamilton Depression Scale (HDS), and to correlate negatively with psychomotor retardation. Gjerris *et al.* (1987*a*) noted a significant negative correlation between somatic anxiety and hypochondriasis on the HDS and CSF epinephrine levels in depressed patients. Nordin (1988) reported a negative correlation of sadness on the Montgomery-Asberg Depression Rating Scale, with MHPG levels.

There have also recently been a number of reports combining the CSF data with other biological markers. Banki *et al.* (1983*b*) found dexamethasone suppression test (DST) non-suppressors to have a lower CSF HVA, but this was not disease-specific and was found with DST non-suppressors in both depression (nonsignificantly) and in alcohol dependence (highly significant).

Serotonin (5-HT)

Many investigators have detected low concentrations of the 5-HT metabolite 5-HIAA in the CSF of manic and of depressed patients (Post and Goodwin, 1974*b*; Coppen, 1976; Banki, 1977; Asberg *et al.*, 1984*a,b*).

Involvement of indoleamine systems in the affective disorders has been suggested largely again by pharmacological and by animal studies. It has been considered that there may be denervation-like induced alterations in serotonin receptors which may underlie affective illness (see Siever *et al.*, 1984 for review). The majority of CSF studies have centred around the serotonin metabolite 5-hydroxyindolacetic acid (5-HIAA) as an indicator of central serotonergic turnover. These studies have been plagued by some of the same methodological issues as the catecholamine studies and by the question of the central origin of 5-HIAA in lumbar CSF, discussed earlier. Overall, most studies looking at 5-HIAA have reported lower levels in depression compared to controls. There have again, however, been many inconsistencies between studies (Gjerris, 1988*a,b*).

5-HIAA has been found to be decreased, using the probenecid technique, in a number of investigations and it appears to be further reduced with antidepressant therapy (Post and Goodwin, 1978). The serotonin precursors L-tryptophan and 5-hydroxytryptophan (5-HTP), conversely, will elevate 5-HIAA levels in the CSF (Takahashi *et al.*, 1975). Low levels of 5-HIAA appear to persist with recovery (van Praag, 1980*b*). Banki (1984) found CSF 5-HIAA levels to be independent of drug response, but lower levels tended to predict more relapses in their depressed patients. Banki *et al.* (1981) also reported low 5-HIAA levels to correlate positively with somatisation and retardation, and negatively with anxiety and agitation using the HDS. Sedvall *et al.* (1980) have also noted low concentrations of 5-HIAA, as well as of HVA, to be related to an increased risk for depressive disorders amongst family members.

Assessment of suicide risk and violent behaviour

Certainly the most widely studied issue in CSF studies in affective illness has been the relationship of 5-HIAA levels to suicide risk. Asberg *et al.* (1976) reported a bimodal distribution of 5-HIAA CSF levels in a population of depressed patients. They found that those with lower concentrations (less than 15 µg/l) were more likely to commit suicide than those with higher levels. They were also more likely to use violent means. Post *et al.* (1980*b*) found a similar bimodel distribution in male but not in female depressed patients.

Those depressed patients most prone to suicide, particularly those using violent methods, tend to demonstrate particularly low levels of CSF 5-HIAA (Asberg *et al.*, 1976; van Praag, 1982; Montgomery and Montgomery, 1982). The use of zimelidine, which inhibits 5-HT reuptake, has been reported to reduce suicidal thoughts in depressed patients (Montgomery and Montgomery, 1982). Post-mortem analysis of hind-brain tissue of persons commiting suicide also shows reduced levels of 5-HIAA (Coppen, 1976). These results may have important implications for the detection of at-risk suicidal patients and for the choice of antidepressant treatment of these patients (Asberg *et al.*, 1976; Montgomery and Montgomery, 1982; van Praag, 1982). Asberg *et al.* (1984*a*) noted that their findings of decreased CSF-5-HIAA and HVA in their drug-free depressed patients persisted after excluding the suicidal patients and did not differ significantly between unipolar and bipolar patients. They also suggest that such a disturbance in central 5-HT activity could indicate a predisposition toward depression. Asberg *et al.* (1984*a*) and van Praag (1982) have pointed out since low CSF 5-HIAA levels are associated with anxiety and suicide in depressed patients and with aggressive behaviour in nondepressed persons, this would be compatible with the classical psychoanalytical idea of depression as "aggression turned inwards."

Decreased CSF levels of 5-HIAA have also been associated with impulsive and aggressive behaviours in a variety of situations besides in depressive illness. This index of diminished central serotonergic activity may then be indicative of a general increased vulnerability to self-destructive and aggressive behaviour. This may reflect a disinhibitory state secondary to a loss of the modulatory effect of the 5-HTergic system. Brown *et al.* (1979) found low CSF 5-HIAA in habitually violent military men showing impulsive violent behaviours. Bioulac *et al.* (1980) also noted low CSF 5-HIAA amongst XYY criminal offenders who had committed arson and other impulsive-aggressive offences. Linnoila *et al.* (1983*a*) have also reported low 5-HIAA in habitually impulsive homicidal offenders with antisocial personality disorder, but normal CSF 5-HIAA levels in homicidal offenders who had committed premeditated, nonimpulsive, homicidal acts. The same group (Virkkunen *et al.*, 1987) also found low CSF 5-HIAA levels in arsonists. Also, patients with Lesch-Nyhan Syndrome who exhibit self-mutilating behaviour may have low 5-HIAA levels (van Praag, 1986) and low levels have also been observed in patients with alcoholism and borderline personality disorder, related to suicide attempts. Ninan *et al.* (1984) reported decreased CSF 5-HIAA levels in a group of suicidal schizophrenic patients compared to non-suicidal schizophrenics. These studies all suggest that decreased central serotonergic metabolism is not a disease-specific phenomena for depression, but may well be an indicator of impulsivity and/or aggression towards self or others.

Roy *et al.* (1988) have suggested that this deficiency of serotonin metabolism, associated with violent and suicidal behaviour, could relate to serotonergic deficits predisposing individuals to disturbances of glucose metabolism. They noted a tendency in violent and impulsive offenders towards reactive hypoglycaemia on glucose tolerance testing with a significantly lower glucose nadir and a longer duration of hypoglycaemia. This appeared to relate to truancy, stealing, crimes against property, multiple sentences, and sleep disturbances. They point out that lesions of the suprachiasmatic nucleus in rats will abolish circadian rhythms of sleep and cause enhanced insulin secretion after glucose loading. They speculate that, since the suprachiasmatic nucleus has a major serotonergic input, the decreased 5-HT metabolism apparent in impulsive violent offenders may relate, via this mechanism, to affect sleep patterns and glucose metabolism, predisposing them to violent outbursts, suicide attempts and alcohol abuse.

CSF 5-HIAA studies thus have potential clinical value in prediction of suicide and violent behaviour. One should note, however, that decreased CSF 5-HIAA concentrations are not a constant feature in depression, (seen in only about 30% of depressed patients), and that there is substantial overlap in 5-HIAA levels between patients and healthy controls (Virkkunen, 1988). It may however be helpful in distinguishing subgroups of depression and individuals at risk for suicide. Asberg *et al.* (1987) points out that low CSF 5-HIAA levels in suicide attempters are associated with a 20% mortality from suicide within a year, and therefore suggests that routine spinal taps may be helpful in clinical management of these patients. The low sensitivity and specificity of this test does not, however, justify routine LP in suicidal patients. As lumbar puncture is an invasive procedure, requires hospitalisation and standardised procedures, and also requires that the patient not be taking antidepressants at the time of lumbar puncture, further research into other potential markers of serotonin function (e.g. platelet MAO activity, and REM sleep eye movement activity) and to other possible biological correlates of suicide (e.g. dexamethasone suppression test) would certainly seem more practical in routine clinical assessment. The interested reader is referred to the extensive reviews of Asberg *et al.* (1987), Brown and Goodwin (1986), and Ricci and Wellman (1990).

Prediction of treatment response

CSF 5-HIAA concentrations may also be of use in choosing antidepressant therapy (Post and Goodwin, 1974*a*; Banki, 1977; van Praag, 1979, 1982). Several investigators have suggested therapeutic applications of CSF 5-HIAA levels in predicting treatment response and prognosis of affective disorders. A study by Banki (1977) indicated that low pretreatment levels of 5-HIAA in CSF were associated with a poor therapeutic response to amitriptyline, a tricyclic which appears to act more on catecholamine than indoleamine systems. Post and Goodwin (1974*a*), however, observed that imipramine and amitriptyline significantly lower the amount of 5-HIAA that accumulates in CSF following transport blockade by probenecid. This would seem to indicate that these tricyclic antidepressants act by decreasing central serotonin turnover. Van Praag (1979) also found low 5-HIAA concentrations in a subgroup of depressive patients who responded to therapy with either 5-HTP or clomipramine. They found that persistently low CSF 5-HIAA levels were associated with a higher depression rate than "normoserotonergic" patients. Low 5-HIAA levels in CSF have also been associated with ECT treatment, monoamine oxidase inhibitors, lithium carbonate therapy, a reduced nortriptyline response and peribedil therapy (Post and Goodwin, 1974*b*; Post *et al.*, 1978*b*, 1980*b*).

Though CSF 5-HIAA levels do not seem to be clearly related to severity of affective illness (Banki, 1977), Traskman-Bendz *et al.* (1984) demonstrated 5-HIAA to increase after therapy and recovery in depressed patients. Low pretreatment levels of CSF 5-HIAA have also been found to be predictive of therapeutic response to zimeldine (Aberg-Wistedt *et al.*, 1981) and to imipramine (Maas *et al.*, 1982) and high CSF 5-HIAA has been reported to be predictive of benefit from treatment with NE blockers (Traskman-Bendz *et al.*, 1979).

CSF levels of 5-HIAA thus appear to have some potential clinical value in delineating subgroups of depressive patients, and perhaps in prediction and evaluation of therapeutic response. There are still, however, some discrepancies between studies addressing this issue (Asberg *et al.*, 1984*a,b*; Gjerris, 1988*a,b*).

Van Praag *et al.* (1990) argue that the serotonin abnormalities do not appear to be linked to a particular syndromal subtype of depression, but rather to particular psychopathological dimensions that may occur in depression as well as in other psychiatric illnesses. Evidence of decreased

5-HT activity has been found in a number of psychiatric disorders and does not appear to be disorder-specific, but rather may relate to particular functional abnormalities, i.e. hypoactivity/inertia, increased aggression/anxiety and anhedonia. In contrast to the classical nosological approach of biological psychiatry viewing psychiatric disorders each with its own causation, symptomatology and course, they suggest that a dysfunction-oriented approach to altered serotonin metabolism in biochemical and psychopharmacological research may be more fruitful. Meltzer (1990) has reviewed the biochemical and pharmacological data implicating the role of serotonin in depression.

Gamma aminobutyric acid (GABA)

Goodnick et al. (1980) found no significant differences in CSF GABA in patients with either unipolar or bipolar affective disorders compared to normal controls with corrections for age differences. Post et al. (1980b) also did not note a significant difference in either manic or depressed patients, compared to normal controls, although one of their patients did show levels significantly elevated in the manic phase of illness compared to the depressive phase. Faull et al. (1978), using mass spectrometry, also found levels in a bipolar patient to be in the range of other patients with tardive dyskinesia, HD, and schizophrenia.

More recent studies, however, have demonstrated significantly lower levels of CSF GABA in acutely depressed subjects (Gold et al., 1980a; Kasa et al., 1982; Berrettini et al 1983; Gerner et al., 1984a). CSF GABA levels do not appear to differ, however, in mania or in euthymic bipolar patients and Berrettini et al. (1986) suggest that CSF GABA is a state-dependent marker of affective illness. Pharmacological and biopsy studies have recently provided increasing evidence for the "GABA hypothesis" of depression. Honig et al. (1988) have found cortical tissue GABA levels to correlate negatively with depression in refractory depressive patients undergoing stereotactic subcaudate tractotomy. Lloyd et al. (1987) have reviewed the pharmacological data in support of the GABA hypothesis of depression. They point out that the most consistent of the effects of antidepressants and ECT are the down-regulation of beta-adrenergic binding and the up-regulation of $GABA_b$ binding. These more recent CSF studies thus do tend to support the biopsy and pharmacological evidence implicating a role for GABA in affective illness.

Other amino acids

Goodnick et al. (1980) measured CSF concentrations of 32 amino acids in patients with unipolar and bipolar affective disorders before and after probenecid administration. Bipolar patients tended to have higher mean concentrations of all amino acids, but when corrections for age differences were made, only the group differences for tyrosine were significant.

Protein

Pitts *et al.* (1990) have recently reported increased CSF total protein in nine of 24 patients with depression, eight of which were male, compared to 17 healthy controls. They suggest that depression is associated with increased blood-brain barrier permeability and possibly broad-band CSF immunoglobulin synthesis, particularly in males.

Prostaglandins (PGs)

Gerner and Merrill (1983) found no difference in CSF total PGE between manic or depressed patients and normal controls. Linnoila *et al.* (1982), however, measured CSF concentrations of PGE2, PGF2α, and 6-keto-PGF1α in seven unipolar and five bipolar depressed patients and in 11 schizophrenics. They found markedly elevated levels of PGE2 in their female subjects with unipolar depression. These results were not observed in either of the other two groups. They postulated that PGE2 could induce depressive symptoms in these patients by antagonizing the effects of central NE on the second messenger system, since it is thought to do this in peripheral beta-adrenergic receptors.

Opioid peptides

Prior to the introduction of ECT and tricyclic therapy, opium was widely used for its antidepressant effects, the so-called "laudanum cure" (Frecska and Davis, 1991). Gerner *et al.* (1982) noted depressed patients to exhibit transient increases in energy, sociability and interest in other patients and activities after beta-endorphin infusion. There have also been a number of other studies using opioid agonists showing transient improvement in depression, but clinical trials using opiate antagonists have not shown any consistent effect on mood. These studies have been reviewed by Frecska and Davis (1991) and by Berger *et al.* (1986).

Observations of the psychotomimetic properties of opiates has led to speculation of elevated endogenous opioids in mania. Lindstrom *et al.* (1978) reported higher levels of CSF opioid-like compounds in manic patients. Terenius and Nyberg (1986) also detected elevation of an endorphin-like fraction in the CSF of some bipolar depressed patients. Pickar *et al.* (1982*b*) did not find differences in either CSF opioid activity or in beta-endorphin immunoreactivity in manic and depressed patients compared to normal controls. They did, however, note higher levels of CSF opioid activity in four bipolar patients during the manic phase of their illness when compared to their depressive phase.

Post *et al.* (1984*b*) noted no significant differences in CSF levels of opioid binding beta-endorphin in manic or depressed patients compared to controls. They did note opioid binding activity to correlate with the severity of anxiety in depressed patients, suggesting a possible depressive subtype. Interestingly, amongst the normal volunteers, those with the highest self-rated anxiety levels had the lowest levels of CSF opioids. Rubinow *et al.* (1981) found a positive correlation of CSF opioid activity in depressed patients with urinary free cortisol, suggesting a link between opioid activity and hypothalamic-ptuitary-adrenal (HPA) axis dysfunction in major depression.

Thus CSF studies of opioid peptide have not clearly elucidated their role in affective illness, but it appears that they may relate to mania, to anxiety and to HPA axis dysfunction. Further study measuring specific opioid peptides should help to clarify these issues.

Somatostatin

Somatostatin is a tetradecapeptide which is thought to have a number of depressant behavioural properties. It exerts its effects on various neurotransmitter systems implicated in affective illness, stimulating the synthesis and turnover of DA, NE, and 5-HT after intraventricular injection (Gold *et al.*, 1982).

Rubinow *et al.* (1983*a,b*) measured CSF somatostatin in 47 patients with affective illness and in 39 normal subjects. They found somatostatin concentrations to be significantly lower in drug-free depressed patients compared to either controls or to recovered patients. Values for patients in improved and manic states were intermediate between normal and depressed patients. No correlation with severity of the illness was noted. CSF somatostatin correlated positively with CSF 5-HIAA and negatively with CSF NE. CSF levels of GABA and HVA did not correlate with somatostatin levels. A negative correlation with duration of sleep in these patients was also noted.

There have to date been six studies confirming decreased CSF levels of somatostatin in depressive illness (see reviews of Post *et al.* 1988, Vecsei and Widerlov, 1988*b*, and Rubinow *et al.* 1991). The decreased levels of somatostatin appear to be a state-related marker for depression and do not appear to persist in the recovered state or in the manic state. Of particular note is the study of Rubinow (1986) relating low CSF somatostatin with escape from dexamethasone suppression in both depression and schizophrenia. Somatostatin has an inhibitory influence over the secretion of adrenocorticotrophic hormone (ACTH), presumably at the level of adenylate cyclase. The low CSF somatostatin in depression may thus partially explain the hypercortisolism seen in some 50% of depressed patients (Rubinow, 1986). There has been only one post mortem study (Charlton *et al.*, 1988) to date, looking at somatostatin immunoreactivity and receptors in cortical tissue from depressed patients and finding no clear alteration of cortical somatostatin function in affective illness. Nonetheless the consistency of the CSF studies certainly speaks for a role for this neuropeptide in affective illness. Now that the somatostatin gene has been isolated and sequenced (Shen and Rutter, 1984) there exists the possibility of a molecular genetic approach to altering somatostatin function (Rubinow *et al.*, 1991). Further investigations with somatostatin agonists and antagonists may also prove fruitful (Rubinow *et al.*, 1991).

Corticotrophin-releasing factor (CRF)

A number of studies have demonstrated increased CSF levels of corticotrophin-releasing factor (Banki *et al.*, 1987; Widerlov *et al.*, 1988) as well as a blunted ACTH response to exogenously administered CRF (Gold *et al.*, 1986) in depression. Gold *et al.* (1986) suggest that the hypercortisolism seen in depression and blunted ACTH response to CRF may be related to increased endogenous CRF secretion. Post *et al.* (1988) suggest that CRF stimulation may be a useful clinical test in the differential diagnosis between depression and Cushing's disease, as patients with primary depression who may be obese and/or hirsute with high cortisol levels may be difficult to differentiate from early Cushing's disease. Patients with Cushing's disease tend to have an exaggeration of the ACTH response to CRF, in contrast to depressed patients. Post *et al.* also point out some of the animal studies linking maternal deprivation to hyperactivity of the HPA axis in adult life, and linking CRF to appetite and to sexual and motor behaviours. This then may provide a physiological basis for some of the dynamic formulations of depressive illness.

Other neuropeptides

Other neuropeptides measured in CSF in affective illness include the finding of decreased levels of oxytocin in manic patients compared to depressed patients (Gold *et al.*, 1980b); increased CSF substance P levels (Rimon *et al.*, 1984); increased CSF vasopressin in manic patients and normal CSF levels of vasopressin in depression (Sorensen *et al.*, 1985); decreased levels of delta-sleep inducing peptide in depression (Lindstrom *et al.*, 1985); normal CCK levels in depression (Gerner and Yamada, 1982) and decreased levels of CCK in bipolar patients (Verbanck *et al.*, 1984); decreased neuropeptide

Y (Widerlov *et al.*, 1988*a*) as well as normal CSF neuropeptide Y levels (Berrettini *et al.*, 1987*b*) in depression; decreased CSF VIP levels in nonendogenous type depression (Gjerris and Rafaelsen, 1984); decreased CSF levels of immunoreactive calcitonin in manic patients compared to normal volunteers and to other bipolar patients (Carman *et al.*, 1984); and increased diazepam-binding inhibitor immunoreactivity in depressed patients (Barbaccia *et al.*, 1986).

The significance of these neuropeptide alterations in affective illness remains to be clarified. The interested reader is referred to the extensive review of Post *et al.* (1988).

Calcium

Jimerson *et al.* (1979) studied CSF electrolytes in psychiatric patients and noted CSF calcium levels to be positively correlated with symptom severity in depression. In four bipolar patients, levels were higher during depressive episodes than during mania. Mean CSF concentrations did not, however, differ significantly from neurological controls or from other psychiatric patients. Various other studies of CSF calcium have noted both normal and elevated levels in depression. These are reviewed by Jimerson *et al.* (1980).

Carman *et al.* (1984) have also noted significant state-related shifts in CSF calcium in patients over time, showing an inverse relationship to level of activation or excitement (lowest in mania or catatonic excitement, highest in catatonic stupor or in bipolar depression, and intermediate in euthymia). They suggest that these shifts in calcium could provide a possible explanation for other monoaminergic and neuroendocrinological findings accompanying bipolar mood changes.

S-adenosylmethionine (SAM)

S-adenosylmethionine is an important methyl donor involved in a number of important reactions in the CNS, linked to folate and vitamin B12 metabolism as well as to methylation reactions with a variety of neurotransmitters, polyamines, phospholipids and proteins. Bottiglieri *et al.* (1990) have demonstrated significantly lower CSF levels of SAM in severely depressed patients compared to neurological controls. They also demonstrated that the administration of SAM, orally or i.v., shows a significant antidepressant effect and that its administration is associated with a significant rise in CSF SAM, providing a rational basis for its role as an antidepressant. This has has now been looked at in a number of trials. Carney *et al.* (1989) have suggested that SAM may be related to the postulated "switch mechanism" suggested to play a role for bipolar patients "switching out" of a depressed phase. They noted nine of 11 bipolar patients treated with SAM to "switch" into an elevated mood state (hypomania, mania or euphoria). The "switchers" showed an increase in CSF HVA, suggesting a possible link between SAM and dopaminergic mechanisms for the switch.

Conclusion

The CSF studies of the catecholamines and their metabolites have been extremely variable and have not shown any consistent support for the catecholamine hypotheses of affective illness. CSF studies of the 5-HT metabolite 5-HIAA have been more promising in delineating subgroups of patients in depression, possible prediction or monitoring of treatment response to various antidepressants, and in predicting suicide risk. The low levels of CSF 5-HIAA associated with increased suicide risk do not appear to be disease-specific for depression but rather more likely relate to impulsivity and aggression in a large number of psychiatric conditions. CSF levels of GABA, calcium, somatostatin, and other neuropeptides have been suggested as possible state-related markers in affective illness and the increased CSF CRF levels observed in depression appear to be related to the hypercortisolism observed in many patients. The study of neuropeptides in the CSF has advanced dramatically over the last decade and it appears will lead to major revisions of the classical catecholamine and indoleamine theories of affective illness.

Attention Deficit Disorder

Attention deficit disorder (ADD) or minimal brain dysfunction (MBD) is a common childhood disorder characterised by impaired perception and attention, hyperexcitability, motor difficulties, difficulty in impulse control and often hyperactive behaviour. CSF studies of ADD have focused primarily on metabolites of the catecholamines and serotonin. Evidence supporting a link between ADD and CNS biogenic amine metabolism stems largely from investigations of the actions of the stimulant drugs such as methylphenidate and dextroamphetamine used in treating ADD. Further evidence is provided by several animal studies and investigations of plasma DBH, platelet MAO activity, and urinary amine metabolites in children with ADD (See review of Hunt et al., 1982).

Shetty and Chase (1976) studied CSF levels of HVA and 5-HIAA in 23 MBD children with hyperactivity. They found no significant difference in either metabolite compared to age-matched controls considered to be free of CNS disease. Administration of dextroamphetamine caused a marked reduction in HVA and a slight increase in 5-HIAA. This decline in CSF

HVA correlated closely with the degree of clinical improvement. They suggest that the hyperkinetic behaviour patterns in these children may be due to an increase in dopaminergic mechanisms and that d-amphetamine may act by diminishing the synthesis and release of brain DA. These conclusions may be premature without examining the CSF HVA levels in amphetamine-treated controls. The changes in HVA and 5-HIAA seen with treatment could also be interpreted as reflecting a feedback inhibition of DA activity with an inhibitory serotonergic compensation (Hunt *et al.* 1982; Shaywitz *et al.* 1980).

Shaywitz *et al.* (1977) used the probenecid loading technique in studying CSF HVA and 5-HIAA in six boys with MBD. These subjects differed somewhat from those of Shetty and Chase in that only three had a history of childhood hyperactivity. CSF concentrations of HVA correlated with probenecid levels. They found CSF HVA concentrations per unit of probenecid were significantly lower than in their neurological and psychiatric controls. CSF 5-HIAA levels were not significantly different. These results suggest that a diminished central DA turnover may play a role in MBD.

More recently, Kruesi *et al.* (1990*a*) looked at CSF levels of HVA, 5-HIAA, and the NE metabolite MHPG in 29 children in adolescence with disruptive behaviour disorders, 21 of which fulfilled the criteria for attention deficit disorder, and the eight remaining patients having histories compatible with a probable diagnosis of attention deficit disorder. They noted no significant differences in CSF HVA or MHPG, but noted those with disruptive behaviour disorders to have significantly lower CSF 5-HIAA levels compared to their control group children with obsessive-compulsive disorder (OCD). They noted a significant negative correlation between CSF 5-HIAA levels and the Diagnostic Interview for Children and Adolescents (DICA) aggression score and expressed emotionality (EE) of the patient towards their mother. They noted no significant correlations between 5-HIAA levels and measures of impulsivity. Their study controlled or statistically corrected for CSF aliquot, age, height, season, time of day, LP site and diet and used high pressure liquid chromatography with electrochemical detection (HPLC-EC), in contrast to the earlier paediatric studies which were less well controlled and used the less sensitive fluorometric assay technique. Although one might question the appropriateness of using patients with childhood OCD as a contrast group, the study of Kruesi *et al.* is interesting in view of the adult studies relating low levels of CSF 5-HIAA with various measures of impulsivity and aggression.

The same group (Kruesi *et al.*, 1990*b*) also reported lower levels of CSF somatostatin in ten patients with disruptive behaviour disorder relative to children with OCD. They suggest that this may relate to the differences seen between these two groups in CSF 5-HIAA levels, since somatostatin appears important in the regulation of serotonin. They further speculate that this decrease in somatostatin may be related to the observation that children with disruptive behaviour disorders are more mesomorphic, as somatostatin is known to inhibit the release of growth hormone. They thus suggest that the increases in bone and muscle mass observed in these children are due to a loss of inhibition of growth hormone resulting from the decreased somatostatin activity.

Panic Disorder

There have been relatively few CSF studies of panic disorder compared to other areas of psychiatry. Noradrenergic, serotonergic, and GABAergic systems, lactate, carbon dioxide, and various neuropeptides have all been implicated in the pathogenesis of panic attacks, largely stemming from pharmacological studies. These have recently been reviewed by Malison and Price (1991) and the pharmacological aspects of panic disorder have recently been reviewed by Cox *et al.* (1991). The anxiogenic effects of the α-2 adrenoceptor antagonist yohimbine and the anxiolytic properties of α-2 agonists thought to act on the locus coeruleus have pointed to noradrenergic dysregulation in panic disorder (Malison and Price, 1991).

CSF studies of the norepinephrine metabolite MHPG have not, however, been found to differ from controls. George *et al.* (1990) and Lepola *et al.* (1990) have both reported CSF levels of MHPG not differing from controls. George *et al.* studied panic disorder in alcoholics, compared to alcoholics without panic disorder and to controls and found no difference in CSF levels of HVA, 5-HIAA, MHPG or diazepam-binding inhibitor, but did find increased levels of CSF beta-endorphin in subjects with panic disorder. Lepola *et al.* studied 34 patients with panic disorder and 10 neurological controls, and found no differences in CSF levels of HVA, 5-HIAA, MHPG, somatostatin or beta-endorphin. They did, however, note a modest correlation between total anxiety scores and CSF MHPG.

Eriksson *et al.* (1989) and Pitkanen *et al.* (1989) have both noted increased levels of CSF beta-endorphin in patients with panic disorder compared to controls. Eriksson found no effect of antidepressant treatment on CSF beta-endorphin levels, although they had a dramatic clinical effect. Anton *et al.* (1989) have also looked at prostaglandin E in the CSF of patients with agoraphobia and panic attacks and in controls, finding no difference between the groups.

The CSF studies of panic disorder have been too small and too few to draw any firm conclusions. They have not, however, generally given support to the noradrenergic and serotonergic hypotheses of panic disorder, but several studies have shown increased levels of beta-endorphin which do not appear to be related to treatment response.

Obsessive-compulsive Disorder (OCD)

CSF studies of obsessive-compulsive disorder (OCD) have focused on the serotonin metabolite 5-hydroxyindolacetic acid (5-HIAA). Interest in serotonin metabolism in OCD has been generated primarily by the pharmacological effects of serotonin reuptake inhibitors in its treatment. The role of serotonin and other biological factors in OCD has been reviewed by Insel et al. (1990) and by Turner et al. (1985).

Thoren and colleagues (1980) looked at CSF levels of 5-HIAA, as well as the dopamine metabolite HVA and the norepinephrine metabolite MHPG, in 24 patients with OCD and compared these with 37 paid healthy volunteer controls. The patients were treated with clomipramine, nortriptyline, or placebo in a double-blind fashion. They found no significant difference in the amine metabolites prior to treatment. They did find high CSF 5-HIAA pre-treatment levels to relate to clomipramine responsiveness in the OCD group. They also found a significant correlation between the obsessive symptoms and a reduction of CSF 5-HIAA levels in the clomipramine group, after treatment. The reduction in 5-HIAA thus appeared to be associated with treatment response and was also related to plasma clomipramine concentrations in a U-shaped manner, with both very low and very high concentrations of clomipramine associated with a smaller reduction of 5-HIAA than intermediate concentrations. They thus concluded that the anti-obsessional effect of clomipramine is related to its serotonin uptake inhibition as reflected in the CSF 5-HIAA levels.

Insel et al. (1985) found CSF 5-HIAA levels to be 30% higher in one cohort of eight patients with OCD, compared to 23 healthy volunteer controls. They used the more specific 5-HT uptake inhibitor zimelidine and found that, although it caused a significant reduction in CSF 5-HIAA, it was clinically ineffective. They also noted a decrease in 5-HIAA with desipramine and with clomipramine, and all three drugs decreased CSF MHPG but had negligible affects on CSF HVA. They interpreted these results as indicating that 5-HT reuptake blockade alone is not sufficient for the anti-obsessional response in OCD.

Thus, although there are some inconsistencies between these two studies, both seem to indicate a state of increased serotonin turnover. In the study of Thoren et al. this was evident only in their patients who responded to clomipramine. Furthermore, both studies seem to indicate that the effect of serotonin reuptake inhibitors is related to a decrease in CSF 5-HIAA and that this inhibition of serotonin uptake may be necessary for treatment response (but perhaps not the whole story explaining treatment response) in these patients.

More recently Altemus et al. (1992) noted no difference in CSF 5-HIAA, HVA or MHPG compared to normal controls but found significantly increased CSF arginine vasopressin (AVP) and corticotrophin releasing factor (CRF). They suggest that overactivity of these systems could relate to the perseverative behaviours, attention difficulties and exaggerated grooming behaviours seen in OCD.

Swedo *et al.* (1992) studied 43 children with OCD and found an association of CSF 5-HIAA with clomipramine response similar to that seen in Thoren *et al.*'s adult study. They also looked at CSF levels of AVP and found them to correlate negatively with OCD symptoms. Dynorphin (1-8), oxytocin, HVA, ACTH, MHPG and CRF levels did not significantly relate to OCD symptoms, but oxytocin levels did correlate positively with depressive symptoms.

In summary, CSF studies in OCD have confirmed the role of serotonin in the treatment response of these patients, but the relationship of serotonin turnover to OCD symptoms is still not clear. They have also implicated a role for AVP, and perhaps oxytocin and CRF. The finding of increased CSF AVP in the adult study of Altemus *et al.* (1992) and the negative correlation of AVP with OCD symptoms in Swedo *et al.*'s paediatric study suggest a possible difference between adult and childhood forms of OCD. It is interesting to note, however, that a subgroup of "checkers" in the latter study was also noted to have increased CSF AVP, perhaps indicating that certain subgroups of patients with OCD may be defined by biochemical and clinical parameters.

Autism

Autism is a pervasive developmental disorder which affects cognitive, language and social aspects of development. Biochemical investigation of autism has been limited largely to investigation of body fluids and there have been very few post-mortem studies done. The most consistent finding to date has been that of hyperserotonemia in some 25% of autistic children, which may in some cases be familial (Cook, 1990).

CSF studies in autism have been generally made difficult by the lack of true normal control children in these studies. Cohen *et al.* (1974) examined CSF levels of the dopamine metabolite homovanillic acid (HVA), and the serotonin metabolite 5-hydroxyindoleacetic acid (5-HIAA), using probenecid. They found post-probenecid CSF 5-HIAA levels in autistic children to be intermediate between levels of medicated epileptic children and "atypical development" children. Both the atypical and autistic groups were found to have elevated CSF HVA compared to the treated epileptic children. Cohen *et al.* (1977), in a follow up study, noted no differences however in CSF HVA or 5-HIAA among autistic, non-autistic psychotic, aphasic, and cognitively impaired children compared to a contrast group of paediatric patients. The only significant difference noted between the diagnostic groups post-probenecid was a lower 5-HIAA level in autistic children compared to non-autistic, early onset psychotic children.

More recently, Winsberg *et al.* (1980) have reported normal CSF HVA and 5-HIAA levels and Gillberg *et al.* (1983) and Gillberg and Svennerholm (1987) have reported increased CSF HVA levels in autism. Anderson *et al.* (1988) has also recently reported normal CSF levels of indoleacetic acid (IAA). Normal levels of the NE metabolite MHPG have been reported by Young *et al.* (1981) and by Gillberg *et al.* (1983).

CSF studies of DA, NE, and 5-HT metabolites in autism have thus produced conflicting results. Anderson (1987) has reviewed the urine, plasma, and CSF monoamine studies in autism, concluding that most of the studies of catecholamines and their metabolites in body fluids have not shown any differences between autistic and the control subjects, with the exception of abnormal platelet 5-HT function in a subgroup of autistic children.

Two studies have looked at opioids in the CSF of autistic children. Gillberg *et al.* (1985) found increased CSF endorphin fraction II in 20 autistic children. Ross *et al.* (1987) also have found increased CSF beta-endorphin levels in six autistic children. These findings are particularly interesting in view of the frequently reported diminished sensitivity to pain and frequent self-injurious behaviour seen in autistic children which may be associated with increased endorphin activity. Frecska and Davis (1991) suggest that an autoaddiction mechanism may be a possible explanation for the self-abusiveness seen in autism. They review the trials of opiate antagonists which have shown some initially promising results in autistic children with self-abusive behaviour.

Young *et al.* (1987) and Cook (1990) have reviewed the neurobiological aspects of autism.

Anorexia Nervosa

Anorexia nervosa is a psychosomatic disorder with a remarkable interplay between psychodynamic, physiological, social, and cultural factors. Patients with anorexia nervosa have been found to have abnormalities in the hypothalamic-pituitary-adrenal (HPA) axis, serotonergic, nora-drenergic, and dopaminergic systems, as well as of thyroid, gonadotrophic hormones, and various neuropeptides. Since diet has a marked effect on central neurotransmitters, and as the neurochemical changes in anorexia nervosa may vary according to the state of weight loss in a given patient, it is often difficult to assess what role these changes play in the aetiology of this disorder. Here we will focus on the CSF studies of serotonin, catecholamines and the neuropeptides in anorexia nervosa.

Serotonin and catecholamines

The noradrenergic system, in particular the α-2 receptors, appear to be involved physiologically in the regulation of feeding behaviour. Application of norepinephrine to the paraventricular nucleus of the hypothalamus (PVN) may bring on feeding behaviours in otherwise satiated animals, and similarly, the α-2 receptor agonist clonidine appears to elicit a preferential increase in appetite for carbohydrate, at the expense of protein. This will occur physiologically with the onset of the active period (nocturnal cycle) in the rat. Activation of the locus coeruleus, the main noradrenergic system in the brain, is associated with anxiety and its activity may be decreased by starvation with a possible subsequent reduced anxiety (Fava *et al.*, 1989; Leibowitz, 1989).

Serotonin (5-HT) in general is believed to act antagonistically with the α-2 noradrenergic system. Pharmacological studies show that activation of central 5-HT1B and possibly 5-HT1C as well as 5-HT2 receptors will inhibit food intake, whereas activation of 5-HT1A receptors will enhance feeding behaviours (Samanin and Garattini, 1989). Leibowitz (1989, 1990) has proposed that norepinephrine and serotonin interact antagonistically in the medial hypothalamus to control carbohydrate and protein ingestion. As mentioned above, norepinephrine will stimulate the first meal in the active period of animals which is generally rich in carbohydrate and, as a result, there is increased tryptophan absorption and a surge in 5-HT activity. Serotonin then will act through the "satiety" centres in the hypothalamus to inhibit the carbohydrate meal and to turn the animal's preference toward protein for the following meal. Serotonergic activity exhibits a circadian rhythm characterised by a peak at the beginning of the active cycle when carbohydrate intake has been stimulated by norepinephrine, and may be triggered by the increased tryptophan availability and by the deficits in energy stores at that time. Serotonin will thus induce carbohydrate satiety and switch the animal's preference toward protein intake.

The pharmacological evidence along with the observed decreases in plasma tryptophan, urinary 5-HIAA, platelet serotonin-binding and the frequent association of anorexia nervosa with depression and obsessive-compulsive disorder (also apparently involving 5-HT) have all given strong evidence for the role of serotonin in anorexia nervosa. The role of serotonin in eating disorders has been reviewed by Samanin and Garattini (1989) and by Leibowitz (1990).

Dopaminergic regulation of eating behaviours appears to be linked to the endorphins. Low doses of dopamine and dopamine agonists will stimulate feeding, whereas higher doses will inhibit feeding. This presumably occurs through the parafornical lateral hypothalamus. The fact that dopamine stimulation of feeding can be inhibited by naloxone suggests its link to the opioid system (Fava *et al.*, 1989).

CSF studies

Kaye *et al.* (1984*a*,*b*) studied eight women admitted underweight to a weight restoration program, and measured CSF levels of the dopamine metabolite homovanillic acid (HVA), the 5-HT metabolite 5-hydroxyindoleacetic acid (5-HIAA), and norepinephrine (NE) before treatment and in the same patients a few weeks after weight restoration, as well as in long term weight recovered anorectic women who had maintained a continuously stable weight for a minimum of six months before the study.

The underweight anorectics had a 30% decrease in CSF HVA and a 20% decrease in CSF 5-HIAA, both of which returned to normal shortly after weight recovery. CSF levels of NE, however, were similar to that of normal subjects in both the underweight anorectics and in those who had recently restored their weight. The long term weight recovered anorectics, however, had a 50% decrease in CSF NE compared to controls. They suggest that central 5-HT and DA metabolism are associated with the loss of weight in anorexia nervosa, but that the changes in NE metabolism may be a trait-dependent neurotransmitter alteration that may have been obscured by the state-related changes in the underweight state and immediately after weight recovery. Kaye *et al.* controlled for activity level and the aliquot of CSF used for analysis and the patients were all of similar age and height. They did not control for amino acid content of the diet prior to lumbar puncture, but did measure serum concentrations of monoamine precursor amino acids.

Gerner *et al.* (1984*b*) measured CSF, tyrosine, tryptophan, 5-HIAA, MHPG, HVA, GABA, choline and calcium in 33 anorexic and 14 normal controls. They found the only significant difference between groups was a lower tyrosine level in the anorexic patients. CSF levels of the NE metabolite MHPG were non-significantly higher in the anorexics. The study was controlled for diet with all subjects on a modified low monoamine diet and for activity levels. CSF HVA was positively correlated with percentage of ideal body weight and choline was negatively correlated with anorexia ratings. Nineteen of the anorexic patients also had a diagnosis of secondary depression and within this group, the depression ratings and anorexia ratings were positively correlated with each other. In view of the finding of low CSF tyrosine, which is a precursor for both dopamine and norepinephrine, it is interesting that the respective metabolites HVA and MHPG were not significantly altered and that tyrosine, HVA and MHPG were not significantly correlated in any group.

Kaye *et al.* (1984*a*) reported further data on their 16 anorexic patients, dividing them into bulimic and non-bulimic groups and reporting on both their baseline and post-probenecid CSF metabolite levels. They found that CSF 5-HIAA accumulation, corrected for probenecid concentration, was increased in non-bulimic anorexic patients after weight recovery, compared with bulimic anorexic patients. They suggest that this may be indicative of increased serotonin metabolism in non-bulimic anorexic patients causing appetite suppression particularly of carbohydrate intake, and that these patients may thus differ both clinically and physiologically from bulimic anorexic patients. This group has also recently reported decreased CSF 5-HIAA and HVA in a group of 11 women with bulimia nervosa (Jimerson et al., 1992).

Jimerson et al. (1990) have reviewed the precursor, metabolite and pharmacological studies of serotonin in anorexia nervosa.

Neuropeptides

Corticotrophin-releasing hormone (CRH) and adrenocorticotrophic hormone (ACTH)

Patients with anorexia nervosa consistently show hypothalamic-pituitary adrenal (HPA) abnormalities, particularly resistance to dexamethasone suppression and hypercortisolism even more severe than that seen in depressed patients. These observations, along with the observation that the central administration of CRH to rats will reduce food intake, induce hyperactivity and decrease LH secretion (all phenomena which appear to occur in anorexia nervosa) have led several investigators to investigate the role of this neuropeptide in anorexia.

Hotta et al. (1986), administered i.v. synthetic ovine CRH in 13 patients with anorexia nervosa and measured the concentrations of the immunoreactive CRH in the CSF of seven of them, as well as mean basal levels of plasma ACTH and cortisol. The mean basal plasma cortisol levels were higher than that of aged-matched normal female controls. The response to CRH injection of plasma ACTH and cortisol was significantly lower in the anorexic patients. The CSF concentration of CRH in the seven anorexic patients was markedly higher than that of control subjects with cervical spondylosis. They postulate that the hypercortisolaemia, the diminished response to i.v. CRH, as well as perhaps the appetite suppression and suppression of reproductive functions, could relate to increased secretion of CRH in the CSF in anorexia nervosa.

Kaye et al. (1987) also measured the CSF levels of CRH in patients with anorexia nervosa when they were underweight and after restoration of weight. They also found significantly elevated CSF CRH levels in anorexic patients who were underweight and hypercortisolaemic, with both pituitary-adrenal function and CSF CRH levels normalising after weight recovery. CSF CRH levels correlated significantly with depression ratings in weight corrected patients, compatible with other studies showing increased CRH secretion in the depressed phase of primary affective disorder. They suggest that hypersecretion of CRH may be a defect associated with both anorexia nervosa and depression and may account for many of the vegetative features overlapping in both disorders. Gold *et al.* (1986) have noted that despite normalisation of the apparent defect in CRH secretion on restoration of weight, normal weight anorexics may continue to show a markedly attenuated ACTH response to CRH. They suggest that depression and anorexia nervosa have a similar pathophysiology of hypercortisolism and, as they frequently have overlapping symptoms and family histories, that these two disorders may lie on a pathophysiologic continuum.

Gwirtsman *et al.* (1989), of the same group, measured CSF levels of ACTH as well as CSF, plasma and urine free cortisol levels in 16 patients with anorexia nervosa, 14 patients with bulimia, and 11 healthy aged-matched women volunteers. Underweight anorexic patients showed increased levels of CSF, plasma, and urine free cortisol which declined after restoration of weight. Anorexics and controls had similar levels of cortisol-binding globulin. CSF ACTH levels were significantly low in the underweight anorexics and returned to normal after weight recovery, while the plasma levels of ACTH were noted to be normal. Their group of bulimic patients had normal levels of ACTH and cortisol on admission, but significantly decreased CSF levels of ACTH following one month of abstinence from binge-purge episodes in the hospital. The bulimics with higher CSF ACTH levels tended to have larger decreases following the period of abstinence. They suggest that the decreased CSF ACTH in these patients could be a response to the negative feedback of cortisol or may be related to depletion of pro-opiomelanocortin as a result of hyper-secretion of CRF. As weight loss may act as an activator of the HPA axis, one cannot entirely exclude the possibility that these findings are related to starvation and weight loss. However, the authors point out that the anorexic patients were not in a phase of acute starvation at the time of LP and that the amount of weight loss before hospitalisation did not correlate with any other biochemical variables.

Arginine vasopressin

Vasopressin has also been implicated in eating disorders, as anorexic patients often have polyuria and defects in urinary concentration. Vasopressin has been reported to have a variety of behavioural effects (McDonald and Krishnan, 1991). Gold *et al.* (1983) measured baseline CSF levels of vasopressin, as well as plasma vasopressin response to intravenous hypertonic saline, in patients with anorexia before and after restoration of their weight loss. Abnormal vasopressin response to hypertonic saline was observed in all four of their subjects studied before correction of their weight loss, and these defects persisted in the three patients that were studied three to four weeks following recovery of body weight. Two of these patients were studied six months after recovery and these abnormalities were noted to be absent then. Normal responses were also noted in five of seven other patients studied at least six months after recovery. The abnormalities in osmoregulation of plasma arginine vasopressin tended to be associated with an absolute increase in CSF arginine vasopressin or a reversal of the normal CSF/plasma ratio of arginine vasopressin (< 1.0).

Oxytocin

Oxytocin has been postulated to act as a "brake" on the HPA axis. CSF oxytocin levels have been reported to be low in patients with anorexia nervosa and diminished central oxytocin may disinhibit the HPA axis and produce amenorrhoea. Oxytocin has been linked to the sensation of satiety and luteinising hormone (LH) release is also dependent upon oxytocin (Pedersen, 1991).

Neurotensin

Neurotensin appears to have significant interactions with dopaminergic systems and has been related to a number of behaviours (Levant *et al.* (1991). Nemeroff *et al.* (1989) looked at CSF levels of neurotensin in anorexia nervosa and a variety of other neuropsychiatric illnesses, finding CSF levels of neurotensin to be unaltered in anorexia nervosa.

Neuropeptide Y (NPY) and peptide YY (PYY)

Neuropeptide Y is one of the most abundant peptides in neurons in both the peripheral and central nervous systems. It has been shown to co-localise with serotonin, epinephrine, and norepinephrine. The paraventricular nucleus (PVN) of the hypothalamus, which as mentioned above is a primary site of action for epinephrine and norepinephrine, receives a rich innervation of NPY-IR nerve endings. Injection of neuropeptide Y (NPY) and its related peptide YY (PYY) directly into the PVN will induce a dose-dependent feeding response in rats. NPY will also preferentially stimulate carbohydrate intake in rats, has its biggest response at the onset of the active (nocturnal) cycle in the rat, and will stimulate the release of corticosterone and vasopressin, similar to the effects of norepinephrine (Leibowitz, 1989). NPY exhibits some reciprocal antagonistic interractions with the α-2 noradrenergic receptors of the PVN. There is also some animal evidence suggesting a relationship between NPY, the onset of puberty, and the transition towards the development of adult eating patterns in young females (Leibowitz, 1989).

Peptide YY appears to be approximately three times as potent as neuropeptide Y in stimulating feeding. Both NPY and PYY may override mechanisms of satiety and body weight control. NPY induced stimulation of feeding appears to be more potent than that of any pharmacological agent previously tested and also appears to be very long-lasting. These effects have been observed in various mammalian species and appear not to be mediated through its interactions with noradrenergic, dopaminergic or opioid systems (Widerlov et al., 1991).

Kaye et al. (1990) measured NPY and PYY in the CSF of anorectic and bulimic patients compared to healthy volunteers. The CSF NPY level was increased in the underweight anorectic patient group. It was also elevated in many of the anorectic patients after regaining their weight. In the long term weight-restored anorectic patient group, those with amenorrhoea or oligo-amenorrhoea had elevated CSF NPY. The CSF levels of PYY were significantly elevated in the normal weight bulimic patient group who had been abstinent from binge eating for a period of a month, both when compared with themselves while actively binge eating and vomiting as well as when compared to the control group of healthy volunteers. They postulated that neuropeptide Y may be important in several aspects of anorexia nervosa, particularly menstrual dysregulation, and that PYY may be a contributor to a drive to overfeed in normal weight bulimic patients.

Opioids

The interaction of the opioid peptides with appetite regulation appears to be a complex one. In general, opioid agonists tend to decrease feeding behaviour while opioid antagonists increase feeding. However, this is somewhat dependent upon the species being tested and on the specific opioid receptors being acted on. Naloxone and naltrexone are both reported to reduce food intake and for that reason have been tried in the treatment of bulimia to decrease binge eating behaviours.

There is also evidence to suggest that anorexia may be related to an increase in endogenous opioids suppressing appetite. Marrazzi and Luby (1989) have postulated that anorexia nervosa may be an auto-addiction, with opioids being released during an initial period of dieting that then will make the patient "high" on dieting and, thus, "addicted" to it. The stress of self-induced vomiting may also bring on a similar euphoria in some patients, presumably mediated by endogenous endorphin release. The opioids may then act by increasing food intake to correct the starvation, resulting in bingeing. Marrazzi and Luby, as well as others, have reported some initially promising results using opioid antagonists in the treatment of anorexia nervosa.

Gerner and Sharp (1982) noted no difference in the beta-endorphin immunoreactivity in the cerebospinal fluid of moderately underweight anorexic patients compared to normal controls.

Kaye et al. (1982), however, found increased levels of CSF opioid activity by radio receptor assay in underweight anorexic patients compared to the same patients after restoration of their weight and compared to normal controls. They also examined a group of chronic anorexic patients who were not severely underweight and had normal levels of CSF opioid activity. They suggest that the increased opioid activity may be a compensatory response to weight loss and thus decrease metabolic rate. This could simultaneously bring about the preoccupation with food.

Kaye *et al.* (1987) have subsequently reported decreased CSF beta-endorphin and other pro-opiomelanocortin-related peptides in underweight anorexic patients, normalising after restoration of their weight. They suggested that a reduction of these pro-opiomelanocortin peptides is a result of weight loss and malnutrition in these patients.

The apparent discrepancy between these studies is probably best explained by the methodological differences between them and by the higher weight of Gerner and Sharp's patients. The earlier studies of Gerner and Sharp, and Kaye *et al.* (1982) used radio receptor assays studying total opioid activity. The more recent study of Kaye *et al.* (1987) used a radio immunoassay which looks at specific peptides of the opioid family (Frecska and Davis, 1991). Frecska and Davis suggest that the pituitary-ACTH-beta-endorphin hyperactivity in anorexia nervosa contributes to the metabolic changes and endocrinologic abnormalities, whereas the behavioural aspects (food refusal) may relate to the decreased hypothalamic pro-opiomelanocortin function with a dissociation between the pituitary and hypothalamic pro-opiomelanocortin systems.

8. CSF in Systemic Illness Affecting the CNS

Uraemia

CSF findings in uraemic patients include elevated pressure (possibly related to congestive heart failure and increased central venous pressure), pleocytosis, elevated urea (proportional to the rise in serum values) and increased protein (Fishman, 1980). The CSF levels of chloride and nonprotein nitrogen reflect the alterations in serum levels (Tourtellotte and Shorr, 1982). Sullivan *et al.* (1980) have also detected raised concentrations of CSF tryptophan and 5-HIAA in uraemic encephalopathy, suggesting that abnormal central serotonin metabolism may play a role in aetiology of the encephalopathy. CSF 5-HIAA was noted to decrease moderately following dialysis. Sperschneider *et al.* (1982) also found increased tryptophan concentrations in post-mortem CSF specimens of uraemic patients and detected the presence of "middle molecular weight substances" (peptides of 500-5000 daltons) in both the serum and CSF. These middle molecular weight substances have been implicated in the pathogenesis of uraemic neuropathy and encephalopathy. Increased CSF levels of phosphate have also been implicated in the twitching movements seen in uraemic encephalopathy.

Hypertension

There is considerable evidence linking central catecholamine metabolism, particularly norepinephrine, to the pathogenesis of hypertension. Some of this evidence was discussed earlier in the section on catecholamines in the CSF. Those regions of the CNS implicated in the regulation of arterial blood pressure, e.g. the nucleus tractus solitarii, nucleus dorsalis motorius/nervi vagi, the hypothalamus, and the intermediolateral cell columns, are innervated by noradrenergic neurons and destruction of these neurons has been shown to prevent certain types of hypertension in animals (Scriabine *et al.*, 1976). The antihypertensive effects of clonidine and methyldopa are also thought due to their actions on central alpha-adrenergic receptors (Scriabine *et al.*, 1976).

Increased concentrations of both norepinephrine (Lake *et al.*, 1980*a*, 1981*a*; Major *et al.*, 1984), and its principal metabolite methoxyhydroxy-phenylglycol (MHPG) (Saran *et al.*, 1978) have been detected in the CSF of patients with hypertension. The fact that younger hypertensives have the highest CSF NE levels suggests that CSF NE is highest early in the development of hypertension (Major et al., 1984). Furthermore both substances correlate directly with the severity of the hypertension (Saran et al., 1978, Major et al., 1984). Investigations into the role of peripheral noradrenegic function are more controversial. Both increased (Esler et al., 1977) and normal (Lake et al., 1980a, 1981a; Major et al., 1984) concentrations of plasma norepinephrine in hypertensives have been reported. Further CSF studies of catecholamines and their metabolites may help elucidate their role in the development of essential hypertension.

Involvement of the renin-angiotensin system has also been implicated in the regulation of blood pressure and the pathogenesis of hypertension. Ito et al. (1980) found both plasma and CSF levels of angiotensinogen to be elevated in hypertensive patients, though neither correlated significantly with arterial pressure. They also demonstrated differences in the immunological and chemical nature of these, suggesting the CSF angiotensinogen to be of central origin.

Alcoholism

Acute alcoholic intoxication results in an increase in the CSF cell count, protein, and pressure, as well as detectable amounts of ethanol and acetaldehyde which are capable of penetrating the blood-CSF barrier (De Jong, 1979; Poso et al., 1981). The CSF in chronic alcoholism and the alcohol withdrawal states may include the above findings as well as alterations in acid-base balance, lactate, urate, neurotransmitter metabolites, opiate-like alkaloids, neuropeptides, and cyclic nucleotides.

CSF lactate and acid base changes

Chronic alcoholics may exhibit a significant CSF acidosis which is not associated with systemic acidosis and persists for several weeks after the last drink (Carlen et al., 1980). This acidosis may be at a level usually associated with severe morbidity in normal patient populations, yet the alcoholic may remain ambulatory and retain fairly normal mental capabilities (Wilkinson and Carlen, 1982). Brooks and Adams (1975) studied alcoholics who had recently undergone withdrawal seizures and found no difference in CSF acid-base status compared to control values. They did note, however that CSF lactate was markedly increased in these patients. Patients with delirium tremens of recent onset without withdrawal seizures show evidence of a mixed metabolic and repiratory alkalosis in both CSF and arterial blood samples as well as increased lactate in both (Brooks, 1980). A marked elevation of CSF lactate (> 3.0 mEq/l) occurring shortly after a seizure may indicate a prolonged course of delirium tremens in alcoholic patients (Brooks, 1980).

Uric acid

CSF uric acid is markedly elevated in alcoholic withdrawal states (Carlsson and Dencker, 1973). This increase may be a reflection of altered nucleic acid catabolism or merely a nonspecific result of the increased CSF protein (Fishman, 1980).

Serotonin (5-HT)

Beck *et al.* (1983) reported that, although acute ethanol ingestion in normal subjects will lower CSF tryptophan levels (the amino acid precursor of 5-HT), chronic alcoholics have high CSF tryptophan levels suggesting altered 5-HT metabolism in alcoholics. Banki (1981) reported decreased levels of the 5-HT metabolite 5-HIAA in recently abstinent (after 4-8 days) female alcoholics. CSF levels of the 5-HT precursor tryptophan did not differ from those of neurologic controls, indicating that these findings were not due to insufficient tryptophan availability. The 5-HIAA levels correlated inversely with number of days of abstinence. These results are in agreement with a similar study by Ballenger *et al.* (1979). Zarcone *et al.* (1977) also found CSF 5-HIAA levels to decrease significantly in chronic alcoholics after one day of alcohol ingestion. Orenberg *et al.* (1976) also noted 5-HIAA to decrease in seven of 11 alcoholic subjects after ethanol ingestion. They also noted the changes in 5-HIAA paralleled those of cAMP. Banki (1981) suggested that a deficiency of central indoleamines may be linked to development of dependence and to the increased frequency of depression seen in alcoholics, particularly following abstinence.

These findings suggesting decreased 5-HT metabolism are interesting in view of the pharmacological studies showing zimelidine, a 5-HT reuptake inhibitor, may decrease alcohol consumption in both human and rat studies (see review of Tabakoff and Hoffman, 1987). 5-HTergic systems thus appear to play an important role in ethanol-induced reinforcement and may well be amenable to pharmacological modulation (Tabakoff and Hoffman, 1987).

A study by Banki and Molnar (1981*b*) of 14 male alcoholics with delirium tremens found both CSF 5-HIAA and tryptophan significantly elevated compared to neurologic controls. The CSF 5-HIAA concentrations correlated with severity of delirium tremens, and with symptoms of disorientation and hallucinations. They suggested that central 5-HT metabolism was increased via positive feedback in order to overcome central receptor hypoactivity. In contrast, Fujimoto *et al.* (1983) found no variation from controls of 5-HIAA in patients with alcohol withdrawal delirium or with minor asymptomatic withdrawal.

Martin *et al.* (1989) looked at CSF somatostatin and CSF 5-HIAA concentrations in patients with Korsakoff's psychosis (KP) and dementia associated with alcoholism (DAA). They found treatment with fluvoxamine, a 5-HT reuptake blocker, improved episodic memory in patients with Korsakoff's psychosis and these improvements were correlated with the decreased levels observed in CSF 5-HIAA levels in these patients. They also noted low CSF somatostatin levels in patients with DAA, within the range reported for Alzheimer's and Parkinson's disease. Although their study was a small one, it has some interesting possible implications for the role of serotonin in alcoholic amnestic disorder.

Ballenger *et al.* (1979) have suggested that alcoholics may have pre-existing low CNS 5-HT levels which may be transiently increased with ethanol ingestion, but that 5-HT levels will, with repeated drinking, be further depleted thus resulting in a "vicious cycle", continually trying to make up for their central 5-HT deficit. Diminished central serotonin turnover, as reflected by low CSF 5-HIAA levels, is associated with impulsivity, suicide and aggression towards self and others in a number of psychiatric conditions besides alcoholism and may be a trait related phenomenon (Asberg *et al.* 1987; Brown and Goodwin, 1986; Ricci and Wellman, 1990). This diminished 5-HT turnover in alcoholism may well then relate to the impulsive violent behaviour towards themselves and towards others seen in alcoholism and may be amenable to modification with 5-HTergic drugs (Roy *et al.* 1987). Roy *et al.* (1990c), however, recently did not find any difference in CSF 5-HIAA levels between alcoholics who had a history of suicide attempts and those who had not, compared to healthy volunteers, although they point out that only five of the 20 alcoholics in their study had made a violent suicide attempt. This may be important as CSF 5-HIAA levels appear to relate more clearly to violent than to nonviolent attempts. Linnoila *et al.* (1989) looked at CSF 5-HIAA levels in 54 violent offenders with alcoholism and found that 35 of their subjects with alcoholic fathers had lower CSF 5-HIAA levels and were more impulsive than those without alcoholic fathers. They suggest that low 5-HIAA levels in the CSF may delineate a subgroup of alcoholics compatible with the type II alcoholism inherited from fathers to sons, suggested by adoption studies and associated with aggressive and impulsive behaviour. Limson *et al.* (1991) have recently found a significant negative correlation between CSF 5-HIAA and lifetime aggression scores in alcoholics.

Gamma aminobutyric acid (GABA)

Increased, decreased, and normal brain GABA concentrations as a result of acute alcohol administration have all been reported (Colangelo and Jones 1982). Goldman *et al.* (1981) found CSF levels of GABA in alcoholics without seizures to be significantly higher than in either alcoholics with seizures or in controls. Alcoholics with withdrawal seizures had levels similar to control values. They suggested that alcohol withdrawal seizures may be related to a decreased affinity of central GABA receptors. The finding of increased GABA levels in alcoholics without seizures could then represent a compensation for this decreased affinity, preventing the occurrence of seizures.

Norepinephrine (NE)

Though acute ethanol administration has no significant effect on steady state levels of brain NE, the turnover rate of NE is affected in a variety of ways in different regions of the brain (Noble and Tewari, 1977; Colangelo and Jones, 1982). Major *et al.* (1980, 1984) studied CSF dopamine beta-hydroxylase (DBH), the enzyme which converts DA to NE, in chronic alcoholics and related low levels to personality disorders in these patients. They also found that low levels of CSF DBH were associated with susceptibility to adverse disulfiram reactions.

Several studies have demonstrated increased CSF NE or its metabolites in alcoholics. Hawley *et al.* (1981*b*) showed CSF NE to be higher in alcoholics during acute withdrawal than after recovery from withdrawal and higher in both when compared to neurologic controls. Borg *et al.* (1981) have reported elevated levels of CSF MHPG, the major metabolite of NE, in both withdrawal and in acute intoxication, suggesting increased central noradrenergic activity. Following acute intoxication CSF MHPG declined successively at one and three weeks of abstinence. Blood alcohol levels correlated significantly with the CSF MHPG concentrations during intoxication. Alcohol ingestion in healthy volunteers also increased CSF MHPG levels. They thus suggest that alcohol acts to enhance NE activity in both alcoholics and nonalcoholic subjects. Sjoquist *et al.* (1981) also reported similar effects of alcohol intoxication on CSF MHPG concentrations. Fujimoto *et al.* (1983) found CSF MHPG to correlate with the severity of withdrawal symptoms and to be markedly elevated in severe alcohol withdrawal.

Hawley *et al.* (1985) measured CSF and plasma levels of MHPG during alcohol withdrawal and found increased CSF MHPG levels relating to the alcohol withdrawal state, which they calculated to be of central origin. These CSF levels correlated positively with blood pressure, tremor, heart rate, decreased appetite and sweating. They postulate that the increased CSF NE and MHPG in alcohol withdrawal may relate to these symptoms of sympathetic hyperactivity and could be a compensatory response to a subsensitivity of or related to damage to α-2 adrenoreceptors. This could then be one possible explanation for the therapeutic effects of clonidine, an α-2 agonist, in ethanol withdrawal.

Dopamine (DA)

Alcohol dependence, withdrawal, and tolerance have all been linked to dopaminergic mechanisms by various animal and pharmacological studies (Tabakoff et al., 1980; Colangelo and Jones, 1982).

CSF studies of HVA in withdrawal states have shown some conflicting results. Banki and Molnar (1981) found CSF HVA, the major DA metabolite, to be elevated in alcoholics with delirium tremens. HVA concentrations correlated closely with symptoms of motor agitation. In contrast, Fujimoto et al. (1983) found CSF HVA levels to be decreased in alcohol-withdrawal delirium. Banki (1981) showed CSF HVA levels to correlate with severity of withdrawal symptoms in recently abstaining (within 4 days) alcoholics but found no difference in concentrations compared to neurologic controls.

Several studies have also looked at the effects of acute alcohol ingestion on DA metabolites in alcoholics. A study by Zarcone et al. (1977) noted increases in CSF HVA in three chronic alcoholic subjects, decreases in five, and no change in one following one day of alcohol ingestion. However, no overall significant difference in HVA levels was found. Orenberg et al. (1976) also noted no consistent pattern of change in CSF HVA in alcoholics following the drinking of ethanol. Ballenger et al. (1979) similarly found no significant differences in CSF HVA levels in alcoholics in the immediate post-intoxication period or during abstinence compared to controls.

Major et al. (1977) measured CSF HVA levels in drug-free and disulfiram-treated alcoholics compared to age-matched controls with a diagnosis of personality disorder. They found CSF HVA levels to be significantly lower following treatment with disulfiram suggesting that this was due to the inhibiting effect of disulfiram on the enzyme aldehyde dehydrogenase (ADH) which breaks down DA to HVA. They speculated that in addition to the well known peripheral effects of disulfiram, it may also have direct central effects and that this inhibition of aldehyde dehydrogenase could increase aldehyde intermediaries of DA, leading to the formation of the morphine-like alkaloid tetra-hydropapaveroline (THP). They hypothesise that this alteration of DA metabolism could then account for some of the therapeutic effects and central side-effects of disulfiram.

Catecholamine-derived alkaloids

The condensation of biogenic amines with acetaldehyde (a direct metabolite of ethanol) or other aldehydes may cause the formation of isoquinoline alkaloids related to naturally occurring plant alkaloids thought to be morphine precursors (Noble and Tewari, 1977; Cohen, 1971). These compounds have been implicated in the aetiology of alcohol dependence. Salsoline and salsolinol are two such compounds formed from the condensation of DA and acetaldehyde. Borg *et al.* (1980) detected salsoline and salsolinol in the CSF of alcoholics, both after a heavy alcoholic binge and after one week of abstention, using gas chromatography-mass spectrometry (GC-MS). Marked individual variations in concentration were noted and several subjects had no detectable levels. Sjoquist *et al.* (1981) also detected minor amounts of salsolinol as well as methylated salsinol in the CSF of hospitalized alcoholics also using GC-MS. These compounds were detectable within the first week following long-standing intoxication but not after.

The hypothesis that alcoholism could be related to the endogenous formation of opiate alkaloids via amine-aldehyde condensation is an intriguing possibility. Myers (1985) has reviewed the human and animal data relating to this. There is also evidence that these aldehyde adducts are responsible for some of the acute alcohol withdrawal symptoms in addition to their suggested role in dependence (see review of Airaksinen and Peura, 1987).

Neuropeptides

Genazzani *et al.* (1982) studied pro-opiocortin-related peptides in the CSF of alcoholics and found three-fold lower levels of beta-endorphin and four-fold higher concentrations of ACTH compared to normal controls. They suggested that a central deficiency of beta-endorphin may exist in alcoholics through a feedback inhibition by isoquinolines or other mechanisms. This could play an important role in alcohol dependence mechanisms. Savoldi *et al.* (1983) also found decreased CSF beta-endorphin levels and increased CSF ACTH levels in chronic alcoholics, as well as unaffected beta-lipotrophin levels.

CSF levels of somatostatin, corticotrophin-releasing hormone (CRF) and corticotrophin (ACTH), and galanin levels have not been shown to differ from controls in alcoholics maintaining abstinence for at least three weeks before sampling (Roy *et al.*, 1990a,b). Adinoff *et al.* (1990) have, however demonstrated a blunted response to ovine CRH in nine of 11 alcoholics measured at one and three weeks of abstinence, compared to controls measuring plasma and CSF levels of CRH and corticotrophin. Alcoholics then, particularly in the withdrawal state, appear to have significant hypothalamic-pituitary-adrenal (HPA) axis dysfunction and Adinoff *et al.* suggest that repeated withdrawal episodes could cause a progressive exacerbation of hypercortisolism related to adrenal hypertrophy.

Cyclic nucleotides

Since the cyclic nucleotides are thought to play an important role in the modulation of the effects of neurotransmitters, alterations in cAMP and cGMP have been implicated in alcohol dependence and tolerance (Noble and Tewari, 1977; Zimmer *et al.*, 1982). Weitbrecht and Cramer (1980) studied cyclic nucleotides in rat CSF and noted decreases in both cAMP and cGMP after acute ethanol administration. Zarcone *et al.* (1977) also found CSF cAMP to decrease in chronic alcoholics following one day of alcohol ingestion, as did Orenberg *et al.* (1976). Hawley *et al.* (1981*a*) noted no difference in cAMP or cGMP in CSF samples taken from alcoholics during acute alcohol withdrawal compared to samples taken from the same patients during convalescence. In contrast, Zimmer *et al.* (1982) found reduced CSF cAMP levels in acute delirium tremens which did not change two weeks later following recovery. Concentrations of cGMP were elevated in acute delirium tremens and further increased two weeks later. Both cAMP and cGMP thus appear to decrease as an acute effect of alcohol ingestion, but there are some conflicting results in the studies looking at withdrawal states in alcoholism.

Conclusion

CSF studies in alcoholism have helped elucidate some of the biochemical mechanisms suggested by the pharmacological and animal studies. CSF studies of the serotonin metabolite 5-HIAA have shown some inconsistencies, but have generally indicated decreased serotonin turnover as reflected in diminished levels of CSF 5-HIAA. This may relate to the pathogenesis of dependency itself and possibly to the impulsive and aggressive behaviours associated with alcoholism. It may well also relate to a subgroup of alcoholics consistent with type II alcoholism and may have some potential therapeutic implications for these patients. CSF studies of GABA have indicated that this neurotransmitter may be important in the pathogenesis of withdrawal seizures in alcoholics and studies of norepinephrine and its metabolite MHPG have shown that their elevation in CSF is associated with the withdrawal state and may relate to withdrawal symptoms. CSF studies in alcoholism have provided some preliminary evidence for the hypothesis that acetaldehyde-amine condensation products forming isoquinoline alkaloids may relate to the pathogenesis of alcohol dependence, although these studies require replication and further investigations to make any conclusions. The CSF studies of neuropeptides have given some evidence for a deficiency-state of beta-endorphin in alcoholics and for HPA axis dysfunction.

Systemic Lupus Erythematosus

Systemic lupus erythematosus is a generalised autoimmune disorder associated with the production of multiple autoantibodies, the most well known being antinuclear antibodies. Multi-organ involvement is seen with organs being affected by various types of vasculopathy including vasculitis. It is most common in young females (15 to 35 years of age). For the purpose of verifying the diagnosis, criteria have been established which usually require the presence of a positive test for antinuclear antibodies and at least four cardinal manifestations such as skin abnormalities (butterfly rash, discoid lesions, photosensitivity), arthritis, pleuritis or pericarditis, neurologic abnormalities, haematologic abnormalities, renal involvement, fever, lymphadenopathy and myalgias. Other laboratory support for the diagnosis includes the presence of hypocomplementaemia, positive LE cell test, increased serum gamma globulin, positive tests for rheumatoid factor, biological false positive tests for syphilis, and circulating anticoagulants.

Neuropsychiatric disorders appear early in the course of SLE in over half the cases, and rarely may constitute presenting symptoms (Feinglass *et al.,* 1976). Patients may present with stroke, seizures, delirium, dementia, coma, psychosis, affective disorders, movement disorders, myelopathy, and neuropathy. It is now well established that there are multiple mechanisms for these neuropsychiatric manifestations of SLE, including thromboembolism (usually in association with antiphospholipid antibodies), metabolic derangements and, less frequently, vasculitis or intracerebral haemorrhage. A possible role for antineuronal antibodies in producing non-focal symptoms of neuropsychiatric SLE (altered mental states, generalised seizures, and the presence of these antibodies appears to be a marker for such cases of diffuse central nervous system (CNS) SLE.

Multiple spinal fluid abnormalities are frequently present when SLE affects the CNS. Understanding these abnormalities may greatly help clinicians in determining the mechanism of CNS injury and guide therapy. For example, abnormal intrathecal immunoglobulin production or blood-brain barrier disturbance found by CSF exam might suggest that a patient's psychosis is due to active autoimmune processes of SLE rather than steroids.

Cellularity and total protein

The most typical abnormalities of CSF seen on routine studies in neuropsychiatric lupus (or "cerebral lupus") are mild pleocytosis and slight elevation of total protein concentration (Johnson and Richardson, 1968). Lymphocytes predominate, but are occasionally outnumbered by neutrophils (Gibson and Myers, 1976). Clinicians must avoid complaisance when CSF shows these typical findings, seen in about half the cases, since often infectious processes, e.g. chronic and acute meningitis due to a variety of organisms, occur in these patients (Ellis and Verity, 1979). Thus appropriate cultures and repeat CSF analysis may be needed. Occasionally patients will present with a picture of aseptic meningitis consisting of headache, meningismus, and CSF pleocytosis without identifiable cause other than lupus.

Increased CSF protein concentration may be due to inflammation, other mechanisms which disrupt the blood-brain barrier, or intrathecal production of immunoglobulins. Reports have differed concerning the frequency of disturbance of the blood-brain barrier, measured as a ratio of serum to CSF albumin, but such disturbance is probably common (Zvaifler and Bluestein, 1982; Ernerudh et al., 1985). The possibility of disturbance of the blood-CSF barrier at the choroid plexus is still debated. Although deposits of immunoglobulin are found in the choroid plexus in cerebral lupus, this may be a very non-specific abnormality found in a number of disease states (Boyer et al., 1980).

CSF immunoglobulins

Investigations into the pathology of lupus have long focused on autoantibodies in the serum, and CSF studies have been similar. Evidence for tissue injury due to immune complex formation and vasculitis in systemic lupus make it tempting to propose similar mechanisms of injury in cerebral lupus. However, only a small percentage of autopsy specimens have shown cerebral vasculitis (Ellis and Verity, 1979). Vascular abnormalities other than vasculitis, consisting of endothelial proliferation, subendothelial hyalin deposits, perivascular lymphocytosis, and diffuse microinfarcts (possibly due to thrombosis), are common. Thus ischaemia seems likely to contribute to neuropsychiatric lupus, and this is further supported by cerebral perfusion studies. Evidence for neuronal dysfunction due to antineuronal antibodies has also been sought. Antineuronal antibodies, as defined by a variety of assays have indeed been demonstrated by a number of investigators.

Early successes in demonstrating antineuronal antibodies involved using neuroblastoma cell lines and immunofluorescent techniques (Bluestein *et al.*, 1981). Multiple studies verified the positive findings of these early investigators, and a wide variety of assays involving multiple neural antigens have been developed. Some of these assays are now commercially available, but their accuracy is questionable. Bluestein has continued to study a large number of patients with cerebral lupus, and finds antineuronal antibody activity in about 80% of cases (Bluestein, 1988). These antibodies, primarily IgG, are found less often in groups of patients with focal neurologic symptoms, and are rarely seen in lupus patients without neuropsychiatric symptoms. Antineuronal antibodies appear to be concentrated in the CSF as compared to serum.

Examination of CSF for concentration of IgG, both as absolute concentration and expressed as an "IgG index" is widely available. Elevation of the IgG index is correlated with the presence of cerebral symptoms in multiple studies (Zvaifler and Bluestein, 1982; Winfield *et al.*, 1983). In serial studies of individual patients, the IgG index also correlates with the presence of cerebral symptoms (Hirohata *et al.*, 1985). Bluestein has noted that increases in the IgG index may be due to local production of IgG, depressed CSF albumin (seen frequently), or accumulation of IgG locally due to binding to neuronal elements (Bluestein, 1988). The CSF IgM index may be a more sensitive indicator than the IgG index for active CNS disease, being elevated in 100% of cases of CNS lupus in one series (Hirohata *et al.*, 1985) and the IgA index is also generally elevated in CNS lupus. The clinical usefulness of these indices clearly deserves more study as they appear to be helpful indicators of disease activity as well as of response of the CNS lesions to treatment (Hirohata *et al.*, 1985).

Oligoclonal bands are also seen frequently in the CSF in cerebral lupus (Ernerudh *et al.*, 1985), but probably are a less frequent finding than in multiple sclerosis. Their significance, other than the fact that they are found in patients with cerebral symptoms, is unknown.

Miscellaneous considerations

A variety of other abnormalities suggesting disturbance of immune function have been reported in CSF studies in lupus, but their clinical significance remains to be defined. CSF complement levels may be low in active disease, but deterioration of complement is rapid and this makes a practical assay tenuous.

Subarachnoid haemorrhage has been reported in many patients with lupus. This is usually in the absence of aneurysm, and is often associated with the presence of vasculitis (Ellis and Verity, 1979). This should be considered when spinal fluid appears xanthochromic or when excess red blood cells are present.

Opening pressure is usually normal. When elevations of opening pressure are found, pseudotumour cerebri (or benign intracranial hypertension) should be considered and other pathology appropriately ruled out. Several cases of intracranial hypertension have been reported in lupus, and steroid withdrawal is often suspected to be contributory. In patients with lupus nephropathy, hypervitaminosis A should also be considered as a cause of pseudotumour cerebri.

Glucose concentration is rarely decreased in neuropsychiatric lupus, and again pathology other than lupus should be considered when this is found (Abel et al., 1980).

Concluding remarks

Although the abnormalities of cerebrospinal fluid mentioned above are generally nonspecific (with the possible exception of some of the antineuronal antibody assays), these abnormalities may be very helpful when placed within the context of a specific patient with cerebral lupus. A frequent diagnostic dilemma is the patient with SLE on steroids who presents with acute psychosis. Such a patient may have contributing metabolic disturbances. In this case a spinal fluid revealing a high IgG or IgM index and mild pleocytosis is highly suggestive of cerebral lupus.

The studies mentioned in this review primarily involved patients with generalised symptoms of cerebral lupus (generalised seizures, psychosis, coma, other altered mental states), and it is this group of patients which frequently display abnormalities of the blood-brain barrier and immunoglobulin abnormalities in the spinal fluid. It is interesting to note that this group of patients also display diffuse abnormalities on electro-encephalography and tests of cerebral metabolism and cerebral perfusion. Unfortunately, many studies of neuropsychiatric lupus have not attempted to distinguish patient groups which may constitute important clinical subsets in terms of CSF profiles. Future studies should consider certain focal neurological disorders associated with lupus separately from those with diffuse abnormalities.

Hepatic Encephalopathy

The CSF in hepatic encephalopathy generally shows increases in protein, ammonia, glutamine, and alpha-ketoglutaramate. The pressure is usually normal except in the acute fulminant forms of hepatic encephalopathy where there is brain oedema and severe intracranial hypertension (see review of Fishman, 1992 pp. 320-322). The most useful clinical parameter to follow in hepatic encephalopathy is the CSF glutamine although it may also be elevated in patients with liver disease without hepatic encephalopathy (Zacarias et al., 1971). Other amino acids are also elevated in the CSF and there is evidence for both a non-specific increase in BBB permeability and for selective stimulation of neutral amino acid transport systems across the BBB (Cascino *et al.*, 1982). The increased CSF glutamine, however probably relates to the increased ammonia and results from glutamate metabolism (Zacarias *et al.*, 1971).

There have been alterations found in the CSF metabolites of catecholamines, serotonin, histamine and GABA in hepatic encephalopathy, and false transmitters have also been hypothesised to play a role in its pathogenesis (Borg *et al.*, 1982). The finding of increased quinolinic acid in the CSF and frontal cortex of patients with hepatic coma suggests also a role for excitotoxicity (Moroni *et al.*, 1986). The finding by several investigators of an increased concentration of the neuropeptide diazepam binding inhibitor (DBI) correlating with disease activity, and the amelioration of some manifestations of hepatic encephalopathy with benzodiazepine receptor antagonists suggests a role for this "endogenous benzodiazepine" as well as for GABA (Mullen *et al.*, 1990; Jones *et al.*, 1989; Rothstein *et al.*, 1989*a,b*). As levels of DBI are not elevated in patients with liver disease not associated with mental status changes or in patients with non-hepatic encephalopathy, these findings could have both diagnostic and therapeutic potential.

9. Current and Future Clinical Utility of Cerebrospinal Fluid in Neurology and Psychiatry

The preceding chapters have discussed many hundreds of laboratory tests that can be performed on cerebrospinal fluid. Table 9.1 summarises the practice parameters for lumbar puncture in adults and children for both diagnostic and therapeutic purposes as defined by the Quality Standards Subcommittee of the American Academy of Neurology (AAN) (single asterisks), their relative sensitivity and specificity as defined by the Health and Public Policy Committee of the American College of Physicians (ACP) (double asterisks), and some of the new more promising indications discussed in the previous chapters here. As the study of CSF continues to blossom, and as the political and financial realities of health care are changing, it is becoming more important to realise the clinical potential and limitations of laboratory testing. The committees of the ACP (1986), AAN (1993), and Fishman (1992, pp. 345-352) have addressed some of these controversial issues. Table 9-1 addresses the current clinical indications, non-indications, potential indications, and contraindications for lumbar puncture.

Currently, the major indication for lumbar puncture in neurology and psychiatry is to exclude CNS infection. Recent years have seen exciting advances discussed in earlier chapters. Immunological tests including countercurrent immunoelectrophoresis (CIE), enzyme-linked immuno-sorbent assays (ELISA), and organism-specific antibody indices (OSAI) are becoming more and more clinically useful. CIE and ELISA are being used more frequently in the detection of bacterial antigens and OSAI has been looked at in coccidioides meningitis, cryptococcal meningitis, cystericercosis cerebri, CMV meningoencephalitis, HIV infection, HIV encephalopathy, *Rochalimeae henselae* infection, HSV encephalitis, mumps meningitis, neuroborreliosis, neurobrucellosis, neurosyphilis, rubella meningoencephalitis, SSPE, toxoplasmosis, tropical spastic paraparesis, and varicella meningoencephalitis, among others (see Peter, 1993 for review). Perhaps the most exciting new technology in CNS infections, however, is the polymerase chain reaction (PCR) which promises to be able to quickly measure specific viral, bacterial, and fungal nucleic acids and antigens, and specific genetic markers. It has been looked at thus far in tuberculous meningitis, HIV infection, *R.henselae* infection,

arbo- and echovirus infections, *toxoplasma gondii* infection, neuroborreliosis, and HSV encephalitis. Its major drawback at this time appears
to be that it may be too sensitive and subject to cross-contamination.

In addition to these advances, there are also some promising potential
diagnostic markers for Alzheimer's disease, C-J disease, amyloid
angiopathy, and the lysosomal storage diseases among others. The greatest
need for the future, however, in CSF studies is that of clinically useful
markers in psychiatric and neuropsychiatric illness. The study of CSF
neurotransmitters and peptides has produced some exciting insights into
subcategories of neuropsychiatric illness and into disease mechanisms, but
more work needs to be done in finding clinically useful diagnostic CSF
markers and predictors of treatment response in this growing field.

TABLE 9.1. *Lumbar puncture practice parameters (see text for discussion of specific
    tests).*

I *Diagnostic Lumbar Puncture in Adults*
  A. Diseases detected with high sensitivity and high specificity**
     *1. Bacterial meningitis [CSF profile, gram stain, CIE, ELISA]
     *2. Tuberculous meningitis [CSF profile, acid fast stain, culture, PCR]
     *3. Fungal meningitis [CSF profile, microscopy, culture, cryptococcal anti-
        gen, OSAI]
  B. Diseases detected with high sensitivity and moderate specificity**
     *1. Viral meningitis [CSF profile, antibody titre increases, culture, OSAI,
        PCR; currently most of these studies are still of epidemidogical interest
        and not of clinical utility]
     *2. Subarachnoid haemorrhage [xanthochromia, RBCs, CSF D-dimer; L.P.
        indicated only if CT scan is not diagnostic or if meningitis suspected]
     *3. Multiple sclerosis [IgG index, oligoclonal bands, MBP]
     *4. Neurosyphilis [positive reagin test is diagnostic]
     *5. Infectious polyneuritis [CSF profile, increased protein]
      6. Paraspinal abscess [CSF of limited specificity in parameningeal infection
        and abscess; better evaluated by neuroimaging]
  C. Diseases detected with moderate sensitivity and high specificity**
     *1. Meningeal malignancy [pleocytosis, ↑ protein, ↓ glucose, cytology, CSF
        tumour markers]
  D. Diseases detected with moderate sensitivity and moderate specificity**
      1. Intracranial haemorrhage [better evaluated by neuroimaging; CSF may
        be useful if amyloid angiopathy suspected]
     *2. Viral encephalitis [CSF profile, culture, OSAI, PCR; viral antibodies
        identified for HSV, CMV, Arboviruses (Eastern equine, La Crosse,
        Western equine, St. Louis), influenza viruses A and B, LCM, adenovirus,
        echovirus, coxsackie A and B, measles, varicella-zoster, and mumps]
      3. Subdural haematoma [not an indication for LP; best evaluated with
        neuroimaging]

TABLE 9.1 *Cont.*

E. Other recognised indications for L.P.

*1. Cysticercosis, toxoplasmosis, and rickettsia infections [produce an eosinophilic pleocytosis; OSAI in cysticercosis and toxoplasmosis; PCR in toxoplasmosis]

*2. Amebic infections [culture, phase-contrast microscopy, CSF profile]

*3. Lyme borreliosis [CSF profile, *B.burgdorferi* antibodies, PCR]

*4. Aseptic meningitis [non-specific pleocytosis and ↑ protein; clues to specific diagnoses include large endothelial cells in Mollaret's meningitis, epithelioid cells in neurosarcoidosis, eosinophilia with immunoglobulin elevation in chemical and drug hypersensitivity meningitis, and fat droplets or keratin in craniopharyngioma, epidermoid or dermoid rupture]

*5. Inflammatory polyneuropathies [↑ protein, immunoglobulins]

*6. Brain tumours [non-specific changes for most tumours, better evaluated with neuroimaging; some specific markers, e.g. human chorionic gonadotrophin for metastatic trophoblastic and germ cell; and alpha-fetoprotein for germ cell tumours]

*7. Paraneoplastic syndromes [Purkinje cell antibodies (PCA, Yo) in paraneoplastic cerebellar degeneration associated with gynecologic and breast cancer; neuronal nuclear (NNA, Hu) antibodies in subacute sensory neuropathy and paraneoplastic encephalomyelitis associated with small cell lung cancer]

*8. Pseudotumour cerebri [requires LP to comfirm ↑ pressure and to exclude meningitis]

*9. Normal pressure hydrocephalus [may sometimes be helpful in prediction of response to shunting]

*10. Septic cerebral emboli [produces early pleocytosis]

*11. Systemic lupus erythematosus [↓ C4 levels, ↑ IgG, IgA, and IgM indices]

*12. Hepatic encephalopathy [↑ CSF glutamine]

*13. Subacute sclerosing panencephalitis (SSPE) [elevated measles antibodies can be diagnostic]

*14. Rubella panencephalitis [elevated virus-specific antibodies can be diagnostic]

F. Some diseases with newer diagnostic tests or tests of uncertain sensitivity and specificity

1. Stroke [better evaluated with neuroimaging; LP indicating only if SAH suspected and CT non-diagnostic, where CNS vasculitis is suspected, when tuberculous meningitis or other CNS infection is suspected, if septic cerebral emboli is suspected, in young patients with unexplained strokes, and in patients with AIDS or with positive serum syphilis serology]

2. HIV infection [LP indicated to exclude concomitant infection; β-2-microglobulin and other markers for HIV dementia have been proposed but await confirmation; HIV Ag and Ab of limited clinical utility]

3. Herpes simplex encephalitis [HSV-specific antibody index elevated but negative result does not exclude diagnosis; PCR is promising]

4. Tropical spastic paraparesis [elevated HTLV-1 antibody index]

5. Alzheimer's disease [decreased amyloid β-protein precursor]

6. Creutzfeldt-Jakob disease ['prion-associated proteins']

TABLE 9.1 *Cont.*
  7. Amyloid angiopathy [cystatin C, amyloid β-protein]
  8. Neurosarcoidosis [CSF angiotensin converting enzyme]
  9. Seizures [indicated only to exclude an acute CNS infection, or bleed despite a normal CT scan]
  10. Vitamin-deficiency states [B12, other levels]

II *Therapeutic Lumbar Puncture in Adults*
  A. Infections
    *1. Bacterial meningitis [requires intrathecal therapy only if cultures remain positive after 72 h of therapy, or if ventriculitis present]
    *2. Coccidioidomycosis and refractory cryptococcal, candidal, or histoplasmal meningitis [intrathecal amphotericin B]
  B. Neoplastic disease
    *1. Leukaemic meningitis [methotrexate and cytarabine]
    *2. Leptomeningeal lymphoma
    *3. Meningeal carcinomatosis [with breast carcinoma]
  *C. Postoperative Pain [low doses of morphine]
  *D. Headaches from increased intracranial pressure without a mass lesion [may give temporary relief of symptoms]

III *Relative Contraindications to Lumbar Puncture in Adults and Children (see text for discussion)*
  † A. Increased intracranial pressure with a mass lesion or ventricular obstruction
  † B. Complete spinal subarachnoid block
  † C. Coagulation defects
  † D. Local infection at the site of lumbar puncture
  † E. Bacteraemia [very occasionally associated with secondary meningitis – see discussion in Chapter 4]

IV *Diagnostic Lumbar Puncture in Children*
  *A. Meningitis [CSF changes may be less specific and findings initially normal in children; secondary meningitis related to bacteraemia at time of LP may be more common in children]
  *B. Other infections [as with adults; most show non-specific changes except for antibody titres in SSPE, measles, rubella, and progressive rubella panencephalitis]
  *C. Febrile seizures [only if clinical evidence of meningitis is present; likelihood of meningitis increased with focal seizures or abnormal neurologic findings; in infants less than 12 months, clinical signs of meningitis may be absent and LP generally indicated; ages 12-24 months LP indicated only if any question of meningitis; age >24 months, clinical signs more reliable]
  *D. Intracranial haemorrhage in neonates [xanthochromia]
  *E. Pseudotumour cerebri [requires measurment of ↑ CSF pressure for diagnosis]
  *F. Lead encephalopathy [↑ pressure, ↑ protein, pleocytosis]
  *G. CNS neoplasia [as with adults]
  H. Diseases with newer diagnostic tests of uncertain sensitivity and specificity.
    1. Lysosomal storage diseases [specific glycosphingolipids, see text for discussion of individual storage diseases]

TABLE 9.1 *Cont.*

V *Therapeutic Lumbar Puncture in Children*
  *A. Neoplastic diseases [warrants intrathecal therapy more commonly in children]
    1. Prophylaxis of the spread of acute leukaemia and lymphoma
    2. Therapy of medulloblastoma less successful
  *B. Refractory infections of the CNS
  *C. Increased intracranial pressure without mass lesion [repeated LP may be effective therapy in some children]
    *.1 Pseudotumour cerebri
    *2. Following haemorrhage or meningitis
  *D. Spinal anaesthesia [to avoid bronchopulmonary dysplasia and respiratory distress in children born prematurely undergoing surgery]
  *E. Pain control [intrathecal morphine]

VI *Incidental Lumbar Puncture in Adults and Children*
  *A. Indicated for myelography [same precautions and contraindications apply]

VII *Neuropsychiatric Conditions under Investigation* where there is, as yet, no clinical indication for lumbar puncture; includes but not limited to the following: Parkinson's disease, Huntington's chorea, dystonia, migraine, narcolepsy and hypersomnia, epilepsy, Tourette syndrome, schizophrenia, affective illness, attention deficit disorder, panic disorder, obsessive-compulsive disorder, autism, anorexia nervosa, uraemia, hypertension, alcoholism.

---

* = Recognised indications of the Quality Standards Subcommittee of the American Academy of Neurology (1993). (*Neurology*, **43**, 625-627).
** = As defined by the Health and Public Policy Committee of the American College of Physicians (1986).
† = Recognised (relative) contraindications of the Quality Standards Subcommittee of the American Academy of Neurology (1993).
OSAI = Organism-specific antibody index [see Peter (1993, pp. 179-181) for review]:

$$OSAI = \left[\frac{\text{Organism-specific Ig in CSF}}{\text{Total Ig in CSF}} \right] \div \left[\frac{\text{Organism-specific Ig in serum}}{\text{Total Ig in serum}} \right]$$

PCR = polymerase chain reaction.
Note: some of the newer diagnostic tests listed in this table are not at the time of publication readily available commercially and have not been specifically addressed by either the AAN or ACP committees. The clinician is advised to check with his/her local laboratory for commercial availablitity of specific tests.
CSF Profiles (appearance, cell count, protein, glucose, pressure) are outlined in Table 6.1 for specific illnesses.

References

Abel, T., Gladman, D.D. and Urowitz, M.B. (1980). Neuropsychiatric lupus. *Journal of Rheumatology*, **3**, 325-332.

Aberg-Wistedt, A., Jostell, K., Ross, S. and Westerland, D. (1981). Effects of zimelidine and desipramine on serotonin and noradrenaline uptake mechanisms in relation to plasma concentrations and to therapeutic effects during treatment of depression. *Psychopharmacology*, **74**, 297-305.

Abramson, J.S., Hampton, K.D. Babu, S. Wasilauskas, B.L. and Marcon, M.J. (1985). The use of C-reactive protein from cerebrospinal fluid for differentiating meningitis from other central nervous system diseases. *Journal of Infectious Diseases*, **151** (5), 854-858.

Ackermann, R., Rehse-Kupper, B., Gollmer, E. and Schmidt, R. (1988). Chronic neurologic manifestations of erythema migrans borreliosis. *Annals of the New York Academy of Science*, **539**, 16-23.

Adams, R.D. and Petersdorf, R.G. (1980). Pyogenic infections of the central nervous system. *In* "Principles of Internal Medicine". (Eds K.J. Isselbacher *et al.*). pp. 19-60. McGraw-Hill, New York.

Adams, R. and Victor, M. (1985). "Principles of Neurology". McGraw-Hill, New York.

Addy, D.P. (1987). When not to do a lumbar puncture. *Archives of Diseases in Childhood*, **62**, 873-875.

Adinoff B., Martin, P.R., Bone, G.H.A., Eckardt, M.J., Roehrich, L., George, D.T. *et al.* (1990). Hypothalamic-pituitary-adrenal axis functioning and cerebrospinal fluid corticotropin releasing hormone and corticotropin levels in alcoholics after recent and long-term abstinence. *Archives of General Psychiatry*, **47**, 325-330.

Adinolfi, M., Beck, S.E., Haddad, S.A. and Seller, M.J. (1976). Permeability of the blood-cerebrospinal fluid barrier to plasma proteins during foetal and perinatal life. *Nature*, **259**, 140-141.

Agid, Y., Taguet, H., Cesselin, F., Epelsbaum, J. and Javoy, F. (1986). Neuropeptides and Parkinson's Disease. *Progress in Brain Research*, **66**, 107-116.

Ahlskog, J., Kelly, P. van Heerden, J. *et al.* (1990). Adrenal medullary transplantation into the brain for treatment of Parkinson's Disease: clinical outcome and neurochemical studies. *Mayo Clinic Proceedings*, **65**, 305-328.

Ahonen, A., Myllyla, V. and Hokkanen, E. (1978). Measurement of reference values for certain proteins in CSF. *Acta Neurologica Scandinavica*, **57**, 358-365.

AIDS Task Force, American Academy of Neurology. (1989). Human immunodeficiency virus (HIV) infection and the nervous system. *Neurology*, **39**, 119-122.

Airaksinen, E.M. and Leino, E. (1982). Decrease of GABA in the CSF of patients with progressive myoclonus epilepsy and its correlation with the decrease of 5-HIAA and HVA. *Acta Neurologica Scandinavica*, **66**, 666-672.

Airaksinen M.M. and Peura, P. (1987). Mechanisms of alcohol withdrawal syndrome. *Medical Biology*, **65**, 105-112.

Akil, H. and Liebeskind, J. (1975). Monoaminergic mechanisms of stimulation-produced analgesia. *Brain Research,* **94,** 279-296.

Al-Kassab, S. and Olsen, T.S. (1982). The serum-albumin/CSF-albumin ratio and the Ig G-Index in various neurological diseases. *Acta Neurologica Scandinavica,* **65,** (Suppl 90) 264-265.

Alafuzoff, I., Adolfsson, R., Bucht, G. and Winblad, B. (1983). Albumin and immunoglobulin in plasma and cerebrospinal fluid, and blood-cerebrospinal fluid barrier function in patients with dementia of Alzheimer type and multi-infarct dementia. *Journal of the Neurological Science,* **60,** (3) 465-72.

Albrecht, P., Boone, E., Torrey, E., Hicks, J., and Daniel, N. (1980). Raised CMV antibody level in CSF of schizophrenic patients. *Lancet,* **ii,** 769-72.

Albrecht, P., Tourtellotte, W., Hicks, J.T., Sato, H. Boone, E. and Potvin, A. (1983). Intra-blood-brain barrier measles virus antibody synthesis in MS patients. *Neurology,* **33,** 45-50.

Albright, A., Marton, L., Lubich, W. and Reigel, D. (1983). CSF polyamines in childhood. *Archives of Neurology,* **40,** (4) 237-240.

Alfredsson, G., Bjerkenstedt, L., Edman, G. *et al.* (1984). Relationships between drug concentrations in serum and CSF, clinical effects and monoaminergic variables in schizophrenic patients treated with sulpiride or chlorpromazine. *Acta Psychiatrica Scandinavica,* **69,** (Suppl 311) 49-74.

Alom, J., Galard, R., Catalan, R., Castellanos, J.M. Schwartz, S. and Tolosa, E. (1990). Cerebrospinal fluid neuropeptide Y in Alzheimer's disease. *European Neurology,* **30,** 207-210.

Altemus, M., Pigatt, T., Kalogeras, K.T. *et al.* (1992). Abnormalities in the regulation of vasopressin and CRF secretion in OCD. *Archives of General Psychiatry,* **49,** 9-20.

Alter, M., Yamoor, M. and Harshe, M. (1974). Multiple sclerosis and nutrition. *Archives of Neurology,* **31,** 267-272.

Alvord, E., Hruby, S., C. Shaw, and Slimp, J. (1984*a*). MBP and its antibodies in the CSF in experimental allergic encephalomyelitis, multiple sclerosis and other diseases. *In* "Immunological and Clinical Aspects of Multiple Sclerosis". (Eds R. Gansette and P. Delmotte). pp. 39. MTP Press, Hingham, MA.

Alvord, E.C. Jr., Hruby, S., Shaw, C.M. and Slimp, J. (1984*b*). Myelin basic protein and its antibodies in the cerebrospinal fluid in experimental allergic encephalomyelitis, multiple sclerosis and other diseases. *Progress in Clinical Biological Research,* **146,** 359-363.

Anderson, G.M. (1987). Monoamines in autism: an update of neurochemical research on a pervasive developmental disorder. *Medical Biology,* **65,** 67-74.

Anderson, G.M., Bowers, M.B., Roth, R.H., Young, J.G., Hrbek, C.C. and Cohen, D.J. (1983). Comparison of high-performance liquid chromatographic, gas chromatographic – mass spectrometric, and fluorometric methods for the determination of homovanillic acid and 5-hydroxyindoleacetic acid in human cerebrospinal fluid. *Journal of Chromatography,* **277,** 282-286.

Anderson, G.M., Ross, D.L., Klykylo, W., Feibel, F.C. and Cohen, D.J. (1988). Cerebrospinal fluid indoleacetic acid in autistic subjects. *Journal of Autism and Developmental Disorders,* **18,** 259-262.

Angrist, B., Sathananthan, G., Wilk, S. and Gershon, S. (1974). Amphetamine psychosis: behavioral and biochemical aspects. *Journal of Psychiatric Research,*

11, 13-23.

Ansseau, M. and Reynolds, III. C.F. (1988). Neuropeptides and sleep. *In* "Neuropeptides in Psychiatric and Neurological Disorders". (Ed. C.B. Nemeroff), Chapter 8. Johns Hopkins University Press, Baltimore.

Anton, R.F., Ballenger, J.C., Lydiard, R.B., Laraia, M.T., Howell, E.F. and Gold, P.W. (1989). CSF Prostaglandin-E in agoraphobia with panic attacks. *Biological Psychiatry*, **26**, 257-264.

Appleman, M.E., Marshall, D.W., Brey, R.L., Houk, R.W., Beatty, D.C. *et al.* (1988). Cerebrospinal fluid abnormalities in patients without AIDS who are seropositive for the human immunodeficiency virus. *Journal of Infectious Diseases*, **158**, (1) 193-199.

Arieff, A.I. (1989). Acid-base balance in specialised tissues: central nervous system. *In* "The Regulation of Acid-Base Balance". (Eds D.W. Seldin and G. Biebisch). Chapter 6 Raven Press Ltd, New York.

Arnason B.G.W. (1984). Acute inflammatory demyelinating polyradicu-loneuropathies. *In* "Peripheral Neuropathy". 2nd Edn. (Eds P.J. Dyck, P.K. Thomas, E.H. Lambert and R. Burge), pp. 2050-2100. W.B. Saunders, Philadelphia.

Arnon, R., Kelley, R., Schumaker, V.N. and Fahey, J.L. (1979). Idiotype antiidiotype complexes in cerebrospinal fluids of multiple sclerosis patients. *Journal of the Neurological Sciences*, **43**, 149-156.

Asberg, M., Traskman, L. and Thoren, P. (1976). 5-HIAA in the CSF: A biochemical suicide predictor? *Archives of General Psychiatry*, **33**, 1193-1197.

Asberg, M., Bertilsson, L. and Martensson, B. (1984*a*). CSF monoamine metabolites, depression and suicide. *In* "Frontiers in Biochemical and Pharmacological Research in Depression". (Eds E. Usdin *et al.*), pp. 87-95. Raven Press, New York.

Asberg, M., Bertilsson, L., M'artensson, B., Scalia-Tomba, G.P., Thoren, P. and Traskman-Bendz, L. (1984*b*). CSF monoamine metabolites in melancholia. *Acta Psychiatrica Scandinavica*, **69**, (3) 201-219.

Asberg, M., Schalling, D., Traskman-Bendz, L. and Wagner, A. (1987). "Psychobiology of Suicide, Impulsivity, and Related Phenomena. Psychopharmacology: The Third Generation of Progress". (Ed. Herbert Y. Meltzer), pp. 655-668. Raven Press, New York.

Asbury, A.K. (1984). Uremic neuropathy. *In* "Peripheral Neuropathy". 2nd Edn. (Eds P.J. Dyck, P.K. Thomas, E.H. Lambert and R. Burge). pp. 1811-1825. W. B. Saunders, Philadelphia.

Asbury, A.K. and Cornblath, D.R. (1990). Assessment of current diagnostic criteria for Guillain-Barré syndrome. *Annals of Neurology*, **27**, (Suppl) S21-S24.

Asher, D.M., Gibbs, C.J. and Gajdvsek, D.C. (1985). Subacute spongiform encephalopathies: slow infections of the nervous system. *Clinical and Microbiological Newsletter*, **7**, 129-136.

Assies, J., Shellekens, A. and Touber, J. (1978). Prolactin in human CSF. *Journal of Clinical Endocrinology and Metabolism*, **46**, 576-586.

Austin, J.H. (1958). Recurrent polyneuropathies and their corticosteroid treatment. *Brain*, **81**, 157-192.

Bady, B., Vital, C., Brudon, F., Lapras, J., Kopp, N., and Trillet, M. (1988). Peripheral neuropathies simulating amyotrophic lateral sclerosis. *Review of*

Neurology, **144**, 710-715.

Bagdy, G. *et al.* (1984). Decrease of CSF dopamine, its metabolites, and noradrenalin after withdrawal of chronic neuroleptic treatment in schizophrenic patients. *Psychiatry Research*, **12**, 177-78.

Bagdy, G., Perenyi, A. *et al.* (1985) Decrease in dopamine, its metabolites and noradrenaline in cerebrospinal fluid of schizophrenic patients after withdrawal of long-term neuroleptic treatment. *Psychopharmacology*, **85**, 62-64.

Bagdy, G., Perenyi, E. *et al.* (1988). Effect of adjuvant reserpine treatment on catecholamine metabolism in schizophrenic patients under long-term neuroleptic treatment. *Journal of Neural Transmission*, **71**, 73-78.

Bailey, E.M., Domenico, P. and Cunha, B.A. (1990). Bacterial or viral meningitis? Measuring lactate in CSF can help you know quickly. *Postgraduate Medicine*, **88**, 217-223.

Bakay, L. (1956). "The Blood-Brain Barrier". C. Thomas Rollister, Springfield, Illinois.

Baker, L.L. (1983). Headache due to spontaneous low spinal fluid pressure. *Minn. Medicine*, **66**, 325-328.

Baker, H.F., Ridley, R.M., Crow, T.J. and Tyrrell, D. A. (1989). A re-investigation of the behavioural effects of intracerebral injection in marmosets of cytopathic cerebrospinal fluid from patients with schizophrenia or neurological disease. *Psychiatric Medicine*, **19**, 325-329.

Bakke, O.M., Guldberg, H.C. and Schreiner, A. (1974). Acid monoamine metabolites of CSF in meningitis and encephalitis. *Acta Neurologica Scandinavica*, **50**, 146-152.

Balhuizen, J.C., Bots, G., Schaberg, A. and Bosman, F. (1978). Value of CSF cytology for the diagnosis of malignancies in the central nervous system. *Journal of Neurosurgery*, **48**, 747-753.

Ballenger, J.C., Goodwin, F.K., Major, L.F. and Brown, G.L. (1979). Alcohol and central serotonin metabolism in man. *Archives of General Psychiatry*, **36**, 224-227.

Ballenger, J.C., Post, R.M. and Goodwin, F.K. (1983). Neurochemistry of CSF in normal individuals: relationship between biological and psychological variables. *In* "Neurobiology of Cerebrospinal Fluid 2". (Ed. J.H. Wood). pp. 143-156.

Bamworth, A. (1941). Chronische Lymphozytare Meningitis, entzundliche Polyneuritis und Rheumatismus. *Archiv Psychiatrische Nervenkrankheit*. **11**, 281 376.

Banik, N.L. and Hogan, E.L. (1983). CSF enzymes in neurological disease. *In* "Neurobiology of Cerebrospinal Fluid 2". (Ed. J.H. Wood). pp. 205-232.

Banki, C.M. (1977). Correlation of anxiety and related symptoms with CSF 5-HIAA in depressed women. *Journal of Neural Transmission*, **41**, 135-143.

Banki, C.M. (1981). Factors influencing monoamine metabolites and tryptophan in patients with alcohol dependence. *Journal of Neural Transmisson*, **50**, 89-101.

Banki, C.M. (1984). Some clinical and biochemical predictors of outcome in depression. *In* "Frontiers in Biochemical and Pharmacological Research in Depression". (Eds E. Usdin *et al.*). pp 147-151. Raven Press, New York.

Banki, C.M. and Molnar, G. (1981a) The influence of age, weight and body weight on CSF amine metabolites and tryptophan in women. *Biological Psychiatry*, **16**,

753-76.

Banki, C. and Molnar, G. (1981*b*). CSF Amine Metabolites in Delirium Tremens. *Psychiatric Clinics*, **14**, 167-177.

Banki, C.M., Vojnik, M. and Molmar, C. (1981). CSF amine metabolites, tryptophan and clinical parameters in depression. Background variables. *Journal of Affective Disorders*, **3**, 81-89.

Banki, C.M., Arato, M. and Papp, Z. (1983*a*). Cerebrospinal fluid biochemical examinations: do they reflect clinical or biological differences? *Biological Psychiatry*, **18**, 1033-1044.

Banki, C.M, Arat'o, M., Papp, Z. and Kurcz, M. (1983*b*). The effect of dexamethasone on cerebrospinal fluid monoamine metabolites and cortisol in psychiatric patients. *Pharmacopsychiatria*, **16**, (3) 77-81.

Banki, C.M., Vojnik, M., Papp, Z., Balla, K.Z. and Arato, M. (1985). Cerebrospinal fluid magnesium and calcium related to amine metabolites, diagnosis, and suicide attempts. *Biological Psychiatry*, **20**, 163-171.

Banki C.M., Bissette, G., Arato, M., O'Connor, L. and Nemeroff, C.B. (1987). CSF corticotropin-releasing factor-like immunoreactivity in depression and schizophrenia. *American Journal of Psychiatry*, **144**, (7) 873-877.

Barbaccia, M.L., Costa, E., Ferrero, P., Guidotti, A. *et al.* (1986). Diazepam-binding inhibitor. A brain neuropeptide present in human spinal fluid: studies in depression, schizophrenia, and Alzheimer's disease. *Archives of General Psychiatry*, **43**, 1143-1147.

Barbour, A.G., Heiland, R.A. and Howe, T.R. (1985). Heterogeneity of major proteins in Lyme disease Borreliae: a molecular analysis of North American and European isolates. *Journal of Infectious Diseases*, **152**, (3) 478-484.

Bareggi, S.R., Francceshi, M., Bonini, L., Zecca, L. and Smirne, S. (1982). Decreased CSF concentrations of HVA and GABA in Alzheimer's disease. *Archives of Neurology*, **39**, 709-712.

Baringer J.R. and Townsend, J.J. (1984). Herpes virus infection of the peripheral venous system. *In* "Peripheral Neuropathy". 2nd Edn. (Eds P.J. Dyck, P.K. Thomas, E.H. Lambert and R. Burge). pp. 1941-54. W. B. Saunders, Philadelphia.

Barkai, A.I. and Nelson, H.D. (1987). Alterations by antidepressants of cerebrospinal fluid formation and calcium distribution dynamics in the intact rat brain. *Biological Psychiatry*, **22**, 892-898.

Barkhof, F., Frequin, S., Hommes, O. *et al.* (1992). A correlative triad of gadolinium – DTPA MRI, EDSS, and CSF-MBP in relapsing multiple sclerosis patients treated with high-dose iv methylprednisolone, *Neurology*, **42**, 63-67.

Barrie M., and Jowett, A. (1967). A pharmacological investigation of cerebrospinal fluid from patients with migraine. *Brain*, **90**, 785-794.

Barthold, S.W., Moody, K.D., Terwilliger, G.A., Duray, P.H., Jacoby, R.O. and Steere, A.C. (1988). Experimental Lyme arthritis in rats infected with *Borrelia burgdorferi*. *Journal of Infectious Diseases*, **157**, (4) 842-846.

Bartleson, J.D., Swanson, J.W. and Whisnant, J.P. (1981). A migrainous syndrome with cerebrospinal fluid pleocytosis. *Neurology*, **31**, 1257-1262.

Bass, N.H, and Lundborg, P. (1976). Transport mechanisms in the cerebrospinal fluid system for removal of acid metabolites from developing brain. *Advances in Experimental Medicine and Biology*, **69**, 31-40.

Bastron, J.A. (1984). Neuropathy in diseases of the thyroid and pituitary glands. *In* "Peripheral Neuropathy". 2nd Edn. (Eds P.J. Dyck, P.K. Thomas, E.H. Lambert, and R. Burge). pp. 1833-46. W. B. Saunders, Philadelphia.

Batnitzky, S., Keucher, T.R., Mealey, J. and Campbell, R.L. (1977). Iatrogenic intraspinal epidermoid tumors. *Journal of the American Medical Association,* **237,** (2) 148-150.

Bauer, J.D. (1982) *In* "Clinical Laboratory Methods". pp. 754-761. C.V. Mosby, St Louis.

Bauer, K. and Kornhuber, J. (1987). Blood-cerebrospinal fluid barrier in schizophrenic patients. *European Archives of Psychiatry and Neurological Science,* **236,** 257-259.

Bauer, H., Poser, S. and Ritter, G. (1980). "Progress in Multiple Sclerosis Research". Springer-Verlag, New York.

Baumgarten, A. (1987). Viral antigen detection in CSF. *In* "Advances in CSF Protein, Research and Diagnosis". (Ed. E.J. Thompson). pp. 129-149. MTP Press Ltd, Lancaster.

Baumhefner, R.W. and Tourtellotte, T.W. (1985). Cellular immunology in multiple sclerosis – a review through 1984. *In* "Concepts in Immunopathology". Vol 2. (Eds J.M. Cruse and R.E. Lewis Jr). pp. 151-188. Organ Based Autoimmune Diseases. Karger, New York.

Beal, M. and E. Bird (1988). Neuropeptides in Huntington's disease. *In* "Neuropeptides in Psychiatric and Neurological Disorders". (Ed. C. Nemerof). pp. 137-55 . Johns Hopkins University Press, Baltimore.

Beal, M.F., Mazurek, M.F., Tran, V.T., Chattha, G., Bird, E.D. and Martin, J.B. (1985). Reduced numbers of somatostatin receptors in the cerebral cortex in Alzheimer's disease. *Science,* **229,** 289-291.

Beck, O., Borg, S. and Sedvall, G. (1983). Tryptophan levels in human cerebrospinal fluid after acute and chronic ethanol consumption. *Drug and Alcohol Dependence,* **12,** (3) 217-22.

Beckmann, H., Lang, R.E. and Gattaz, W.F. (1985). Vasopressin-oxytocin in cerebrospinal fluid of schizophrenic patients and normal controls. *Psychoneurendocrinology,* **10,** (2) 187-191.

Bell, C. (1802). "The Anatomy of the Brain". Whittingham Press, London.

Bell, W.E., Joynt, R.J. and Sahs, A.L. (1960). Low spinal fluid pressure syndromes. *Neurology,* **10,** 512-521.

Belmaker, R.H., Ebstein, R.P., Biederman, J., Stern, R., Berman, M. and van Praag, H.M. (1978). The effect of L-Dopa and propanolol on human CSF cyclic nucleotides. *Psychopharmacology,* **58,** 307-310.

Benson, K.L., Zarcone Jnr, V.P., Faull, K.F., Barchas, J.D. and Berger, P.A. (1988*a*). REM sleep eye movement activity and CSF concentrations of 5-hydroxyindoleacetic acid in psychiatric patients. *Psychiatry Research,* **8,** 73-78.

Benson, C.A., Harris, A.A. and Levin, S. (1988*b*). Acute bacterial meningitis: general aspects. *In* "Handbook of Clinical Neurology". Vol 8. (52) Microbial Disease, (Ed. A.A. Harris). (Chapter 1). Elsevier Science Publishers, B.V.

Berg, B., Gardsell, P. and Skansberg, P. (1982). CSF lactate in the diagnosis of meningitis: diagnostic value compared to standard biochemical methods. *Scandinavian Journal of Infectious Diseases,* **14,** 115.

Berger, B., Tassin, J.P., Rancurel, G. and Blane, G. (1980). Catecholamines in innervation of the human cerebral cortex in pre-senile and senile dementia. Histochemical and biochemical studies. *In* "Enzymes and Neurotransmitters in Mental Disease". (Eds E. Usdin *et al.*). pp. 317-328. John Wiley and Sons, New York.

Berger, M.P., and Paz, J. (1976). Diagnosis of cryptococcal meningitis. *Journal of the American Medical Association*, **236**, 2517-2518.

Berger, P.A. and Nemeroff, C.B (1987). Opioid peptides in affective disorders. *In* "Psychopharmacology: the Third Generation of Progress". (Ed. H. Y. Meltzer). pp. 637-646. Raven Press, New York.

Berger, P.A., Watson, S.J., Akil, H. and Barchas, J.D. (1986). Investigating opioid peptides in schizophrenia and depression. *In* "Neuropeptides in Neurologic and Psychiatric Disease". (Eds. J.B. Martin and J.D. Barchas). Raven Press, New York.

Bering, E.A. (1974). The cerebrospinal fluid and the extracellular fluid of the brain. *Federal Proceedings*, **33**, 2061-2063.

Berkowitz, R.S., Osathanondh, R., Goldstein, D.P., Martin, P.M., Mallampati, S.R. and Datta, S. (1981). CSF human HCG levels in normal pregnancy and choriocarcinoma. *Surgery, Gynecology and Obstetrics*, **153**, 687-689.

Berretini, W., Nurberger, J., Hare, T. *et al.* (1983). Reduced plasma and CSF GABA in affective illness: effect of lithium carbonate. *Biological Psychiatry*, **18**, 185.

Berretini W.H., Nurnberger Jr, J.I., Hare, T.A., Simmons-Alling S. and Gerson, E.S. (1986). CSF GABA in euthymic manic-depressive patients and controls. *Biological Psychiatry*, **21**, 842-844.

Berrettini, W.H., Nurnberger, J.I., Zerbe, R.L., Gold, P.W., Chrousos, G.P. and Tomai, T. (1987a). CSF neuropeptides in euthymic bipolar patients and controls. *British Journal of Psychiatry*, **150**, 208-212.

Berrettini, W.H., Doran, A.R. Kelsoe, J., Roy, A. and Pickar, D. (1987b). Cerebrospinal fluid neuropeptide Y in depression and schizophrenia. *Neuropsychopharmacology*, **1**, (1) 81-83.

Berry, H. and J. Steiner (1979). L-Glutamine increases CSF GABA in a patient with Huntington's disease. (Abst). *Neurology*, **29**, 535.

Bichat, M.F.X. and Traite, D. (1802). "Anatomie descriptive". 3rd Vol. Paris.

Bickerstaff, E.R. (1980). "Neurological Examination in Clinical Practice". Blackwell Publishers, London.

Bigner, S.H. and Johnston, W.W. (1981a). The cytopathology of cerebrospinal fluid II: metastatic cancer, meningeal carcinomatosis and primary CNS neoplasms. *Acta Cytologica*, **25**, 461-479.

Bigner, S.H. and Johnston, W.W. (1981b). The cytopathology of cerebrospinal fluid I: non-neoplastic conditions. *Acta Cytologica*, **25**, 335-353.

Bioulac, B., Benezech, M., Renaud, B. *et al.* (1980). Serotonergic dysfunction in the 47 XYY syndrome. *Biological Psychiatry*, **15**, 917-23.

Bishchoff A. (1963). "Die Diabetische Neuropathie". G. Thieme, Stuttgart.

Bissette, G. and Nemeroff, C.B. (1988). The role of neuropeptides in the pathogenesis and treatment of schizophrenia. *In* "Neuropeptides in Psychiatric and Neurological Disorders". Chapter 3. (Ed. C.B. Nemeroff). Johns Hopkins University Press, Baltimore.

Bissette, G. and Nemeroff, L.B. (1990). III. CSF CRF concentrations in other neuropsychiatric and endocrine disorders. *In* "Corticotropin-Releasing Factor: Basic and Clinical Studies of a Neuropeptide". (Eds B. De Souza and C.B. Nemeroff). CRC Press, Boca Raton, Florida.

Bissette, G., Nemeroff, C.B. and MacKay, A.V.P. (1986*a*). Neuropeptides and schizophrenia. *In* "Progress in Brain Research". (Eds P.C. Emson, M.N. Rossor and M. Tohyama). pp. 161-174. Elsevier Science Publishers, B.V.

Bissette, G., Widerlov, E., Walleus, H., Karlsson, I., Eklund, K., Forsman, A. and Nemeroff, C.B. (1986*b*). Alterations in cerebrospinal fluid concentrations of somatostatinlike immunoreactivity in neuropsychiatric disorders. *Archives of General Psychiatry,* **43**, 1148-1151.

Bito, L.Z. and Wallenstein, M.C. (1977). Transport of prostaglandins across the blood-brain and blood-aqueous barriers and the physiological significance of these absorptive transport processes. *Experimental Eye Research,* **25**, (Suppl) 229-243.

Bjerkenstedt, L., Edman, G., Hagenfeldt, L., Sedvall, G. and Wiesel, A. (1985). Plasma amino acids in relation to cerebrospinal fluid monoamine metabolites in schizophrenic patients and healthy controls. *British Journal of Psychiatry,* **147**, 276-282.

Block, W. (1992). Personal communication, (October) Reference Electrophoresis Laboratory, Inc., Behesda, MD.

Bloom, F.E. and Segal, D.S. (1980). Endorphins in CSF. *In* "Neurobiology of CSF". (Ed. J.H. Wood). pp. 651-664. Plenum Press.

Bluestein, H.G. (1988). Nervous system disease in systemic lupus erythematosus. *Immunology-Allergy Clinics of North America,* **8**, 315-329.

Bluestein, H.G., Williams, G.W. and Steinberg, A.D. (1981). Cerebrospinal fluid antibodies to neuronal cells: Association with neuropsychiatric manifestations of systemic lupus erythematosus. *American Journal of Medicine,* **70**, 240-246.

Bodansky, O. (1975). "Biochemistry of Human Cancer". Academic Press, New York,

Böddinghaus, B., Rogall, T., Flohr, H., Blocker, E. and Bottger (1990). Detection and identification of mycobacteria by amplification of rRNA. *Journal of Clinical Microbiology,* **28**, 1751-1759.

Bogden, J.D. and Troiano, R.A. (1978). Plasma calcium, copper, magnesium and zinc concentrations in patients with the alcohol withdrawal syndrome. *Clinical Chemistry,* **24**, (9) 1553-1556.

Bogden, J.D., Troiano, R.A. and Joselow, M.M. (1977). Copper, zinc, magnesium, and calcium in plasma and cerebrospinal fluid of patients with neurological diseases. *Clinical Chemistry,* **23**, (3) 485-489.

Bohlen, P., Huot, S. and Palfreyman, M. (1979). The relationship between GABA concentrations in brain and CSF. *Brain Research,* **167**, 297-305.

Bohmer, T., Kjekshus, J. and Vaagenes, P. (1983). Biochemical indices of cerebral ischemic injury. *Scandinavian Journal of Clinical and Laboratory Investigations,* **43**, 261-265.

Bonadio, W.A. (1988). Bacterial meningitis in children whose cerebrospinal fluid contains polymorphonuclear leukocytes without pleocytosis. *Clinical Pediatrics,* **27**, 198-200.

Bonadio, W.A., Smith, D.S., Metrou, M. and Dewitz, B. (1988). Estimating lumbar-puncture depth in children. *New England Journal of Medicine,* **319**,

952-953.

Bonadio, W.A, Smith, D.S., Goddard, S., Burroughs, J. and Khaja, G. (1990). Distinguishing cerebrospinal fluid abnormalities in children with bacterial meningitis and traumatic lumbar puncture. *Journal of Infectious Diseases*, **162**, 251-254

Bonnet, K.A. (1982). Cyclic nucleotides in the CNS. *In* "Handbook of Neurochemistry". (Ed. A. Lajtha). pp. 257-280. Plenum Press, New York.

Borg, S., Kvande, H. Magnuson, E. and Sjoqvist, B. (1980). Salsolinol and salsoline in CSF of alcoholic patients. *Acta Psychiatrica Scandinavica*, **62**, (Suppl. 286) 171-177.

Borg S., Kvande, H. and Sedvall, G. (1981). Central norepinephrine metabolism during alcohol intoxication in addicts and healthy volunteers. *Science*, **213**, 1135-1137.

Borg J., Warter, J.M., Schlienger, J.R., Imler, M., Marescaux, CC. and Mack, S. (1982). Neurotransmitter modifications in human cerebrospinal fluid and serum during hepatic encephalopathy. *Journal of the Neurological Sciences*, 343.

Borucki, S.J., Nguyen, B.V. Ladoulis, C.T. and McKendall, R.R. (1989). Cerebrospinal fluid immunoglobulin abnormalities in neurosarcoidosis. *Archives of Neurology*, **46**, 270-273.

Boston, P.F., Jackson, P. and Thompson, R.J. (1982). Human 14-3-3 protein: RIA, tissue distribution and CSF levels in patients with neurological disorders. *Journal of Neurochemistry*, **38**, 1475-1482.

Botez, M., Young, S., Bachevalier, J. and Gauthier, S. (1982a). Thiamine Deficiency and CSF 5-HIAA: A preliminary study. *Journal of Neurology, Neurosurgery and Psychiatry*, **45**, 731-733.

Botez, M., Young, S., Bachevalier, J. and Gauthier, S. (1982b). Effect of folic acid and vitamin B12 deficiencies of 5-HIAA in human CSF. *Annals of Neurology*, **12**, 479-484

Bottiglieri, T., Godfrey, P., Flynn, T., Carney, M.W.P., Toone, B.K. and Reynolds, E.H. (1990). Cerebrospinal fluid S-adenosylmethionine in depression and dementia: effects of treatment with parenteral and oral S-adenosylmethionine. *Journal of Neurology, Neurosurgery and Psychiatry*, **53**, 1096-1098.

Bowden, C.L., Huang, L.G., Javors, M.A., Johnson, J.M., Seleshi, E., McIntyre, K., Contreras, S. and Maas. J.W. (1988). Calcium function in affective disorders and healthy controls. *Biological Psychiatry*, **23**, 367-376.

Bowen, D.M. and Davison, A.W. (1980). Biochemistry of Alzheimer's disease. *In* "The Biochemistry of Psychiatric Disturbances". John Wiley, New York.

Bowers, M.B. (1970). 5-HIAA in the brain and ICSF of the rabbit following administration of drugs affecting 5-HT. *Journal of Neurochemistry*, **17**, 827.

Bowers, M.B. (1974a). Lumbar CSF 5-HIAA and HVA in affective syndromes. *Journal of Nervous and Mental Disorders*, **158**, 325-330.

Bowers, M.B. (1974b). Central dopamine turnover in schizophrenic syndromes. *Archives of General Psychiatry*, **31**, 50-54.

Bowers, M.B. (1978a). Serotonin in psychotic states. *In* "Biochemistry of Mental Disorders: New Vistas". (Eds E. Usdin and A.J. Mandell). pp. 191-203. Marcel Dekker, Inc., New York.

Bowers, M.B. (1978b). CSF acid monoamine metabolites in psychotic syndromes:

what might they signify. *Biological Psychiatry*, **13**, (3) 375-383.

Bowers, M.B. Jr. (1984). Family history and CSF homovanillic acid pattern during neuroleptic treatment. *American Journal of Psychiatry*, **141**, (2) 296-8.

Bowers, M.B. (1991). Characteristics of psychotic inpatients with high or low HVA levels at admission. *American Journal of Psychiatry*, **148**, (2) 240.

Bowers, M.B. Jr. and Swigar, M.E. (1987). Acute psychosis and plasma catecholamine metabolites. *Archives of General Psychiatry*, **44**, 190.

Boyer, R.S., Sun, N.C.J., Verity, A., Nies, K.M. and Louie, J.S. (1980). Immunoperoxidase staining of the choroid plexus in systemic lupus erythematosus. *Journal of Rheumatology*, **7**, 645-650.

Bradbury, M. (1979). "The Concept of a Blood-Brain Barrier". John Wiley and Sons, New York.

Bradbury, M.W.B. (1984). The structure and function of the blood-brain barrier. *Federation Proceedings*. **43**, 186-190

Bradbury, M.W.B. and Sarna, G.S. (1977). Homeostasis of the ionic composition of the cerebrospinal fluid. *Experimental Eye Research*, **25**, (Suppl.) 249-257.

Brase, D.A. and Loh, H.H.(1975). Possible role of 5-HT in MBD. *Life Sciences*, **16**, 1005-1016.

Brau, R.H., Garcia-Casti Neiras, S. and Rifkinson, N. (1984). Cerebrospinal fluid ascorbic acid levels in neurological disorders. *Neurosurgery*, **14**, (2) 142-6.

Breasted, J.H. (1930). "The Edwin Smith Surgical Papyrus". University of Chicago Press, Chicago.

Breier, A., Wolkowitz, O.M. *et al.* (1990). Plasma norepinephrine in chronic schizophrenia. *American Journal of Psychiatry*, **147**, 1467-1470.

Bremer, F. (1977). Cerebral hypnogenic centers. *Annals of Neurology*, **2**, 1-6.

Brew, B.J., Bhalla, R.B. Fleisher, M., Paul, M. *et al.* (1989). Cerebrospinal fluid β-2 microglobulin in patients infected with human immunodeficiency virus. *Neurology*, **39**, 830-834.

Brew, B.J., Bhalla, R.B., Paul, M., Gallardo, H., McArthur, J.C., Schwartz, M.K. and Price, R.W. (1990). Cerebrospinal fluid neopterin in human immunodeficiency virus type 1 infection. *Annals of Neurology*, **28**, 556-560.

Briem, H., Hultman, E.H., Kalin, M.E. and Lundbergh, P.R. (1982). Increased total concentrations of amino acids in the CSF of patients with purulent meningitis. *Journal of Infectious Diseases*, **145**, (3) 346-350.

Brinkman, C.J.J., Nillesen, W.M. and Hommes, O.R. (1983). T-Cell subpopulations in blood and cerebrospinal fluid of multiple sclerosis patients – effect of cyclophosphamide. *Clinical Immunology and Immunopathology*, **29**, 341-348.

Brisson-Noel, A, Gicquel, B., Lecossier, D., Levy-Frebault, V., Nassif, X. and Hance, A.J. (1989). Rapid diagnosis of tuberculosis by amplification of mycobacterial DNA in clinical samples. *Lancet*, ii, 1069-1071.

Britton, M., Hultman, E., Murray, V. and Sjoholm, H. (1983). The diagnostic accuracy of CSF analyses in stroke. *Acta Medica Scandinavica*, **214**, 3-13.

Britton, C.B., Miller, J.R. and Jubelt, B. (1989). Acquired immunodeficiency syndrome. *In* "Merritt's Textbook of Neurology". (Ed. L.P. Rowland). Lea and Febiger, Philadelphia.

Brocker, R.J. (1958). Technique to avoid spinal-tap headache. *Journal of the American Medical Association*, **168**, (3) 261-263.

Brody, D., Walkin, A. and Retrosen, J. (1987). Phospholipids and prostaglandin in schizophrenia. *In* "Handbook of Schizophrenia". Vol. 2. (Eds F. Henn and L. De Lisi). pp. 319-336. Elsevier, Amsterdam.

Brook, I., Bricknell, K., Overturf, G. and Finegold, S.M. (1978). Measurement of lactic acid in CSF of patients with infections of the central nervous system. *Journal of Infectious Diseases,* **137,** (4) 384-390.

Brooks, B.R. (1980). Seizure-induced metabolic alterations in human CSF. *In* "Neurobiology of CSF". Vol. 1. (Ed. J.H. Wood). pp. 237-258.

Brooks, B.R. (1989). Nonimmunoglobulin proteins in human cerebrospinal fluid. *In* "The Cerebrospinal Fluid". (Eds R.M. Herndon and R.A. Brumback). Kluwer Academic Publishers, Norwell, MA.

Brooks, B.R. and Adams, R.D. (1975). CSF acid-base and lactate changes after seizures in unanaesthetized man. *Neurology,* **25,** 935-942.

Brooks, B.R., Wood, J.H., Diaz, M., Czerwinski, C., Georges, L. *et al.* (1980). Extracellular cyclic nucleotide metabolism in human CNS. *In* "Neurobiology of CSF". (Ed. J. Wood). pp. 113-140. Plenum Press, New York.

Brown, G.L., and Goodwin., F.K. (1986). Cerebrospinal fluid correlates of suicide attempts and aggression. *Annals of the New York Academy of Science,* **487,** 175-188.

Brown, G., Goodwin, F., Ballenger, J. *et al.* (1979). Aggression in human correlates with CSF amine metabolites. *Psychiatry Research,* 1, 131-139.

Brown, G.B., Smythies J.R. and Morin, R.D. (1983). Endogenous halluncinogens in CSF: measurement and meaning. *In* "Neurobiology of CSF". (Ed. J.H. Wood). pp. 173-178. Plenum Press, New York.

Brown, J.K. (1976). Lumbar puncture and its hazards. *Developmental Medicine and Child Neurology,* **18,** 803-16.

Bruce, O.A. (1980). Cerebrospinal fluid pressure dynamics and brain metabolism. *In* "Neurobiology of CSF". (Ed. J.H. Wood). pp. 351-364. Plenum Press, New York.

Brumback, R. (1989*a*). Anatomic and physiologic aspects of the CSF space. *In* "The Cerebrospinal Fluid". (Eds R. Herndon and R. Brumback). pp.15-43. Kivwer Academic Publishers, Boston.

Brumback, R. (1989*b*). Collecting cerebrospinal fluid. *In* "The Cerebrospinal Fluid". (Eds R.M. Herndon and R.A. Brumback). Kluwer Academic Publishers, Norwell, M.A.

Bukasa, K. S-S., Sindic, C.J.M., Bodeus, M., Burtonboy, G., Laterre, C. and Sonnet, S. (1988). Anti-HIV antibodies in the CSF of AIDS patients: a serological and immunoblotting study. *Journal of Neurology, Neurosurgery and Psychiatry,* **51,** 1063-1068.

Bulat, M. (1974). Monoamine metabolites. *In* "CSF Aromatic Amino Acids in the Brain". CIBA Symposium 22. pp. 243-256. Elsevier, Amsterdam.

Bulat, M. (1977). On the cerebral origin of 5-hydroxyindolacetic acid in the lumbar cerebrospinal fluid. *Brain Research,* **122,** 388-391.

Bulat, M. and B. Zivkovic, (1971). Origin of 5-HIAA in the spinal fluid. *Science,* **173,** 738.

Bulat, M. and Zivkovic, B. (1978). Neurochemical study of the cerebrospinal fluid. Research methods. *In* "Neurochemistry". (Ed. N. Marks). pp. 57-91. Plenum Press, New York.

Bulat, M., Lackovic, Z. Jakupcevic, M. and Damjanov, I. (1974). 5-HIAA in the lumbar fluid: a specific indicator of spinal cord injury. *Science*, **185**, 527-528.

Bullard, D.E. and Schold, S.C. (1985). Tumor markers. *In* "Neurosurgery". (Eds R. Wilkins and S. Rengachary). McGraw-Hill, New York.

Bunzow, J.R., Van Tol, H.H.M., Grandy, D. *et al.* (1988). Cloning and expression of a rat D_2 dopamine receptor cDNA. *Nature*, **336**, 783-787.

Burgdorfer, W., Barbour, A.G., Hayes, S.F., Benach, J.L., Grunwaldt, E. and Davis, J.P. (1982). Lyme disease: a tick borne spirochetosis? *Science*, **216**, 1317-1319.

Buruma, O., Janson, H., den Bergh, F. and Bots, G. (1981). Blood-stained CSF: traumatic puncture or haemorrhage. *Journal of Neurology, Neurosurgery and Psychiatry*, **44**, 144-147.

Busse, O. and Hoffmann, O. (1983). CSF lactate and CT findings in middle cerebral artery infarction. A comparative study. *Stroke*, **14**, (6) 960-39.

Butler, I J., Koslow, S.H., Seifert, Jr. W.E. *et al.* (1979). Biogenic amine metabolism in Tourette syndrome. *Annals of Neurology*, **6**, 37-39.

Butler, I.J., Seifert, W.E. and Enna, S.J. (1980). Huntington's disease: biogenic amines in CSF. *In* "Neurobiology of CSF". (Ed. J.H. Wood). pp. 153-160. Plenum Press, New York.

Butler, A.B., Brooks, W.H. and Netsky, M.G. (1982). Classification and biology of brain tumors. *In* "Neurological Surgery". (Ed. J. Youmans). pp. 2659-2693. W.B. Saunders, Philadelphia.

Caine, E.D. (1985). Gilles de la Tourette's syndrome. A review of clinical and research studies and consideration of future directions for investigation. *Archives of Neurology*, **42**, 393-397.

Calabrese, V.P., Selhorst, J.B. and Harhisom, J.W. (1978). Cerebrospinal fluid infusion test in pseudotumor cerebri. *Annals of Neurology*, **4**, 173

Campbell, A.M.G. and Williams, E.R. (1967). Natural history of Retsum's syndrome in a Gloucestershire family. *British Medical Journal*, **3**, 777-779.

Carbaat, P.A.T. and van Crevel, H. (1981). Lumbar puncture headache: controlled study on the preventive effect of 24 hours' bed rest. *Lancet,* Nov. 21, 1133-1135.

Carlen, P., Kapur, B., Huszar, L., Lee, M., Moddel, G., Singh, R. and Wilkinson, D. (1980). Prolonged CSF acidosis in recently abstinent chronic alcoholics. *Neurology*, **30**, 956-962.

Carlsson, C. and Dencker, S. (1973). CSF uric acid in alcoholics. *Acta Neurologica Scandinavica*, **49**, 39-46.

Carmen, J.S. (1981). Pharmacologic studies of calcium and mood. *In* "Electrolytes and Neuropsychiatric Disorders". (Ed. P.E. Alexander). pp. 295-304. Spectrum, New York.

Carmen, J.S., Wyatt, E.S., Smith, W., Post, R.M. and Ballenger, J.C. (1984). Calcium and calcitonin in bipolar affective disorder. *In* "Neurobiology of Mood Disorders". (Eds R.M. Post and J.C. Ballenger). Chapter 22. Williams and Wilkins, Baltimore.

Carney, M.W.P., Chary, T.K.N. Bottiglieri, T. and Reynolds, E.H. (1989). The switch mechanism and the bipolar/unipolar dichotomy. *British Journal of Psychiatry*, **154**, 48-51.

Carpenter, M.B. (1978). "Core Text of Neuroanatomy". Williams and Wilkins, Co, Baltimore.

Cascino, A., Cangiano, C., Fiaccadori, F. *et al.* (1982). Plasma and cerebrospinal fluid amino acid patterns in hepatic encephalopathy. *Digestive Diseases and Sciences,* **27,** 828-832.

Chad, D.A. Smith, T.W., DeGirolami, U. and K. Hammer (1986). Perineuritis and ulcerative colitis. *Neurology,* **36,** 1377-9.

Chadwick, D. (1981). CSF monoamine metabolites in epileptic patients. *In* "Neurotransmitters, Seizures and Epilepsy". (Ed. P.L. Morselli). pp. 293-298. Raven Press, New York.

Chadwick, D., Hallett, M., Jenner, P. and Marsden, C.D. (1978). Serotonin and action myoclonus: a review. *In* "Neurotransmitter System and their Clinical Disorders". (Ed. N.J. Legg). pp. 151-166. Academic Press, New York.

Chandramuki, A., Allen, P.R.J., Keen, M. and Ivanyi, J. (1985). Detection of mycobacterial antigen and antibodies in the cerebrospinal fluid of patients with tuberculous meningitis. *Journal of Medical Microbiology,* **20,** 239-247.

Chapelon, C., Ziza, J.M., Piette, J.C., Levy, Y., Raguin, G., Wechsler, B. *et al.* (1990). Neurosarcoidosis: signs, course and treatment in 35 confirmed cases. *Medicine,* **69,** (5) 261-276.

Charlton, B.G., Leake, A., Wright, C., Fairbairn, A.F., McKeith, I.G., Candy, J. M. and Ferrier, I.N. (1988). Somatostatin content and receptors in the cerebral cortex of depressed and control subjects. *Journal of of Neurology, Neurosurgery and Psychiatry,* **51,** 719-721.

Chase, T.N. (1980). Neurochemical alterations in Parkinson's disease. *In* "Neurobiology of CSF". (Ed. J.H. Wood). pp. 207-18. Plenum Press, New York.

Chofflon, M., Weiner, H.L. Morimoto, C. and Hafler, D.A. (1989). Decrease of suppressor inducer (CD4 + 2H4+) T cells in multiple sclerosis cerebrospinal fluid. *Annals of Neurology,* **25,** 494-499.

Christiensen, N., Vestergaard, P., Sorensen, T., Rafaelson, O. (1980). CSF adrenaline and noradrenaline in depressed patients. *Acta Psychiatrica Scandinavica,* **61,** 178-182.

Chu, A., Sever, J., Madden, D., Iivanainen, M., Leon, M., Wallen, W., Brooks, B., Lee, Y. and Houff, S. (1983). Oligoclonal Ig G bands in CSF in various neurological diseases. *Annals of Neurology,* **13,** 434-439

Clarke, E., and O'Malley, C. (1968). "The Human Brain and Spinal Cord". University of California Press, Berkeley.

Coe, J.I. (1977). Postmortem chemistry of blood, CSF and vitreous humor. *In* "Forensic Medicine". Vol. 2. (Eds C.G. Tedeschi, W. Eckert and L.G. Tedeschi). pp. 1033-1060. W.B. Saunders, Philadelphia.

Coe, J.I. (1979). Medicolegal autopsies and autopsy toxicology. *In* "Current Methods of Autopsy Practice". (Ed. J. Ludwig). pp. 10-20. W.B. Saunders, Philadelphia.

Cohen A.S. and Rubinow, A. (1984). Amyloid neuropathy. *In* "Peripheral Neuropathy". 2nd Edn. (Eds P.J. Dyck, P.K. Thomas, E.H. Lambert and R. Burge). pp. 1866-98. W. B. Saunders, Philadelphia.

Cohen, G. (1971). Reactions of catecholamines with acetaldehyde to form tetrahydroisoquinolines. *In* "Biological Aspects of Alcohol". (Eds W. McIsaac and P. Creaven). pp. 267-284. University of Texas Press, Austin.

Cohen, R.J. and Allen, G.S. (1980). Effects of subarachnoid blood and spasmodic agents on cerebral vasculative. *In* "Neurobiology of CSF". (Ed. J.H. Wood). pp. 287-301. Plenum Press, New York.

Cohen, S. and Lajtha, A. (1972). Amino acid transport. *In* "Handbook of Neurochemistry". Vol. 7. pp. 543-569.

Cohen, D.J. , B.Shaywitz, A., Johnson, W.T. and Bowers, M.B. (1974). Biogenic amines in autistic and atypical children. *Archives of General Psychiatry*, **31**, 845-853.

Cohen, D.J., Caparulo, B.K., Shaywitz, B.A. and Bowers, M.B. (1977). Dopamine and serotonin metabolism in neuropsychiatrically disturbed children. *Archives of General Psychiatry*, **34**, 545-550.

Cohen, D.J., Shaywitz, B.A. *et al.* (1979). Central biogenic amine metabolism in children with the syndrome of chronic multiple tics of Gilles de la Tourette. *Journal of the American Academy of Child Psychiatry*, **18**, 320-41.

Cohen, S.R., Brooks, B.R., Jubelt, B., Herndon, R. and McKhann, G.M. (1980*a*). Myelin basic protein in CSF: index of active demyelination. *In* "Neurobiology of CSF". (Ed. J.H. Wood). pp. 487-494. Plenum Press, New York.

Cohen, S., Brune, M. , Hernden, R. and McKhann, G. (1980*b*). Diagnostic value of MBP in CSF. *In* "Progress in MS Research". (Eds H. Bauer, *et al.*). pp. 161-167. Springer-Verlag, New York.

Cohen, D.J., Shaywitz, B.A. Young, J.G. and Bowers, M.B. (1980*c*). CSF monoamine metabolites in neuropsychiatric disorders of childhood. *In* "Neurobiology of CSF". (Ed. J.H. Wood). pp. 665-684. Plenum Press, New York.

Colangelo, W. and Jones, D. (1982). The fetal alcohol syndrome: a review and assessment of the syndrome and its neurological sequelae. *Progress in Neurobiology*, **19**, 271-314.

Comings, D.E. (1990*a*). Blood serotonin and tryptophan in Tourette syndrome. *American Journal of Medical Genetics*, **36**, 418-430.

Comings, D.E. (1990*b*). "Tourette Syndrome and Human Behaviour". Hope Press, Duart, CA.

Conly, J.M. and Ronald, A.R. (1983). Cerebrospinal fluid as a diagnostic body fluid. *American Journal of Medicine*, **75**, (Suppl.) 102-108.

Conn D.L. and Dyck, P.J. (1984). Angiopathic neuropathy in connective tissue disease. *In* "Peripheral Neuropathy". 2nd Edn. (Eds P.J. Dyck, P.K. Thomas, E.H. Lambert and R. Burge) pp. 2027-43. W. B. Saunders, Philadelphia.

Controni, G., Rodriguez, W.J., Hicks, J.M., Ficke, M., Ross, S., Friedman, G. and Khan, W. (1977). CSF lactic acid levels in meningitis. *Journal of Pediatrics*, **91**, 379-384.

Cook, E.H. (1990). Autism: review of neurochemical investigation. *Synapse*, **6**, 292-308.

Cook P.T., Davies, M. J. and Beavis, R.E. (1989). Bed rest and postlumbar puncture headache. *Anaesthesia*, **44**, 934.

Coombs, D.W., Maurer, L.H., Cate, C and Pageau, M.G. (1982). CSF β-endorphin and meningeal carcinomatosis. *Archives of Neurology*, **39**, 388.

Cooper, S.J., Leahey, W., Green, D.F. and King, D.J. (1988). The effect of electroconvulsive therapy on CSF amine metabolites in schizophrenic patients. *British Journal of Psychiatry*, **152**, 59-63.

Coovadia Y.M. Dawod, A., Ellis, M.E., Coovadia, H.M. and Daniel, T.M. (1986). Evaluation of adenosine deaminase activity and antibody to mycobacterium tuberculosis antigen 5 in cerebrospinal fluid and the radioactive bromide partition test for the early diagnosis of tuberculous meningitis. *Archives of Diseases in Children,* **61**, 428-435.

Coppen, A. (1976). Indoleamines and affective disorders. *In* "Foundations of Biochemical Psychiatry". (Eds D.S. Segal *et al.*). pp. 222-229. Butterworths, Boston.

Cornblath, D.R. , Asbury, A.K., Albers, J.W. *et al.* (1991). Research criteria for diagnosis of chronic inflammatory demyelinating polyneuropathy (CIDP). *Neurology,* **41**, 617-618.

Corston, R.N., McGale, E., Stonier, C., Aber, G.M. and Hutchinson, E.C. (1981*a*). Abnormalities of CSF amino acids in patients with the Guillain-Barre syndrome. *Journal of Neurology, Neurosurgery and Psychiatry,* **44**, 86-89.

Corston, R.N., McGale, E.H.F., Stonier, C., Hutchinson, E.C. and Aber, G.M. (1981*b*). CSF amino acid concentrations in patients with viral and tuberculous meningitis. *Journal of Neurology, Neurosurgery and Psychiatry,* **44**, 791-795.

Costa, E. and Neff, N.H. (1972). Estimation of turnover rates to study the metabolic regulation of the steady-state levels of neuronal monoamines. *In* "Handbook of Neurochemistry". 4, 45-90 (Ed. A. Lajtha). Plenum Press, New York.

Cowdry, R.W., Ebert, M.H., van Kammen, D.P., Post, R.M. and Goodwin, F.K. (1983). Cerebrospinal fluid probenecid studies: A reinterpretation. *Biological Psychiatry*, **18**, (11) 1287-99.

Cox, B.J., Swinson, R.P. and Endlev, N.J. (1991). A review of the psychopharmacology of panic disorder: individual differences and non-specific factors. *Canadian Journal of Psychiatry*, **36**, (2) 130-138.

Coyle, P.K. and C. Johnson (1983). Optimal detection of oligoclonal bands in CSF by silver stain. *Neurology (NY)* **33**, (11) 1510-2.

Cramer, H. and Schindler, E. (1982). Cyclic nucleotides in CSF of patients with intracranial and spinal tumors. *Acta Neurologica Scandinavica,* **65**, 174-181.

Craven, R.B., Brooks, J.B., Edman, D.C., Converse, J.D., Greenlee, J., Schlossberg, D. *et al.* (1977). Rapid diagnosis of lymphocytic meningitis by frequency-pulsed electron capture gas-liquid chromatography: differentiation of tuberculous cryptococcal, and viral meningitis. *Journal of Clinical Microbiology,* **6**, (1) 27-32.

Crawford, M.A. and Stevens, P. (1981). A study on essential fatty acids and multiple sclerosis. *Progress in Lipid Research,* **20**, 255-258.

Crayton, J.W. (1990). The dopamine hypothesis of schizophrenia – current opinion. *Psychiatry,* **3**, 19-22.

Crone, C. (1986). The blood-brain barrier – a modified tight epithelium. *In* "The Blood Brain Barrier in Health and Disease". (Eds A Suckling *et al.*). pp. 17-40. Ellis Horwood, Chichester.

Crow, T.J. (1980). Molecular pathology of schizophrenia: More than one disease process? *British Medical Journal,* **280**, 66-68.

Crow, T.J. (1987). Two syndromes of schizophrenia as one pole of the continuum of psychosis. A concept of the nature of the pathogen and its gender locus. *In* "Handbook of Schizophrenia". Vol. 2, (Eds F. Henn and L. De Lisi). pp. 17-48. Elsevier Publishers, Amsterdam.

Crow, T.J. and Johnstone, D.C. (1978). Dopaminergic processes in schizophrenia and the mechanism of antipsychotic effects. *In* "Neurotransmitter Systems and their Clinical Disorders". (Ed. N.J. Legg). pp. 207-220. Academic Press, New

York.

Crow, T., Johnstone, D.C., Owens, D. Ferrier, I., MacMillan, J., Parry, R. and Tyrrell, D. (1979). Characteristics of patients with schizophrenia or neurological disorders and virus-like agents in CSF. *Lancet*, i, 842-4.

Csernansky, J.G., Faull, K.F. and Pfefferbaum, A. (1988). Seasonal changes of CSF monoamine metabolites in psychiatric patients: what is the source? *Psychiatry Research*, **25**, 361-363.

Csernansky J.G., King, R.J. *et al.* (1990). 5-HIAA in cerebrospinal fluid and deficit schizophrenic characteristics. *British Journal of Psychiatry*, **156**, 501-507.

Cserr, H.F. (1971). Physiology of the choroid plexus. *Physiological Reviews*, **51**, 273-311.

Cserr, H.F. (1974). Relationship between cerebrospinal fluid and interstitial fluid of the brain. *Federal Proceedings*, **33**, 2075-2078.

Cserr, H.F. (1975). Physiology of the choroid plexus. *In* "The Choroid Plexus in Health and Disease". (Eds M.G. Netsky and S. Shuangshoti). pp. 175-195. University Press of Virginia, Charlottesville.

Cserr, H.F. and Tang, D. (1975). Evidence for bulk flow of cerebral interstitial fluid and its possible contribution to cerebrospinal fluid production. *In* "Intracranial Pressure II". (Eds N. Lundberg, U. Ponten and M. Brock). pp. 24-27. Springer-Verlag, New York

Cserr, H.F., Cooper, D. and Milhorat, T. (1977). Flow of cerebral interstitial fluid as indicated by the removal of extracellular markers from rat caudate nucleus. *Experimental Eye Research*, **25**, (Suppl.) 461-473.

Cunha, L., Goncalres, A.F., Oliveira, C., Dinis, M. and Amaral, R. (1983). HVA in the CSF of Parkinsonian patients. *Canadian Journal of Neurological Science*, **10**, 43-46.

Curzon, G. (1972). Brain amine metabolism in some neurological and psychiatric disorders. *In* "Biochemical Aspects of Nervous Diseases". (Ed. J.N. Cummings). Plenum Press, New York.

Curzon, G. (1973). Involuntary movements other than parkinsonism: biochemical aspects. *Proceedings of the Royal Society of Medicine*, **66**, 873-876.

Curzon, G. (1975). CSF homovanillic acid: an index of dopaminergic activity. *In* "Advances in Neurology". (Eds D. Calne, T. Chase and A. Barbeau). pp. 349-358. Raven Press, New York.

Cutler, N.R. (1987). *In vivo* markers in Alzheimer's disease and related dementias. *In* "Psychopharmacology: The Third Generation of Progress". (Ed. H.Y. Meltzer). Chapter 89, Raven Press, New York.

Cutler, R.W. (1980). Neurochemical aspects of blood-brain-CSF barriers. *In* "Neurobiology of Cerebrospinal Fluid". Vol. 1. (Ed. J.H. Wood). pp. 41-52. Plenum Press, New York.

Cutler, R.W. and Spertell, R.B. (1982). Cerebrospinal fluid: a selective review. *Annals of Neurology*, **11**, 1-10.

D' Souza, G., Mandal, B.K. Hooper, J. and Parker, L. (1978). Lactic acid concentration in CSF and differential diagnosis of meningitis. *Lancet*, i, 579-580.

Dager, S.R., Rainey, J.M., Kenny, M.A., Artru, A.A., Metzger, G.D. and Bowden, D.M. (1990). Central nervous system effects of lactate infusion in primates. *Biological Psychiatry*, **27**, 193-204.

Dalakas, M.C., and Engel, W.K. (1981). Polyneuropathy with monoclonal gammopathy. *Annals of Neurology*, **48**, 383-92.

Dalakas M.C. and Pezeshkpour, G.H. (1988). Neuromuscular diseases associated with human immunodeficiency virus infection. *Annals of Neurology*, **23**, Suppl S38-48.

Dalakas, M.C., Houff, S.A. and Engel, W.K. *et al.* (1980). CSF "monoclonal" bands in chronic relapsing polyneuropathy. *Neurology*, **30**, 864-867.

Dalens, B., Bezou, M., Coulet, M. and Raynaud, E. (1982). CSF cytomorphology in neonates. *Acta Cytologica*, **26**, 395-400.

Daly, J.W. (1977a). The formation, degradation, and function of cyclic nucleotide in the nervous system. *International Review of Neurobiology*, **20**, 105-168.

Daly, J.W. (1977b). "Cyclic Nucleotides in the Nervous System". Plenum Press, New York.

Danguir, J., LeQuan-Bui, K., Elghozi, J., Devynck, M. and Nicolaidis, S.L. (1982). CEC monitoring of 5-hydroxyindolic compounds in the CSF of the rat related to sleep and feeding. *Brain Research Bulletin*, **8**, (3) 293-297.

Daniel T.M. (1987). New approaches to the rapid diagnosis of tuberculous meningitis. *Journal of Infectious Diseases*, **155**, 599-602.

Dans, P.E., Cafferty, L., Otter, S.E. and Johnson, R. J. (1986). Inappropriate use of the cerebrospinal fluid venereal disease research laboratory (VDRL) test to exclude neurosyphilis. *Annals of Internal Medicine*, **104**, 86-89.

Dattwyler, R.J., Thomas, J., Benach, J.L. and Golightly, M.G. (1986). Cellular immune responses in Lyme disease. *Zentralblatt für Bakteriologie, Mikrobiologie und Hygiene*, **263**, 151-159.

Dattwyler, R.J., Volkman, D.J., Halperin, J.J., Luft, B.J., Thomas, J. and Golightly, M.G. (1988). Specific immune responses in Lyme Borreliosis. *Annals of the New York Academy of Sciences*, **539**, 93-102.

Davis, K., Hollister, L., Livesey, J. and Berger, P. (1979). CSF acetylcholinesterase in neuropsychiatric disorders. *Psychopharmacology*, **63**, 155-59.

Davis, K.L. and Goodnick, P.J. (1983). CSF acetylcholinesterase in neuropsychiatric disorders. *In* "Neurobiology of Cerebrospinal Fluid". Vol. 2. (Ed. J.H. Wood). pp. 197-204. Plenum Press, New York.

Davis, K.L., Davidson, M. Mohs, R.C. *et al.* (1984.). Plasma homovanillic acid concentration and the severity of schizophrenic illness. *Science*, **227**, 1601-2.

Davis, K.L., Davidson, M., Yang, R-K., Davis, B.M., Siever, L.J., Mohs, R.C., Ryan, T., Coccaro, E., Bierer, L. and Targum, S.D. (1988). CSF somatostatin in Alzheimer's disease, depressed patients, and control subjects. *Biological Psychiatry*, **24**, 710-712.

Davis, L.E. (1979). Normal laboratory values of CSF during pregnancy. *Archives of Neurology*, **36**, 443.

Davis, L.E. and Schmitt, J.W. (1989). Clinical significance of cerebrospinal fluid tests for neurosyphilis. *Annals of Neurology*, **25**, 50-55.

Davson, H. (1967). "Physiology of the Cerebrospinal Fluid". Little Brown and Company, Boston.

Davson, H. (1972). The cerebrospinal fluid. *In* "Handbook of Neurochemistry". (Ed. A. Lajtha). pp. 23-48. Plenum Press, New York.

Davson, H. (1975). Porous nature of the absorptive mechanism. *In* "Intracranial Pressure II". (Eds N. Lundberg, U. Ponten and M. Brock). pp. 28-34. Springer-Verlag, New York.

Davson, H., Welch, K. and Segal, M. (1987). "Physiology and Pathophysiology of the Cerebrospinal Fluid". Churchill Livingstone, Edinburgh.

De Angelis, L.M. (1981). Intracranial tuberculoma; case report and review of the literature. *Neurology, (Minn)* **31**, 1133-1136.

De Jong, R.N. (1979). "The Neurologic Examination". Harper and Row, New York.

De Lisi, L E. (1984). Is immune dysfunction associated with schizophrenia? A review of the data. *Psychopharmacology Bulletin*, **20**, (3) 509-513.

De Lisi, L. and Wyatt, R. (1987). Endoglandus hallucinogens and other behavioural modifying factors in schizophrenia. *In* "Handbook of Schizophrenia". Vol. 2. (Eds F. Henn and L. De Lisi), pp. 377-390. Elsevier Publishers, Amsterdam.

De Lisi, L., Weinberger, D., Potkin, S., Neckers, L., Shiling, D. and Wyatt, R. (1981). Quantitative determination of immunoglobulin in CSF and plasma of chronic schizophrenic patients. *British Journal of Psychiatry*, **139**, 513-18.

De Reuck, J., de Costa, W. and Van der Eecken, H. (1984). Acid phosphatase activity of CSF cells in multiple sclerosis and related neurological disorders. *In* "Immunological and Clinical Aspects of Multiple Sclerosis". (Eds Gansette and Delmotte). pp. 83-87. MTP Press, Hingham, MA.

De Souza, B., Bissette, G., Whitehouse, P.J., Powers, R.E., Price, D.L., Vale, W.W. and Nemeroff, C.B. (1990). Abnormalities in corticotropin-releasing factor (CRF) in neurodegenerative diseases. *In* "Corticotropin-releasing Factor: Basic and Clinical Studies of Neuropeptide". (Eds B. De Souza and C.B. Nemeroff). CRC Press, Boca Raten, Florida.

De Souza, E.B. (1991). Neurotransmitter receptor imaging techniques. *In* "Neuropeptides and Psychiatric Disorders". (Ed. C.B. Nemeroff). American Psychiatric Press, Washington D.C.

Deane R. and Segal, M.B. (1976). The sodium-dependent absorption of sugars across the choroid plexus of sheep. *Journal of Physiology*, **263**, 274-275.

Degrell, I. and Nagy, E. (1990). Concentration gradients for HVA, 5-HIAA, ascorbic acid and uric acid in cerebrospinal fluid. *Biological Psychiatry*, **27**, 891-896.

Degrell, I, Hellsing, K., Nagy, E. and Niklasson, F. (1989). CSF amino acid concentrations. *Biology Psychiatry*, **26**, 649-650.

Delaney, J. (1979). Spinal fluid aluminum levels in patients with Alzheimer disease. *Annals of Neurology*, **5**, 580-581.

Delaney, P. (1977). Neurologic manifestations in sarcoidosis. *Annals of Internal Medicine*, **87**, 336-345

Delasnerie-Lanpretre, N., Suet-Hubert, C. and Marcelli-Barge, H. (1982). CSF C'2 and HLA system in MS. *Tissue Antigen*, **19**, (1) 79-84.

Delauche, M.C., Clauvel, J.P. and Seligmann, M. (1981). Peripheral neuropathy and plasma cell neoplasias: a report of ten cases. *British Journal of Haematology*, **48**, 383-92.

Den Hartog Jager, W.A. (1980). "Color Atlas of CSF Pathology". Elsevier/North Holland Press, Amsterdam.

Dencker, S. and Malm, U. (1978). Protein pattern of CSF in mental disease. *Acta Psychiatrica Scandinavica*, **203**, Suppl. 105-9.

Deutsch, S.I., Mohs, R.C. Levy, M. I., Rothpearl, A.B. *et al.* (1983). Acetylcholinesterase activity in CSF in schizophrenia, depression, Alzheimer's disease and normals. *Biological Psychiatry*, **18**, (12) 1363-1373.

Diamond, S. and Baltes, B.J. (1973). Headache associated with low spinal pressure syndrome. *Illinios Medical Journal*, **144**, 560-561.

Dieterich M. and Brandt, T. (1988). Incidence of post-lumbar puncture headache is independent of daily fluid intake. *European Archives of Psychiatric and Neurological Science*, **237**, 194-196.

Domer, F.R. and Kaiser, L.R. (1977). Effects of probenecid on methotrexate exchange between the blood and the cerebrospinal fluid. *Archives of International Pharmacodynamics*, **225**, 17-24.

Domschke, W., Dickschas, A. and Mitznegg, P. (1979). CSF β-endorphin in schizophrenia. *Lancet*, i, 1024.

Donald P.R., Malan, C. and Schoeman, J.F. (1987). Adenosine deaminase as a diagnostic aid in tuberculous meningitis. *Journal of Infectious Diseases*, **156**, 1040-1041.

Donaldson, J. and Horak, E. (1982). CSF oestrone in pseudotumor cerebri. *Journal of Neurology, Neurosurgery and Psychiatry*, **45**, 734-736.

Donnan, G.A., Zapf, P., Doyle, A.E. and Bladin, P. (1983). CSF enzymes in lacunar and cortical stroke. *Stroke*, **14**, (2) 266-269.

Doran, A.R., Rubinow, D.R., Roy, A. and Pickar, D. (1986). CSF somatostatin and abnormal response to dexamethasone administration in schizophrenic and depressed patients. *Archives of General Psychiatry*, **43**, 365-369.

Doran, A.R., Boronow, J. *et al.* (1987). Structural brain pathology in schizophrenia revisited. Prefrontal cortex pathology is inversely correlated with cerebrospinal fluid levels of homovanillic acid. *Neuropsychopharmacology*, **1**, (1) 25-31.

Doran, A.R., Rubinow, D.R. *et al.* (1989). Fluphenazine treatment reduces CSF somatostatin in patients with schizophrenia: correlations with CSF HVA. *Biological Psychiatry*, **25**, 431-439.

Dripps, R.D. and Vandam, L.D. (1951). Hazards of lumbar puncture. *Journal of the American Medical Association*, **147**, (12) 1118-21.

Dupont, E., Christensen, S.E., Hansen, A.P., Olivarius, B. and Orskuv, H. (1982). Low CSF somatostatin in Parkinson disease: an irreversible abnormality. *Neurology*, **32**, 312-314.

Dwivedi, C. and Reddy, C.M. (1983). Diagnostic use of cerebrospinal fluid lactic acid levels in meningitis. *Journal of Medicine*, **14**, (5-6) 395-403.

Dyck, P.J. and Arnason, A. (1984). Chronic inflammatory demyelinating polyradiculoneuropathy. *In* "Peripheral Neuropathy". 2nd Edn. (Eds P.J. Dyck, P.C. Thomas, E.H. Lambert and Burge). pp. 2101-2114. W.B. Saunders, Philadelphia.

Dyck P.J., Lais, A.C., Ohta, M. *et al.* (1975). Chronic inflammatory polyradiculoneuropathy. *Mayo Clinic Proceedings*, **50**, 621-637.

Eadie, M.J. and Tyrer, J.H. (1983). "Biochemical Neurology". Alan R. Liss, Inc., New York.

Easton, J.D. (1979). Headache after lumbar puncture. *Lancet*, i, 974-5.

Ebers, G.C. (1984). Cerebrospinal fluid electrophoresis in multiple sclerosis. *In* "The Diagnosis of Multiple Sclerosis". (Ed. C.M. Poser), pp. 179-184. Thienne, New York.

Ebstein, R.P., Freedman, L.S., Lieberman, A., Park, D.H., Pasternack, B., Goldstein, M. and Coleman, M. (1974). A familial study in serum DBH levels in torsion dystonia. *Neurology*, **24**, 684-687.

Ebstein R.P., Biederman, J. *et al.* (1976). Cyclic GMP in the CSF of patients with schizophrenia before and after neuroleptic treatment. *Psychopharmacology*, **51**, 71-74.

Edvinsson, L., Lindvall, M., Owman, C. and West, K. (1983). Autonomic nervous control of CSF production and intracranial pressure. *In* "Neurobiology of CSF". Vol. 2, (Ed. Wood, J.H.). pp. 661-676. Plenum Press, New York.

Edwards, M.S.B., Davis, R.L. and Laurent, J. P. (1985). Tumor markers and cytologic features of cerebrospinal fluid. *Cancer*, **56**, 1773-1777.

Eeg-Olofsson, O., Link, H. and Wigertz, A. (1981). Concentrations of CSF proteins as a measure of blood brain barrier function and synthesis of IgG within the CNS in normal subjects from the age of 6 months to 30 years. *Acta Paediatrica Scandinavica*, **70**, 167-170.

Einstein, E.R. (1982). Proteins of the brain and CSF. *In* "Health and Disease". Charles C. Thomas, Springfield, IL.

Eisenstein, B.I. (1990). The polymerase chain reaction: a new method of using molecular genetics for medical diagnosis. *New England Journal of Medicine*, **322**, (3), 178-183.

Ekstedt, J. (1975). CSF hydrodynamics studied by means of constant pressure infusion technique. *In* "Intracranial Pressure II". (Eds N. Lundberg, U. Ponten, and M. Brock). pp. 35-41. Springer-Verlag, New York.

Elchisak, M.A., Powers, K.H. and Ebert, M.H. (1982). Demonstration of conjugated dopamine in monkey CSF by gas chromatography-mass spectrometry. *Journal of Neurochemistry*, **39**, 726-728.

Eldjarn, L., Try, K., Stokke, O. *et al.* (1966). Dietary effects on serum-phytanic-acid levels and on clinical manifestations in heredopathia atactica polyneuritiformis. *Lancet*, i, 691-693.

Ellis, S.G. and Verity, M.A. (1979). Central nervous system involvement in systemic lupus erythematosus: A review of neuropathologic findings in 57 cases, 1955-1977. *Seminars on Arthritis and Rheumatology*, **8**, 212-221.

Elovaara, I., Iivanainen, M., Poutianinen, E., Valle, S-L., Weber, T., Suni, J. and Lahdevirta, J. (1989). CSF and serum β-2-microglobulin in HIV infection related to neurological dysfunction. *Acta Neurologica Scandinavica*, **79**, 81-87.

Endo, T., Hara, S., Kuriiwa, F. and Kano, S. (1990). Postmortem changes in the levels of monoamine metabolites in human cerebrospinal fluid. *Forensic Science International*, **44**, 61-68.

Eng, R.II.K. and Seligman, S.J. (1981). Lumbar puncture-induced meningitis. *Journal of the American Medical Assoication*, **245**, (14), 1456-1459.

Enna, S., Wood, J. and Snyder, S. (1977a). GABA in human CSF: radioreceptor assay. *Journal of Neurochemistry*, **28**, 1121-1124.

Enna, S.J., Stern, L.Z., Wastek, G.J. and Yamamurura, H.I. (1977b). Cerebrospinal fluid GABA variations in neurological disorders. *Archives of Neurology*, **34**, 683-685.

Enna, S.J., Zeigler, M.G., Lake, L.R., Wood, J.H., Brooks, B.R. and Butler, I.J. (1980). Cerebrospinal fluid GABA: correlation with CSF and blood constituents and alterations in neurological disorders. *In* "Neurobiology of CSF". (Ed. J.H. Wood). pp. 189-196. Plenum Press, New York.

Epstein, M.H., Feldman, A.M. and Brusilow, S.W. (1977). Cerebrospinal fluid production: stimulation by cholera toxin. *Science,* **196**, 1012-1013.

Epstein, L.G., Goudsmit, J.; Paul, D.A., Morrison, S.H., Connor, E.M., Oleske, J.M. and Holland, B. (1987). Expression of human immunodeficiency virus in cerebrospinal fluid of children with progressive encephalopathy. *Annals of Neurology,* **21**, 397-401.

Erickson, D. (1992). Doomsday diagnostic? *Scientific American,* August, 120.

Eriksson, E., Westberg, P., Thuresson, K., Modigh, K., Ekman, R. and Widerlov, E. (1989). Increased cerebrospinal fluid levels of endorphin immunoreactivity in panic disorder. *Neuropsychopharmacology,* **2**, (3) 225-228.

Ernerudh, J., Olsson, T., Lindstrom, F. and Skogh, T. (1985). Cerebrospinal fluid immunoglobulin abnormalities in systemic lupus erythematosus. *Journal of Neurology, Neurosurgery and Psychiatry*, **48**, 807-813.

Ervin, F.R., Palmour, R.M., Young, S.N., Guzman-Flores, C. and Juarez, J. (1989). Voluntary consumption of beverage alcohol by vervet monkeys: population screening, descriptive behaviour and biochemical measures. *Pharmacology, Biochemistry and Behaviour,* **36**, 367-373.

Esler, M., Zweifler, A., Randall, O., Juluis, S. and de Quattro, V. (1977). Agreement among three different indices of sympathetic nervous system activity in essential hypertension. *Mayo Clinic Proceedings,* **52**, 379-382.

Evans, D.L., Stern, R.A., Golden, R.N., Haggerty, Jr, J.J., Perkins, D.O., Simon, J.S. and Nemeroff, C.B. (1991). Neuroendocrine and peptide challenge tests in primary and secondary depression. *In* "Neuropeptides and Psychiatric Disorders". (Ed. C.B. Nemeroff). pp. 15. American Psychiatric Press, Washington D.C.

Extein, I., Roth, R.H. and Bowers, M.B. (1974). Accumulation of ^{3}H-HVA in rabbit brain and CSF following intravenous ^{3}H-LODOPA. *Biological Psychiatry,* **9**, 161-170.

Fahrenkrug, J., Schaffalitzky de Muchadell, O.B. and Fahnenkrug, A. (1977). A VIP in human CSF. *Brain Research,* **124**, 581-584.

Fang, V.S., Fessler, R.G., Rachlin, J.R. and Brown, F.D. (1984). Effect of contrast media on radioimmunoassay of β-endorphin in cerebrospinal fluid. *Clinical Chemistry,* **30**, (2) 311-314.

Farde L., Wiesel, F-A., Hall, H. *et al.* (1987.). No D_2 receptor increase in PET study of schizophrenia. *Archives of General Psychiatry*, **44**, 671-672.

Farde L., Wiesel, F-A., Stone-Elander, S. *et al.* (1990). D_2 dopamine receptors in neuroleptic-naive schizophrenic patients. A positron emission tomography study with [^{11}C] raclopride. *Archives of General Psychiatry,* **47**, 213-219.

Farlow, M., Ghetti, B., Benson, M.D., Farrow, J., van Nostrand, W.E. and Wagner, S.L. (1992). Low CSF concentrations of soluble amyloid β-protein precursor in hereditary Alzheimer's disease, *Lancet,* **340**, 453-54.

Faull, K., DoAmaral, J., Berger, P. and Barchas, J. (1978). Mass spectrometric identification and selected ion monitoring quantitation of GABA in human lumbar CSF. *Journal of Neurochemistry,* **31**, 1119-1122.

Faull, K.F., Guilleminault, C., Berger, P. and Barchas, J. (1983). CSF monoamine metabolites in narcolepsy and hypersomnia. *Annals of Neurology,* **13**, 258-263.

Fava, M., Copeland, P.M., Schweiger, U. and Herzog, D.B. (1989). Neurochemical abnormalities of anorexia nervosa and bulimia nervosa. *American Journal of Psychiatry*, **146**, 963-971.

Feinglass, E.J., Arnet, F.C., Dorsch, E.A. *et al.* (1976). Neuropsychiatric manifestations of systemic lupus erythematosus: diagnosis, clinical spectrum, and relationship to other features of the disease. *Medicine (Baltimore)* **55**, 323-339.

Feldman, A.M., Epstein, M.H. and Brusilow, S.W. (1979). Effect of cholera toxin and prostaglandins on the rat choroid plexus *in vitro*. *Brain Research,* **167**, 119-128.

Felgenhauer, K. (1974). Protein size and CSF composition. *Klinische Wochenschrift,* **52**, 1158-1164.

Felgenhauer, K. (1987). The selectivity of the blood-CSF-barrier under normal and pathological conditions. *In* "Advances in CSF Protein, Research and Diagnosis". (Ed. E.J. Thompson). pp. 35-48. MTP Press Ltd, Lancaster.

Fencl, V. (1971). Distribution of H^+ and HCO_3^- in cerebral fluid. *In* "Ion Homeostatis of the Brain". (Eds S.C. Sorensen and B.K. Siesjo). pp. 175-185. Academic Press, New York.

Feraru, E.R., Aronow, H.A. and Lipton, R.B. (1990). Neurosyphilis in AIDS patients: initial CSF VDRL may be negative. *Neurology*, **40**, 541-543.

Fernandez, E. (1990). Headaches associated with low spinal fluid pressure. *Headache* **30**, 122-128.

Fernstrom, J., Madras, B., Munro, H. and Wurtman, R. (1974). Nutritional control of the synthesis of 5-HT in the brain. *In* "Aromatic Amino Acids in the Brain". CIBA Symposium 22 pp. 153-173. Elsevier, Amsterdam.

Ferrarese, C., Appollonio, I., Frigo, M., Meregalli, S., Piolti, R., Tamma, F. and Frattola, L. (1990). Cerebrospinal fluid levels of diazepam-binding inhibitor in neurodegenerative disorders with dementia. *Neurology*, **40**, 632-635.

Field, E.J. and Joyce. G. (1983). Multiple sclerosis: effect of gamma linolenate administration upon membranes and the need for extended trials of UFAs. *European Neurology*, **22**, 78-83.

Fishman, R.A. (1976). Cerebrospinal fluid. *In* "Clinical Neurology". Vol. 1. Chapter 5, (Eds. A. Baker and L. Baker). pp. 1-40. Harper and Row, New York.

Fishman, R.A. (1980). Cerebrospinal Fluid in Diseases of the Nervous System. W.B. Saunders Company, Philadephia.

Fishman, R.A. (1992). "Cerebrospinal Fluid in Diseases of the Nervous System". 2nd edn. W.B. Saunders, Philadelphia.

Flatten, H., Rodt, S.A., Vamnes, J., Rosland, J. *et al.* (1989). Postdural puncture headache – a comparison between 26- and 29-gauge needles in young patients. *Anaesthesia*, **44**, 147-149.

Fleischer, A.S., Rudman, D.R., Fresh, C.B. and Tindall, G.T. (1977). Con centration of 3,5-cAMP in VCSF of patients following severe head trauma. *Journal of Neurosurgery*, **47**, 517-524.

Flentge, F., Hajonides-van Der Meulen, W.M., Lakke, J.P. and Teelken, A.W. (1984). CSF choline levels in groups of patients with cranial trauma or extrapyramidal disorders. *Journal Neurology, Neurosurgery and Psychiatry*, **47**, (2) 207-9.

Flint Beal, M. and Bird, E.D. (1988). Neuropeptides in Huntington's disease. *In* "Neuropeptides in Psychiatric and Neurological Disorders". Chapter 6. (Ed. C.B. Nemeroff). Johns Hopkins University Press, Baltimore.

Flourens, P. (1858). Memoir of Magendie. *In* "The Way In and the Way Out". (Ed. P. Cranefield). (1974). Chera Publishing Co. New York.

Flowers, D. and Scott, G.M. (1985). How useful are serum and CSF interferon levels as a rapid diagnostic aid in virus infections? *Journal of Medical Virology*, **15**, 35-47.

Folco, G. and Paoletti, R. (eds.) (1978). "Molecular Biology and Pharmacology of Cyclic Nucleotides". Elsevier/North Holland Press, Amsterdam.

Forbes, H.S. and Nason, G.I.(1935). The cerebral circulation. *Archives of Neurology and Psychiatry*, **34**, 533-547.

Foriz, L. (1952). Treatment of mental patients with ADH of the posterior pituitary. *Diseases of the Nervous System*, **13**, 44-47.

Frecska, E. and Davis, K.L. (1991). The opioid model in psychiatric research. *In* "Neuropeptides and Psychiatric Disorders". (Ed. C.B. Nemeroff). pp. 169-192. American Psychiatric Press, Washington D.C.

Frecska, E., Perenyi, A. *et al.* (1985). CSF dopamine turnover and positive schizophrenic symptoms after withdrawal of long-term neuroleptic treatment. *Psychiatry Research*, **16**, 221-26.

Fredrikson, S., Carlander, B., Billiard, M. and Link, H. (1990). CSF immune variables in patients with narcolepsy. *Acta Neurologica Scandinavica*, **81**, 253-254.

French, G.L., Teoh, R., Chan, C.Y., Humphries, M.J., Cheung, S.W. and O'Mahony, G. (1987). Diagnosis of tuberculous meningitis by detection of tuberculostearic acid in cerebrospinal fluid. *Lancet*, ii, 117-119.

French, G.L., Chan, C.Y., Poon, D., Cheung , S.W. and Cheng, A.F.B. (1990). Rapid diagnosis of bacterial meningitis by the detection of a fatty acid marker in CSF with gas chromatography-mass spectrometry and selected ion monitoring. *Journal of Medical Microbiology*, **31**, 21-26.

Frithz, G., Ronquist, G. and Hugosson, R. (1982). Perspectives of adenylate kinase activity and glutathione concentration in CSF of patients with ischemic and neoplastic brain lesions. *European Neurology*, **21**, 41-47.

Fryer-Leibowitz., S. (1989). Hypothalamic neuropeptide Y, galanin and amines: concepts of co-existence in relation to feeding behavior. *Annals of the New York Academy of Sciences*, **575**, 221-235.

Fujimoto, A., Nagao, T., Ebara, T., Sato, M. and Otsuki, S. (1983). Cerebrospinal fluid monoamine metabolites during alcohol withdrawal syndrome and recovered state. *Biological Psychiatry*, **18**, (10), 1141-52.

Fujishiro K., Hagihara, M., Takahashi, A. and Nagatsu, T. (1990). Concentrations of neopterin and biopterin in the CSF of patients with Parkinson's disease. *Biochemical Medicine and Metabolic Biology*, **44**, 97-100.

Fulton, D.S., Levin, V., Lubich, W., Wilson, C. and Marton, L. (1983). Clinical correlations of CSF polyamine levels. *In* "Neurobiology of CSF". Vol 2. (Ed. J.H. Wood). pp. 441-452. Plenum Press, New York.

Furneaux, H.F., Reich, L. and Posner, J. (1990). Autoantibody synthesis in the CNS of patients with paraneoplastic syndromes. *Neurology*, **40**, 1085-1091.

Gaio, J.M., Pollak, P., Hommel, M. and Perret, J. (1987). Clinical and biochemical effects of gamma-vinyl GABA in tardive dyskinesia. *Journal of Neurology, Neurosurgery and Psychiatry*, **50**, 1674-1678.

Gansette, R.E. and Delmotte, P. (eds.) (1984). "Immunological and Clinical Aspects of Multiple Sclerosis". MTP Press Ltd, Hingham, MA.

Garcia-Monco, J.C., Villar, B.F., Alen, J.C. and Benach, J.L. (1990). Borrelia burgdorferi in the central nervous system: experimental and clinical evidence for early invasion. *Journal of Infectious Diseases,* **161**, 1187-1193.

Gardner, D.J., O'Gorman, A.M. and Blundell, J.E. (1989). Intraspinal epidermoid tumour: late complication of lumbar puncture. *Canadian Medical Association Journal,* **141**, 223-225.

Garelis, E. and Sourkes, T.L. (1973). Sites of origin in the central nervous system of monoamine metabolites measured in human cerebrospinal fluid. *Journal of Neurology, Neurosurgery and Psychiatry,* **36**, 625-629.

Garelis, E., Young, S.N., Lal, S. and Sourkes, T.L. (1974). Monoamine metabolites in lumbar CSF: the question of their origin in relation to clinical studies. *Brain Research,* **79**, 1-8.

Garver, D.L., Bissette, G., Yao, J.K. and Nemeroff, C.B. (1991). Relation to CSF neurotensin concentrations to symptoms and drug response of psychotic patients. *American Journal of Psychiatry,* **148**, 484-488.

Gattaz, W., Gattaz, D. and Beckmann H. (1982). Glutamate in schizophrenics and healthy controls. *Archiv für Psychiatrie und Nervenkrankheit,* **231**, 221-225.

Gattaz, W.F., Cramer, H. and Beckmann, H. (1983a). Low CSF concentrations of cyclic GMP in schizophrenia. *British Journal of Psychiatry,* **142**, 288-91, March.

Gattaz W.F., Kattermann, R. Gattaz, D. and Beckmann, H. (1983b). Magnesium and calcium in the CSF of schizophrenic patients and healthy controls: correlations with cyclic GMP. *Biological Psychiatry,* **18**, (8) 935-939.

Gattaz, W.F., Cramer, H. and Beckmann, H. (1984). Haloperidol increases the cerebrospinal fluid concentrations of cyclic GMP in schizophrenic patients. *Biological Psychiatry* **19**, (8) 1229-1235.

Gattaz, W.F., Roberts, E. and Beckmann, H. (1986a). Cerebrospinal fluid concentrations of free GABA in schizophrenia: no changes after haloperidol treatment. *Journal of Neural Transmission,* **66**, 69-73.

Gattaz, W.F., Rissler, K., Gattaz, D. and Cramer, H. (1986b). Effects of haloperidol on somatostatin-like immunoreactivity in the CSF of schizophrenic patients. *Psychiatry Research,* **17**, 1-6.

Gaukroger, P.B. and Brownridge, P. (1987). Epidural blood patch in the treatment of spontaneous low CSF pressure headache. *Pain,* **29**, 119-122.

Genazzani, A., Nappi, C., Facchinetti, F., Mazzella, G., Parrini, F., Sinforiani, E., Petraglia, F. and Savoldi, F., (1982). Central deficiency of β-endorphin in alcohol addicts. *Journal of Clinical Endocrinology and Metabolism,* **55**, 583-586.

Genazzani, A.R., Nappi, G., Facchinetti, F., Micieli, G., Petraglia, F., Bono, G., Monittola, C. and F. Savoldi, (1984). Progressive impairment of CSF β-EP levels in migraine sufferers. *Pain,* **18**, (2), 127-33.

George D.T., Adinoff, B., Ravitz, B., Nutt, D.J., De Jong, J., Berrettini, W., Mefford, I.N., Costa, E. and Linnoila, M. (1990). A cerebrospinal fluid study of the pathophysiology of panic disorder associated with alcoholism. *Acta Psychiatrica Scandinavica,* **82**, 1-7.

Geracioti, T.D. and Liddle, R.A. (1988). Impaired cholecystokinin secretion in bulimia nervosa. *New England Journal of Medicine,* **319**, (11) 683-688.

Gerhard W., Taylor, A., Wroblewska, Z., Sandberg-Wollheim, M. and Koprowski, H. (1981). Analysis of a predominant immunoglobin population in the cerebrospinal fluid of a multiple sclerosis patient by means of anti-idiotypic hybridonia antibody. *Proceedings of the National Academy of Science, USA*, 78, 3225-3229.

Gerner, R.H. and Merrill, J.E. (1983). Cerebrospinal fluid prostaglandin E in depression, mania, and schizophrenia compared to normals. *Biological Psychiatry*, **18** (5), 565-9. May

Gerner, R.H. and Sharp, B. (1982). CSF β-endorphin-immunoreactivity in normal, schizophrenic, depressed, manic and anorexic subjects. *Brain Research*, **237**, 244-247.

Gerner, R.H. and Yamada, T. (1982). Altered neuropeptide concentrations in cerebrospinal fluid of psychiatric patients. *Brain Research*, **238**, 298-302.

Gerner, R.H., Gorelick, D.A., Catlin, D.H. and Li, C.H. (1982). Behavioral effects of β-endorphin in depression and schizophrenia . *In* "Endorphins and Opiate Antagonists in Psychiatric Research". (Eds N. Shah and A. Donald) pp. 257-270, Plenum Press, New York .

Gerner R.H., Fairbanks, L., Anderson, G.M. *et al.* (1984a). CSF neurochemistry in depressed, manic and schizophrenic patients compared with that of normal controls. *American Journal of Psychiatry*, **141**, (12) 1533-1540.

Gerner, R.H., Cohen, D.J., Fairbanks, L. *et al.* (1984b). CSF neurochemistry of women with anorexia nervosa and normal women. *American Journal of Psychiatry*, **141**, (11) 1441-1444.

Gerner R.H., van Kammen, D. P. and Ninan, P.T. (1985). Cerebrospinal fluid cholecystokinin, bombesin and somatostatin in schizophrenia and normals. *Progress in Neuropsychopharmacology and Biological Psychiatry*, **9**, 73-82.

Geschwind, N. (1977). Insensitivity to pain in psychotic patients. *New England Journal of Medicine* 296, 1480.

Giacobini, E., Becker, R., Elble, R., Mattio T. and McIlhany, M. (1986). Acetylcholine metabolism in brain – is it reflected by CSF changes? *In* "Alzheimer's and Parkinson's Diseases". (Eds A. Fisher, I. Hanin and C. Lachman). pp. 309-316. Plenum Press, New York.

Gibson, B.E., Wedel, D.J., Faust, R.J. and Petersen, R.C. (1988). Continuous epidural saline infusion for the treatment of low CSF pressure headache. *Anaesthesiology*, **68**, (5), 789-791.

Gibson, T. and Myers, A.R. (1976). Nervous system involvement in systemic lupus erythematosus. *Annals of Rheumatological Disorders*, **35**, 398-406.

Gillberg, C. and Svennerholm, L. (1987). CSF monoamines in autistic syndromes and other pervasive developmental disorders of early childhood. *British Journal of of Psychiatry*, **151**, 89-94.

Gillberg, C., L. Svennerholm, and C. Hamilton-Hellberg (1983). Childhood psychosis and monoamine metabolites in spinal fluid. *Journal of Autism and Development Disorder*, **13**, (4), 383-96.

Gillberg, C., Terenius, L. and Lonnerholm, G. (1985). Endorphin acitivity in childhood psychosis. *Archives of General Psychiatry*, **42**, 780-783.

Gjerris, A. (1988a). Baseline studies on transmitter substances in cerebrospinal fluid in depression. *Acta Psychiatrica Scandinavica*, Suppl 346 78.

Gjerris, A., (1988b). Do concentrations of neurotransmitters in lumbar CSF reflect cerebral dysfunction in depression? *Acta Psychiatrica Scandinavica*, (Suppl. 345) **78**, 21-24.

Gjerris, A. and Rafaelsen, O.J. (1984). Catecholamines and vasoactive intestinal polypeptide in cerebrospinal fluid in depression . *In* "Frontiers in Biochemical and Pharmacological Research in Depression". (Ed. E. Usdin *et al.*). pp. 159-60. Raven Press, New York.

Gjerris, A., Rafaelsen, O.J. and Christensen, N.J. (1987*a*). CSF-adrenaline – low in somatizing depression. *Acta Psychiatrica Scandinavica,* **75,** 516-520.

Gjerris, A., Sorensen, A.S., Rafaelsen, O.J., Werdelin, L., Alling, C. and Linnoila, M. (1987*b*). 5-HT and 5-HIAA in cerebrospinal fluid in depression. *Journal of Affective Disorders,* **12,** 13-22.

Gjerris, A., Werdelin, L., Gjerris, F. *et al.* (1987*c*). CSF amine metabolites in depression, dementia, and in controls. *Acta Psychiatrica Scandinavica,* **75,** 619-628.

Gjerris, A., Gjerris, F., Sorensen, P.S., Sorensen, E.B., Christensen, N.J., Fahrenkrug, J. and Rehfeld, J.F. (1988). Do concentrations of neurotransmitters measured in lumbar cerebrospinal fluid reflect the concentrations at brain level? *Acta Neurochirurgica,* **91,** 55-59.

Gjessing, L.R., Gjesdahl, P., Dietrichson, P. and Presthus, J. (1974). Free amino acids in the CSF in old age and in Parkinson's disease. *European Neurology,* **12,** 33-37.

Glass J. and Wertlake, P. (1983). Malignant cells in CSF and their clinical significance. *In* "Neurobiology of Cerebrospinal Fluid". (J.H. Wood). pp. 411-425. Plenum Press, New York.

Gobel, H., Klostermann, H., Lindner, V., Schenkl, S. and Soyka, D. (1989). Vascular reactions in basal cerebral arteries in case of postlumbar puncture headache: a prospective double-blind study. Presented at the Headache Congress, Sydney, Australia, October.

Gold, B.I., Bowers, M., Roth, R. and Sweeny, D.W. (1980*a*). GABA levels in CSF of patients with psychiatric disorders. *American Journal of Psychiatry,* **137,** 362-364.

Gold, P., Goodwin, F.K., Ballenger, J. *et al.* (1980*b*). Central vasopressin function in affective illness. *In* "Hormones and the Brain". (Ed. D. de Wied and P. van Keep). pp. 241-52 . MTP Press, Lancaster.

Gold, P.W., Rubinow, D., Post, R.M. and Goodwin, F.K. (1982). Central peptides in psychiatry illness . *In* " Brain Peptides and Hormones". (Eds R. Collu, *et al.*). Raven Press, New York.

Gold, P.W., Kaye, W., Robertson, G.L. and Ebert, M. (1983). Abnormalities in plasma and cerebrospinal-fluid arginine vasopressin in patients with anorexia nervosa. *New England Journal of Medicine,* **308,** 1117-1123.

Gold, P., Loriaux, D., Roy, A. *et al.* (1986). Response to CRH in the hypercortisolism of depression and Cushing's disease. Pathophysiology and diagnostic implications. *New England Journal of Medicine,* **314,** 1329-35.

Golden, G.S. (1982). Neurobiological correlates of learning disabilities. *Annals of Neurology,* **12,** 409-418.

Goldman, G., L. Volicer, B. Gold, and R. Roth (1981). CSF GABA and cyclic nucleotides in alcoholics with and without seizures. *Alcoholism, Clinical and Experimental Research,* **5,** 431-434.

Goldmann, E.E. (1913). Vital farbung am zentralnervensystem. *Abh. Konpreuss Akad Wiss. Berlin,* (cited by Walker *et al.*) pp. 5-7.

Goldstein, D.A., Romoff, M., Bogin, E. and Massry, S.G. (1979). Relationship between the concentrations of calcium and phosphorous in blood and CSF. *Journal of Clinical Endocrinology and Metabolism*, **49**, 58-62.

Goldstein, G.W. (1979). Relation of potassium transport to oxidative metabolism in isolated brain capillaries. *Journal of Physiology*, **286-295**, 185-195.

Goldstein, G.W. (1988). Endothelial cell-astrocyte interactions. *Annals of the New York Academy of Science*, **529**, 31-39.

Goldstein G.W. and Betz, A.L. (1986). The blood-brain barrier. *Scientific American*, **255**, 74-83.

Gomez S., Davous, P., Faivre-Bauman, A. *et al.* (1986). Acetylcholinesterase activity and somatostatin-like immunoreactivity in LCSF of demented patients. *In* "Alzheimer's and Parkinson's Diseases". (Eds A.Fisher, I. Hanin and C. Lachman). pp. 317-322. Plenum Press, New York.

Goodnick, P.J., Evans, H.E., Dunner, D.L. and Fieve, R.R. (1980). Amino acid concentrations in CSF: effects of aging, depression, and probenecid. *Biological Psychiatry*, **15**, 557-563.

Gordon, E. and Rossanda, M. (1968). The importance of the CSF acid-base status in the treatment of unconscious patients with brain lesions. International Symp. on CSF and CBF. *Scandinavian Journal of Laboratory and Clinical Investigations*, Suppl. 102.

Gordon, E., Perlow, M., Oliver, J., Ebert, M. and Kopin, I., (1975). Origins of catecholamine metabolites in monkey CSF. *Journal of Neurochemistry*, **25**, 347-349.

Goudsmit, J., Paul, D.A., Lange, J.M.A., Speelman, H., van der Noordaa, J. *et al.* (1986). Expression of human immunodeficiency virus antigen (HIV-Ag) in serum and cerebrospinal fluid during acute and chronic infection. *Lancet*, 26 July 177-180.

Gower, D.J., Baker, A.L., Bell, W.O. and Ball, M.R. (1987). Contraindications to lumbar puncture as defined by computed cranial tomography. *Journal of Neurology, Neurosurgery and Psychiatry*, **50**, 1071-1074.

Grant, R., Condon, B., Hart, I. and Teasdale, G.M. (1991). Changes in intracranial CSF volume after lumbar puncture and their relationship to post-LP headache. *Journal of Neurology, Neurosurgery and Psychiatry*, **54**, 440-442 .

Graves, M. (1989). Cerebrospinal fluid infections. *In* "The Cerebrospinal Fluid". Chapter 6. (Eds R.M. Herndon and R.A. Brumback). Kluwer Academic Publishers, Norwell, MA.

Greenfield, J, and Carmichael, E. (1925). "The CSF in Clinical Diagnosis". MacMillan and Co., London.

Greenlee, J.E. (1990). Approach to diagnosis of meningitis – cerebrospinal fluid evaluation. *Infectious Disease Clinics of North America*, **4** (4). 583-595.

Greensher, J, Mofenson, H.C., Borofsky, L.G. and Sharma, R. (1971). Lumbar puncture in the neonate: a simplified technique. *Journal of Pediatrics*, **78**, (6) 1034-1035.

Griauzde, M. and M. Radulovacki (1976). Increase of 5-hydroxyindoleacetic acid and homovanillic acid in cisternal fluid of cats subjected to stress. *Journal of Neurochemistry*, **26**, 1301-1302.

Gribbels E. and Schliep, G. (1970). Diabetische polyneuropathie: problems der diagnostik und nosologie. *Fortschritte der Neurologie-Psychiatrie*, **38**, 369.

Griffin, D.E., McArthur, J.C. and Cornblath, D.R. (1991). Neopterin and interferon-gamma in serum and cerebrospinal fluid of patients with HIV-associated neurologic diseases. *Neurology*, Jan.

Grimaldi, L.M.E., Martino, G.V., Franciotta, D.M., Brustia, R.. Castagna, A., Pristera, R. and Lazzarin, A. (1991). Elevated alpha-tumor necrosis factor levels in spinal fluid from HIV-1-infected patients with central nervous system involvement. *Annals of Neurology*, **29**, 21-25.

Gronhagen-Riska, C. and Selroos, O. (1979). Angiotensin converting enzyme: IV. Changes in serum activity and in lysozyme concentrations as indicators of the course of untreated sarcoidosis. *Scandinavian Journal of Respiratory Diseases*, **60**, 337-44.

Gross, H.A., Lake, C.R., Ebert, M.H. *et al.* (1979). Catecholamine metabolism in primary anorexia nervosa. *Journal of Clinical Endocrinology and Metabolism*, **49**, 805-809.

Grove, J., Schechter, P.J., Tell, G., Rumbach, L., Marescaux, C., Warter, L.M. and Koch-Weser, J. (1982*a*). Artifactual increases in the concentration of free GABA in samples of human cerebrospinal fluid are due to degradation of homocarnosine. *Journal of Neurochemistry*, **39**, 1061.

Grove, J. *et al.* (1982*b*). Concentration gradients of free and total γ-aminobutyric acid and homocarnosine in human CSF. *Journal of Neurochemistry*, **39**, 1618-1622.

Grove, J., Palfreyman, M.G. and Schechter, P.J. (1983). Cerebrospinal fluid GABA as an index of brain GABA activity. *Clinical Neuropharmacology*, **6**, (3), 223-9.

Growdon, J.H. and Logue, M. (1982). Choline, HVA and 5-HIAA levels in cerebrospinal fluid of patients with Alzheimer's disease. *In* "Alzheimer's Disease: A Report of Progress". (Eds S. Corkin *et al.*) Raven Press, New York.

Gschnait, F., Schmidt, B.L. and Luger, A. (1981). Cerebrospinal fluid immunoglobulins in neurosyphilis. *British Journal of Venereal Disease*, **57**, 238-40.

Gu, J., Polak, J., Tapia, Marangos, F. P. and Pearse, A. (1981). Neurone-specific enolase in marked cells: a new, simple and reliable histological marker. *Journal of Pathology*, **134**, 315-316.

Guthrie, S.K., Berrettini, W., Rubinow, D.R. *et al.* (1985). Different neurotransmitter metabolite concentrations in CSF samples from inpatient and outpatient normal volunteers. *Acta Psychiatrica Scandinavica*, **73**, 315-321..

Gwirtsman H.E., Kaye, W.H., George, D.T. *et al.* (1989). Central and peripheral ACTH and cortisol levels in anorexia nervosa and bulimia. *Archives of General Psychiatry*, **46**, 61-69.

Haber, S.N., Kowall, N.W., Vonsattel, J. P. *et al.* (1986). Gilles de la Tourette's syndrome, a postmortem neuropathological and immunohistochemical study. *Journal of Neurological Science*, **75**, 225-241.

Hagberg, B. and Lyon, G. (1981). Pooled European series of hereditary peripheral neuropathies in infancy and childhood. A "correspondence workshop" report of the European Federation of Child Neurology Societies. *Neuropediatrics*, **12**, 4-17.

Hagenfeldt, L., Bjerkenstedt, L., Edman, G., Sedvall, G. and Wiesel, F.A. (1984). Amino acids in plasma and CSF and monoamine metabolites in CSF: interrelationship in healthy subjects. *Journal of Neurochemistry*, **42**, (3) 833-837.

Hallgren, R., Terent, A. and Venge, P. (1982). Lactoferris, lysozyme, and β-2-microglobulin levels in CSF. *Inflammation*, **6**, 291-304.

Hallgren, R., Terent, A. and Venge, P. (1983). Eosinophil cationic protein (ECP). in the CSF. *Journal of Neurological Science*, **58**, 57-71.

Halliburton, W.D. (1917). The possible functions of cerebrospinal fluid. *Proceedings of the Royal Society of Medicine*, Neurology Section 10, part 2, p 1.

Halliday, H.L. (1989). When to do a lumbar puncture in a neonate. *Archives of Disease in Childhood*, **64**, 313-316.

Halliwell, B. (1989). Oxidants and the central nervous system: some fundamental questions. *Acta Neurologica Scandinavica*, **126**, 23-33.

Hallmans, P.G. and Sjostrom, R. (1982). Zinc concentrations in normal and pathological CSF. *Acta Neurologica Scandinavica*, Suppl. 90, **65**, 184-185.

Hallpike J.F. *et al.* (1983). *In* "Multiple Sclerosis, Pathology, Diagnosis and Management". (Eds J.F. Hallpike and W.W. Tourtellotte). pp. 395. Chapman and Hall, London.

Halperin, J. and Heyes, M. (1992). Neuroactive kynurenines in Lyme borreliosis. *Neurology*, **42**, 43-50.

Handler, C.E., Smith, F.R., Perkin, G.D. and Rose, F.C. (1982). Posture and lumbar puncture headache: a controlled trial in 50 patients. *Journal of the Royal Society of Medicine*, **75**, 404-407.

Hansen, K., Cruz, M. and Link, H. (1990). Oligoclonal Borrelia burgdorferi-specific IgG antibodies in cerebrospinal fluid in Lyme neuroborreliosis. *Journal of Infectious Diseases*, **161**, 1194-1202.

Hare, T.A., Manyam, N.V. and Glaese, B.S. (1980). Evaluation of CSF GABA content in neurological and psychiatric disorders. *In* "Neurobiology of CSF". (Ed. J.H. Wood). pp. 171-188. Plenum Press, New York.

Hare, T.A., Wood, J.H., Manyam, B.V., Gerner, R.H., Ballenger, J.C. and Post, R.M. (1982*a*). Central nervous system GABA activity in man. *Archives of Neurology*, **39**, 247-249.

Hare, T., Wood, J., Manyam, B., Gerner, R., Ballenger, J. and Post, R. (1982*b*). CNS GABA activity in man relationship to age and sex as reflected in CSF. *Archives of Neurology*, **39**, (4). 119-123.

Harrington, M.G. and Merril, C.R. (1985). Additional cerebrospinal fluid proteins found in schizophrenia and Creutzfeldt-Jakob disease. *Psychopharmacology Bulletin*, **21**, (3) 361-364.

Harrington, M G., Merril, C.R. and Fuller-Torrey, E. (1985). Differences in cerebrospinal fluid proteins between patients with schizophrenia and normal persons. *Clinical Chemistry*, **31**, (5) 722-726.

Harrington, M.G., Merril, C.R., Asher, D.M. and Gajdusek, D.C. (1986). Abnormal proteins in the cerebrospinal fluid of patients with Creutzfeldt-Jakob Disease. *New England Journal of Medicine*, **315**, (5) 279-283.

Harrison, M.J.G., McAllister, R.H. (1991). Neurologic complications of HIV infection. *In* "Infections of the Central Nervous System". (Ed. H. Lambert) pp. 343-359. B.C. Decker, Philadelphia.

Hartard, C., Spsitzer, K., Kumize, K. *et al.* (1988). Prognostic relevance of initial clinical and paraclinical parameters for the course of multiple sclerosis. *Journal of Neuroimmunology*, **20**, 247-250.

Hartman, E. (1976). Schizophrenia: a theory. *Psychopharmarcology*, **49**, 1-15.

Have, T.R., La Quier, N.W. and Barlow, A.G. (1986). Organisation of genes encoding two outer surface membrane proteins of the Lyme disease agent B.b. within a single transcription unit. *Infection and Immunology*, **54**, 207-212.

Hawley, R., Major, L., Schulman, E., Trocha, P., Takenaga, J. and Catravas, G. (1981*a*). CSF cyclic nucleotides and GABA do not change in alcohol withdrawal. *Life Science*, **28**, 295-299.

Hawley, R., Major, L., Schulman, E. and Lake, R. (1981*b*). CSF levels of norepinephrine during alcohol withdrawal. *Archives of Neurology*, **38**, 289-292.

Hawley, R.J., Major, L.F. Schulman, E.A. and Linnoila, M. (1985). Cerebrospinal fluid 3-methoxy-4-hydroxyphenylglycol and norepinephrine levels in alcohol withdrawal. Correlations with clinical signs. *Archives of General Psychiatry*, **42**, 1056-1062.

Hay, E., Royds, J.A., Davies-Jones, G.A.B., Lewtas, N.A., Timperley, W.R. and Taylor, C.B. (1984). Cerebrospinal fluid enolase in stroke. *Journal of Neurology, Neurosurgery and Psychiatry*, **47**, 724-729.

Hayakawa T., Ushio, Y., Mori, T., Arita, N., *et al.* (1979). Levels in stroke patients of CSF astroprotein, an astrocyte-specific cerebroprotein. *Stroke*, **10**, 685-689.

Hayden, M.R. (1981). "Huntington's Chorea". Springer-Verlag, New York.

Hayward, R.A. Shapiro, M.F. and Oye, R.K. (1987). Laboratory testing on cerebrospinal fluid – a reappraisal. *Lancet*, i, January, 8523.

Health and Public Policy Committee, American College of Physicians (1986) (Position Paper). The diagnostic spinal tap. *Annals of Internal Medicine*, **104**, 880-886.

Hedberg, C.W. and Osterholm, M.T. (1990). Serologic tests for antibody to borrelia burgdorferi – another Pandora's box for medicine. *Archives of Internal Medicine*, **150**, 772-3.

Heikinheimo, M., Wahlstrom, Lehto, V., Barg, B., Hurme, M., and Palo, J. (1982). Pregnancy-specific β-l-glycoprotein-like material in human CSF. *Journal of Clinical Endocrinology and Metabolism*, **55**, (1) 189-192.

Heikkinen, E.R., Myllyla, V.V., Vapaatalo, H. and Hokkanen, E. (1974). Urinary excretion and CSF concentration of cAMP in various neurological diseases. *European Neurology*, **11**, 270-280.

Heilman, K.M., Watson, R.T. and Green, M. (1977). "Handbook of Differential Diagnosis of Neurologic Signs and Symptoms". Appleton-Century-Crofts, New York.

Heipertz, R., Eickhoff, K. and Karstens, K.H. (1979*a*). Magnesium and inorganic phosphate content in CSF related to BBB function in neurological disease. *Journal of Neurological Science*, **40**, 87-95.

Heipertz, R., Eickhoff, K. and Karstens, K.H. (1979*b*). CSF concentrations of magnesium and inorganic phosphate in epilepsy. *Journal of Neurological Science*, **41**, 55-60.

Hempel, K., Dommasch, D. and Brors, W. (1980). Central and peripheral MBP in CSF of MS and other neurological disorders. *In* "Progress in MS Research". (Eds H. Bauer *et al.*). pp. 170-173. Springer-Verlag, New York.

Henriksson, A. and Link, H. (1985). Prolonged IgM response within the central nervous system in lymphocytic meningoradiculitis (Bannwarth's syndrome). *New England Journal of Medicine*, *313*, (19). 1231.

Heritch A.J. (1990). Evidence for reduced and dysregulated turnover of dopamine in schizophrenia. *Schizophrenia Bulletin*, **16**, (4). 605-615.

Hermansen, M.C. and Ellison, P.H. (1982). CSF acid-base balance in newborns. *Annals of Neurology.* **11**, 344-346.

Hernandez, R., Munoz, O. and Guiscafre, H. (1984). Sensitive immunoassay for early diagnosis of tuberculous meningitis. *Journal of Clinical Microbiology,* **20**, 533-535.

Herndon, R. (1989a). A Brief history of the understanding of CSF. *In* "The Cerebrospinal Fluid". (Eds R. Herndon and R. Brumback). pp. 1-13. Academic Publishers, Boston.

Herndon, R.M. (1989b). The medical uses of injection into the cerebrospinal fluid space (intrathecal and intraventricular injection). *In* "The Cerebrospinal Fluid". (Eds R.M. Herndon and R.A. Brumback). Kluwer Academic Publishers, Norwell, MA.

Herndon, R.M. and Brumback, R.A. (1989a). Cytopathology of the cerebrospinal fluid. *In* "The Cerebrospinal Fluid". (Eds R.M. Herndon and R.A. Brumback). Kluwer Academic Publishers, Norwell, MA.

Herndon, R.M. and Brumback, R.A. (1989b). The cytology of cerebrospinal fluid: methods and normal constitutents. *In* "The Cerebrospinal Fluid". (Eds R.M. Herndon and R.A. Brumback). Kluwer Academic Publishers, Norwell, M.A.

Herndon, R.M. and Brumback, R.A. (Eds) (1989c). "The Cerebrospinal Fluid". Kluwer Academic Publishers, Norwell, M.A.

Hershey, C.O., Hershey, L.A. Varnes, A., Vibhakar, S.D., Lavin, P. and Strain, W.H. (1983). Cerebrospinal fluid trace element content in dementia: clinical, radiologic, and pathologic correlations. *Neurology (NY).* **33**, (10). 1350-3.

Hesse, G.W. (1979). Chronic zinc deficiency alters neuronal function of hippocampal mossy fibers. *Science,* **205**, 1005-1006.

Hesser, S. (1976). Two cases of so-called spontaneous aliquorrhea. *Acta Medica Scandinavica,* **170**, 758-768.

Heyes, M.P., Rubinow, D., Lane, C. and Markey, S.P. (1989). Cerebrospinal fluid quinolinic acid concentrations are increased in acquired immunodeficiency syndrome. *Annals of Neurology,* **26**, (2) 275-7.

Heyes, M.P., Mefford, I.N., Quearry, B.J., Dedhia, M. and Lackner, A. (1990a). Increased ratio of quinolinic acid to kynurenic acid in cerebrospinal fluid of D retrovirus-infected rhesus macaques: relationship to clinical and viral status. *Annals of Neurology,* **27**, 666-675.

Heyes, M.P., Gravell, M., London, , Eckhaus, M., Vickers, J., Yergey, J., April, M., Blackmore D. and Markey, S.P. (1990b). Sustained increases in cerebrospinal fluid quinolinic acid concentrations in rhesus macques (*Macaca mulatta*) naturally infected with simian retrovirus type-D. *Brain Research,* **531**, 148-158.

Hilton-Jones, D., Harrad, R.A., Gill. M.W. and Warlow, C.P. (1982). Failure of postural manoeuvres to prevent lumbar puncture headache. *Journal of Neurology, Neurosurgery and Psychiatry,* 45, 743-6.

Hirohata, S., Hirose, S. and Miyamoto, T. (1985). Cerebrospinal fluid IgM, IgA, and IgG indexes in systemic lupus erythematosus. Their use as estimates of CNS disease activity. *Archives of Internal Medicine,* **145**, 1843-1846.

Hiramatsu, M., Fujimoto, N. and Mori, A. (1982). Catecholamine level in CSF of epileptics. *Neurochemistry Research,* 7, 1299-1305.

Hische, E.A.H., Tutarima, J.A., Wolters, E. Ch., van Trotsenburg, L. van Eyk, R.V.W. *et al.* (1988). Cerebrospinal fluid IgG and IgM indexes as indicators of active neurosyphilis. *Clinical Chemistry*, **34**, (4) 665-667.

Hishikawa, Y. (1976) "Sleep Paralysis in Narcolepsy". (Eds C. Guilleminault *et al.*). S.P. Books, New York.

Ho, D.D., T.R. Rota, R.T. Schooley, J.C. Kaplan, J.D. Allan *et al.* (1985). Isolation of HTLV-III from cerebrospinal fluid and neural tissues of patients with neurological syndromes related to the acquired immunodeficiency syndrome. *New England Journal of Medicine*, **313**, (24) 1493-7.

Hochwald, G.M. (1983). Cerebrospinal fluid. *In* "Clinical Neurology". Vol. 1, (Ed. A.B. Baker). Harper and Row, New York.

Hollander, H. and Levy, J.A. (1987). Neurologic abnormalities and recovery of human immunodeficiency virus from cerebrospinal fluid. *Annals of Internal Medicine*, **106**, 692-695.

Hollt, V., Emrich, H., Bergmann, M., Neodophil, N., Dieterle, D., Gurland, H., Nusselt, L., von Zerssen, D. and Herz, A. (1982). 3-Endorphin-like immunoreactivity in CSF and plasma of neuropsychiatric patients. *In* "Endorphins and Opiate Antagonists in Psychiatric Research". (Eds N. Shah and A. Donald). pp. 231-244, Plenum Press, New York.

Honig, A., Bartlett, J.R., Bouras, N. and Bridges, P.K. (1988). Amino acid levels in depression: a preliminary investigation. *Journal of Psychiatric Research*, **22**, (3) pp 159-164.

Hornykiewicz, O. (1982). Brain catecholamines in schizophrenia – a good case for noradrenaline. *Nature*, **299**, 484-86.

Hornykiewicz, O. (1986). Brain noradrenaline and schizophrenia. *Progress in Brain Research*, **65**, 29-39.

Horrobin, D.E., Ally, A.I., Karmali, R., Karmazyn, M., Manku, M. and Morgan, R. (1978). Prostaglandins and schizophrenia: further discussion of the evidence. *Psychological Medicine*, **8**, 43-48.

Horwitz, S.J., Boxerbaum, B. and O'Bell, J. (1980). Cerebral herniation in bacterial meningitis in childhood. *Annals of Neurology*, **7**, (6) 524-529.

Hosobuchi, Y. (1982). Brain and CSF ACTH and their roles in neurologic function. *In* "Brain Peptides and Hormones". (Eds R. Collu *et al.*). pp. 197-205. Raven Press, New York

Hosobuchi, Y. and Bloom, F.E. (1983). Analgesia induced by brain stimulation in man: its effect on release of β-endorphin and adrenocorticotropin into CSF. *In* "Neurobiology of CSF". Vol 2 (Ed. J.H. Wood). pp. 97-106. Plenum Press, New York.

Hotta M., Shibasaki, T., Masuda, A. *et al.* (1986). The responses of plasma adrenocorticotropin and cortisol to corticotropin-releasing hormone (CRH) and cerebrospinal fluid immunoreactive CRH in anorexia nervosa patients. *Journal of Clinical Endocrinology and Metabolism*, **62**, 319-324.

Houston, J.P., Maas, J. W. *et al.* (1986). Cerebrospinal fluid HVA, central brain atrophy, and clinical state in schizophrenia. *Psychiatry Research*, **19**, 207-214.

Huff, F.J., Reiter, C.T., Rosen, J. Peters, J. and van Kammen, D.P. (1988). No effect of haloperidol on cerebrospinal fluid acetylcholinesterase in patients with schizophrenia. *Biology Psychiatry*, **24**, 701-704.

Hunt, R.D., Cohen, D.J., Shaywitz, S.E. and Shaywitz, B.A. (1982). Strategies for study of the neurochemistry of attention deficit disorder in children. *Schizophrenia Bulletin*, **8**, 236-252 .

Hunter, R., Jones, M. and Mallesen, A. (1969). Abnormal CSF total protein and γ-globulin levels in 256 patients admitted to a psychiatric unit. *Journal of Neurological Sciences,* **9,** 11-38.

Inaba, Y., Klatzo, I. and Spatz, M. (Eds) (1985). "Brain Edema". Springer, Berlin.

Insel, T.R., Mueller, E.A., Alterman, I., Linnoila, M. and Murphy, D.L. (1985). Obsessive-compulsive disorder and serotonin: is there a connection. *Biological Psychiatry,* **20,** 1174-1188.

Insel, T.R., Zohar, J., Benkelfat, C. and Murphy, D.L. (1990) Serotonin in obsession, compulsions and the control of aggressive impulses. *Annals of the New York Academy of Sciences,* **600,** 574-585.

Iqbal, A. and Arnason, B.G.W. (1984). Neuropathy of serum sickness. *In* "Peripheral Neuropathy". 2nd Edn. (Eds P.J. Dyck, P.K. Thomas, E.H., Lambert amd R.Burge). pp. 2044-2049. W. B. Saunders, Philadelphia.

Ito, T., Eggena, P., Barrett, J., Katz, D., Metter, J. and Sambhi, M.P. (1980). Studies on angiotensin of plasma and CSF in normal and hypertensive human subjects. *Hypertension,* **2,** 432-436.

Itoh, Y., Enomoto, H., Takagi, K., Obayashi, T. and Kawai, T. (1983). Human microglobulin levels in neurological disorders. *European Neurology,* **22,** 1-6.

Ives, E.R. (1957). Protein content in the CSF of diabetic patients. *Bulletin of Los Angeles Neurological Society,* **22,** 95.

Jackson, A.C. and Johnson, R. T. (1989). Aseptic meningitis and acute viral encephalitis. *In* "Handbook of Clinical Neurology). Vol. 12. (56): Viral Disease (Ed. R.R. McKendall). Elsevier Science Publishers, B.V.

Jaffrey, N., Virmani, V., Ahuja, G. and Jailkhani, B. (1982). Diagnostic significance of free sialic acid in CSF in meningitis. *Journal of Neurology, Neurosurgery and Psychiatry,* **45,** 1070-1071.

Jakupcevic, M., Lackovic, A., Stefoski, D. and Bulat, M. (1977). Nonhomogenous distribution of 5-hydroxyindoleacetic acid and homovanillic acid in the lumbar cerebrospinal fluid of man. *Journal of Neurological Science,* **31,** 165-171.

Javitt, D.C. and Zukin, S.R. (1990). The role of excitatory amino acids in neuropsychiatric illness. *Journal of Neuropsychiatry and Clinical Neuroscience,* **2,** 44-52.

Jennett, B. (1972). Techniques for measuring intracranial pressure. *In* "Intracranial Pressure". (Eds M. Brock and H. Dietz). pp. 365-368. Springer-Verlag, Berlin.

Jeste, D.V., Doongaji, D.R. and Linnoila, M. (1984). Elevated cerebrospinal fluid noradrenaline in tardive dyskinesia. *British Journal of Psychiatry,* **144,** 177-80.

Jibson, M., Faull, K.F. and Csernansky, J.G. (1990) Intercorrelations among monoamine metabolite concentrations in human lumbar CSF are not due to a shared acid transport system. *Biological Psychiatry,* **28,** 595-602.

Jimerson, D.C., Post, R.M., Carman, J.S., van Kammen, D.P., Wood, J.H. Goodwin, F.K. and Bunney, W.E. (1979). CSF calcium: clinical correlates in affective illness and schizophrenia. *Biological Psychiatry,* **14,** 37-51.

Jimerson, D.C., Wood, J.H. and Post, R.M. (1980). CSF calcium: clinical correlates in psychiatric and seizure disorders. *In* "Neurobiology of CSF". (Ed. J.H. Wood). pp. 743-750. Plenum Press, New York.

Jimerson, D.C., Lesem, M.E., Hegg, A.P. and Brewerton, T.D. (1990). Serotonin in human eating disorders. *Annals of the New York Academy of Sciences,* 532-544.

Jimerson, D.C., Lesem, M.D., Kaye, W.H. and Brewerton, T.D. (1992). Low serotonin and dopamine metabolite concentrations in CSF from bulimic patients with frequent binge episodes. *Archives of General Psychiatry*, **49**, 132-138.

Johanssen, B. and Roos, B. (1974). 5-HIAA and HVA in CSF of patients with neurological diseases. *European Neurology*, **11**, 37-45.

Johnson, K.P. (1980). CSF and blood assays of diagnostic usefulness in M.S. *Neurology*, **30**, 106-109.

Johnson, K. and Nelson, B. (1977). Multiple sclerosis – diagnostic usefulness of CSF. *Archives of Neurology*, **2**, 425-31.

Johnson, R.T. and Richardson, E.P. (1968). The neurological manifestations of systemic lupus erythematosus: a clinical pathological study of 24 cases and review of the literature. *Midicine (Baltimore)*, **47**, 337-367.

Johnston, I., Hawke, S., Halmagyi, M and Teo, C. (1991). The Pseudotumour Syndrome. Disorder of cerebrospinal fluid circulation causing intracranial hypertension without ventriculomegaly. *Archives of Neurology*, **48**, 740-747.

Jones, E., Skolnick, P., Gammal, S., Basile, A. and Mullen, K. (1989). The γ-aminobutyric acid A (GABA$_A$) receptor complex and hepatic encephalopathy. *Annals of Internal Medicine*, **100**, 532-546.

Jordan, R.M., Kendall, J.W., Seaich, J.L., Allen, J.P., Paulsen, C.A., Kerber, C.W. and Vanderlaan, W.P. (1976). CSF hormone concentration in the evaluation of pituitary tumors. *Annals of Internal Medicine*, **85**, 49-55.

Jordan, R.M., McDonald, S.D., Stevens, E.A. and Kendall, J.W. (1979). Cerebrospinal fluid prolactin. *Archives of Internal Medicine*, **139**, 208-211.

Jordan, G.W., Statland, B. and Halstead, C. (1983). CSF lactate in diseases of the CNS. *Archives of Internal Medicine*, **143**, (1) 85-87.

Kamaraju, L.S. and Krishnan, K.R.R. (1991). Adrenocorticotropin, interferons and interleukins. *In* "Neuropeptides and Psychiatric Disorders". (Ed. C.B. Nemeroff). pp. 207-224. American Psychiatric Press, Washington D.C.

Kaplan, G. (1967) The psychogenic aetiology of headache post lumbar puncture. *Psychosomatic Medicine*, **29**, (4) 376-379.

Kaplan, S.L. (1983) Antigen detection in cerebrospinal fluid – pros and cons. *American Journal of Medicine*, 109-118.

Karcher, D. and Lowenthal, A. (1987). Electrophoresis of the cerebrospinal fluid proteins and study of brain specific proteins in the cerebrospinal fluid correlated to clinical data. *In* "Advances in CSF Protein, Research and Diagnosis". (Ed. E.J. Thompson). pp. 1-16. MTP Press Ltd, Lancaster.

Kasa, K., Otsuki, S., Yamamoto, M. *et al.* (1982) CSF GABA and HVA in depressive disorders. *Biological Psychiatry*, **17**, 877.

Kaschka, W.P., Theilkaes, L., Eickhoff, K. and Skvarie, E. (1979). Disproportionate elevation of the immunoglobulin G1 concentration in cerebrospinal fluids of patients with multiple sclerosis. *Infection and Immunity*, **26**, 933-941.

Kasik, J.E. (1988). Central nervous system tuberculosis. *In* "Tuberculosis". 2nd Edn. (Ed. D. Schlossberg). pp. 87-97. Springer, New York, Tokyo.

Kassan, S.S. and Kagen, L.J. (1978). Elevated levels of CSF cGMP in SLE. *American Journal of Medicine*, **64**, 732-741.

Kastin, A.J., Banks, W., Zadina, J. and Graf, M. (1983). Brain peptides: the dangers of constricted nomenclatures. *Life Science*, **32**, 295-301.

Katz, R.L., Alappattu, C., Glass, J.P. and Bruner, J.M. (1989). Cerebrospinal fluid manifestations of the neurologic complications of human immunodeficiency virus infection. *Acta Cytologica*, **33**, (2) 233244.

Kaye, E.M., Ullman, M.D., Kolodny, E.H. *et al.* (1992). Possible use of CSF glyco sphingo lipids for the diagnosis and therapeutic monitoring of lysosomal storage diseases. *Neurology*, **42**, 2290-2294.

Kaye, W.H., Pickar, D., Naber, D. and Ebert, M.H. (1982). Cerebrospinal fluid opioid activity in anorexia nervosa. *American Journal of Psychiatry*, **139**, (5) 643-645.

Kaye, W.H., Ebert, M.H. Gwirtsman, H.E. and Weiss, S.R. (1984a). Differences in brain serotonergic metabolism between nonbulimic and bulimic patients with anorexia nervosa. *American Journal of Psychiatry*, **141**, 1598-1601.

Kaye, W.H., Ebert, M.H., Raleigh M. and Lake, C.R. (1984b). Abnormalities in CNS monoamine metabolism in anorexia nervosa. *Archives of General Psychiatry*, 350-355.

Kaye, W.H., Gwirtsman, H.E. George, D.T. *et al.* (1987). Elevated cerebrospinal fluid levels of immunoreactive corticotropin-releasing hormone in anorexia nervosa: relation to state of nutrition, adrenal function, and intensity of depression. *Journal of Clinical Endocrinology and Metabolism*, **64**, 203-208

Kaye W.H., Berrettini, W. Gwirtsman, H. and George, D.T. (1990). Altered cerebrospinal fluid neuropeptide Y and peptide YY immunoreactivity in anorexia and bulimia nervosa. *Archives of General Psychiatry*, **47**, 548-556.

Keir, G. and Thompson, E.J. (1986). Proteins as parameters in the discrimination between different blood-CSF barriers. *Journal of Neurological Sciences*, **75**, 245-253.

Keller, T.L., Halperin, J.J. and Whitman, M. (1992). PCR detection of *Borrelia burgdorferi* DNA in cerebrospinal fluid of Lyme neuroborreliosis patients. *Neurology*, **42**, 32-42.

Kelly, J.J. Jr, Kyle, R.A., Miles, J.M. and Dyck, P.J. (1983). Osteosclerotic myeloma and peripheral neuropathy. *Neurology*, **33**, 202-210.

Keltner, J.L. (1988). Optic nerve sheath decompression. How does it work? Has its time come? *Archives of Opthalmology*. **106**, 1365.

Kemali D., Maj, M., Iorio, G. *et al.* (1985). Relationship between CSF nora-drenaline levels, C-EEG indicators of activation and psychosis ratings in drug-free schizophrenic patients. *Acta Psychiatrica Scandinavica*, **71**, 19-24.

Kennedy, D.H. and Fallon, R.J. (1979). Tuberculous meningitis. *Journal of the American Medical Association*, **241**, 264-268.

Kessler, J.A., Patlak, C.S. and Fenstermacher, J.D. (1976a). Transport of 5-hydroxy-3-indoleacetic acid by spinal cord during subarachnoid perfusion. *Brain Research*, **116**, 471-483.

Kessler, J.A., Fenstermacher, J.D. and Patlak, C.S. (1976b). Homovanillic acid transport by the spinal cord. *Neurology*, **26**, 434-440.

Killingsworth, L.M. (1982). Chemical applications of protein determinations in biological fluids other than blood. *Clinical Chemistry*, **28**, 1093-1102.

Kilpelainen, H., Haloxen, T., Kekoni, J., Molnar, G. and Riekkinen, P. (1980). Acid proteinase, neutral proteinase, and β-glucoronidase activity of CSF in MS *Acta Neurologica Scandinavica*, (Abst.) Suppl. **78**, 39.

Kilpelainen, H., Haloneu, T., Pitkanen, A. and Riekkinen, P.A. (1982). Follow-up study of lysosomal hydrolases in CSF. *Acta Neurologica Scandinavica*, **85**, Suppl.

90 272.

Kim, J.S., Kornhuber, H., Smid-Burgk, W. and Holzmuller, B. (1980). Low CSF glutamate in schizophrenic patients and a new hypothesis of schizophrenia. *Neuroscience Letters*, **20**, 379-82.

Kinnman, J. and Link, H. (1984). Intrathecal production of oligoclonal IgM and IgG in CNS sarcoidosis. *Acta Neurologica Scandinavica*, **69**, 97-106.

Kinnunen, E. and Hillbom, M. (1986) The significance of cerebrospinal fluid routine screening for neurosyphilis. *Journal of the Neurological Sciences*, **75**, 205-211.

Kirch D.G., Kaufmann, C. A. *et al.* (1985). Abnormal cerebrospinal fluid protein indices in schizophrenia. *Biological Psychiatry*, **20**, 1039-1046.

Kirshner, H.S., Tsai, S.L., Runge, V.M. and A.Price, C. (1985). Magnetic resonance imaging and other techniques in the diagnosis of multiple sclerosis. *Archives of Neurology*, **42**, 859-863.

Kirstein, L., Bowers, M. and Heninger, C. (1976). CSF amino metabolites, clinical symptoms, and body movement in psychiatric patients. *Biological Psychiatry*, **11**, (4) 421-34.

Kjeldsberg, C.R. and Krieg, A.T. (1984). CSF and other body fluids. *In* "Clinical Diagnosis and Management by Laboratory Methods". J.B. Saunders, Philadelphia.

Kjeldsberg, C. and Knight, J. (1986). Cerebrospinal fluids. *In* "Body Fluids: Laboratory Examination of Amniotic, Cerebrospinal, Seminol, Serous and Synovial Fluids". American Society Clinical Pathologists Press, Chicago.

Kjellin, K.G. (1983). Xanthochromic compounds in CSF: quantitative spectrophotometry and electromigration. *In* "Neurobiology of CSF". Vol. 2. (Ed. J.H.Wood). pp. 559-570. Plenum Press, New York.

Kjellin, K.G. and Siden, A. (1983). CSF proteins in infectious neurological diseases and Guillain-Barré Syndrome. *In* "Neurobiology of CSF". Vol. 2. (Ed. J.H.Wood). pp. 369-386. Plenum Press, New York.

Kjellin, K.G. *et al.* (1974). Diagnostic significance of CSF spectrophotometry in cerebrovascular diseases. *Journal of Neurological Science*, **23**, 359-69.

Klawans, H.L. (1975). Disorders of the extrapyramidal system. *In* "Biochemistry of Neural Disease". (Ed. M.M. Cohen). pp. 161-184. Harper & Row, New York.

Knigge, K., Morris, M., Scott, D.E., Joseph, S.A., Notter, M., Schock, D. and Krobisch-Dudley, G. (1975). Distribution of hormones by CSF. *In* "Fluid Environment of the Brain". (Eds H.F. Cserr *et al.*). pp. 237-253. Academic Press, New York.

Knight, J.A., Dudek, S.M. and Haymond, R.E. (1981). Early (chemical) diagnosis of bacterial meningitis – CSF glucose, lactate and lactate dehydrogenase compared. *Clinical Chemistry*, **27**, 1431-1434.

Kobatake, K., Shinohara, Y. and Yoshimura, S. (1980). Immunoglobulins in CSF. *Journal of Neurological Science*, **47**, 273-283.

Koetsier, J., van Kamp, G., Luyendijk, L. and Mispelblom Beyer, J. (1984). MBP in CSF detected by an enzyme-immunoassay and its diagnostic value. *In* "Peripheral Neuropathy". 2nd Edn. (Eds P.J. Dyck, P.K. Thomas, E.H. Lambert and R. Burge). pp. 417-420. W. B. Saunders, Philadelphia.

Kohlhepp, W., Kuhn, W. and Kruger, H. (1989). Extrapyramidal features in central Lyme borreliosis. *European Neurology*, **29**, 150-155.

Kohlschutter, A., Reiber, H. and Bauer, H. (1980). MBP in CSF as an indicator of MS process. *In* "Progress in MS Research". (Eds H. Bauer *et al.*). pp. 168-169. Springer-Verlag, New York.

Kolmel, H.W. (1977). "Atlas of CSF Cells". Springer-Verlag, New York.

Komorowski, R.A., Farmer, S.G., Hanson, G.A. and Hause, L.L. (1978). CSF lactic acid in diagnosis of meningitis. *Journal of Clinical Microbiology*, **8**, 89-92.

Konagaya, Y., Konagaya, M. and Takayanagi, T. (1989) Chronic polyneuropathy and ulcerative colitis. *Japanese Journal of Medicine*, **28**, 72-74.

Kopin, I.J., Gordon, E.K., Jimerson, D.C. and Polinsky, R.J. (1983). Relation between plasma and CSF levels of MHPG. *Science*, **219**, 73-75.

Kopin, I., Burns, S. Chieveh, C. and Markey, S. (1986). MPTP-induced Parkinsonian syndromes in humans and animals. *In* "Humans and Animals in Alzheimer's and Parkinson's Diseases". (Eds A Fisher *et al.*). pp. 519-530. Plenum Press, New York.

Korein, J., Cravioto, H. and Leirach, M. (1959). Re-evaluation of lumbar puncture. A study of 129 patients with papilloedema on intracranial hypertension. *Neurology*, **9**, 290-7.

Korf, J., van den Burg, W. and van den Hoofdakker, R. (1983). Acid metabolites and precursor amino acids of 5-HT and DA in affective and other psychiatric disorders. *Psychiatric Clinics*, **16**, 1-16.

Kornblith, P.L., Walker, M.D. and Cassidy, J.B. (1982). Neoplasms of the central nervous system. *In* "Cancer: Principles and Practice of Onocology". (Eds V. DeVita *et al.*). pp. 1181-1253. J.B. Lippincott, Co., Philadelphia.

Kornguth, S.E. (1989). Neuronal proteins and paraneoplastic syndromes. *New England Journal of Medicine,* **321**, 1607-8.

Korpi, E.R., Kaufmann, C., Marnela, K-M. and Weinberger, D.E. (1987). Cerebrospinal fluid amino acid concentrations in chronic schizophrenia. *Psychiatry Research,* **20**, 337-345.

Koslow, S. and Cross, C. (1982). CSF monoamine metabolites in Tourette syndrome and their neuroendocrine implications. *In* "Gilles de la Tourette Syndrome". (Eds A. Friedhoff and T. Chase). pp. 185-197. Raven Press, New York.

Kovacs, K., Bors, L., Tothfalusi, L., Jelencsik, I., Bozsik, G., Kerenyi, L. and Komoly, S. (1989). Cerebrospinal fluid (CSF) investigations in migraine. *Cephalagia*, **9**, 53-57.

Kraemer, G., Hopf, H.L. and Eissner, D. (1987). CSF hyperabsorption: A cause of spontaneous low CSF pressure headache. *Neurology,* (Suppl. 1) **37**, 238.

Kraft, R., Altermatt, H.J. and Nguyen-Tran, Q. (1989). Differential diagnose atypischer plasmazellen im liquor cerebrospinalis. *Deutsche medizinische Wochenschrift*, **114**, 1729-1733.

Krambovitis E., McIllimurray, M.B., Lock, P.E., Hendrickse, W. and Holzel, H. (1984). Rapid diagnosis of tuberculous meningitis by latex particle agglutination. *Lancet*, ii, 1229-1231.

Kremenitzer, M. and Golden, G.S. (1974). Hemiplegic migraine: cerebrospinal fluid abnormalities. *Journal of Pediatrics*, **85**, (1) 139.

Kremzner, L.T., Berl, S., Stellar, S. and Cote, L.J. (1979). Amino acids, peptides and polyamines in cortical biopsies and ventricular fluid in patients with Huntington's disease. *Advances in Neurology*, **23**, 537-546.

Krieg, A.F. (1979). Cerebrospinal fluid and other body fluids. *In* "Clinical Diagnosis and Management by Laboratory Methods". (Ed. J.B. Henry). pp. 635-679, J.B. Saunders, Philadelphia.

Krieger, D.T. (1982). Endorphins and enkephalins. *Disease-a-Month*, **28**, 1-53.

Kruesi, M.J.P., Swedo, S.E., Hamburger, S.D., Potter, W.Z. and Rapoport, J.L. (1988). Concentration gradient of CSF monoamine metabolites in children and adolescents. *Biological Psychiatry*, **24**, 507-514.

Kruesi, M.J.P., Rapoport, J.L., Hamburger, S.D., Hibbs, S.E., Potter, W.Z., Lenane, M. and Brown, G.L. (1990*a*). Cerebrospinal fluid monoamine metabolites, aggression, and impulsivity in disruptive behavior disorders of children and adolescents. *Archives of General Psychiatry*, **47**, 419-426.

Kruesi, M.J.P., Swedo, S., Leonard, H., Rubinow, D. R. and Rapoport, J.L. (1990*b*). CSF somatostatin in childhood psychiatric disorders: a preliminary investigation. *Psychiatric Research*, **33**, 277-284.

Kruger, H., Reuss, K., Pulz, M., Rohrback, E., Pflughaupt, K-W., Martin R. and Mertens, H.G. (1989) Meningoradiculitis and encephalomyelitis due to Borrelia burgdorferi: a follow-up study of 72 patients over 27 years. *Journal of Neurology*, **236**, 322-328.

Kruskall, M.S., Carter, S.R. and Ritz, L.P. (1983). Contamination of CSF by vertebral bone-marrow cells during lumbar puncture. *New England Journal of Medicine*, **308**, 697-700.

Kuberski, T. (1979). Eosinophils in the cerebrospinal fluid. *Annals of Internal Medicine*, **91**, 70-75.

Kumar, V., Giacobini, E. and Markwell, S. (1989). CSF choline and acetylcholinesterase in early-onset vs. late-onset Alzheimer's disease patients. *Acta Neurologica Scandinavica*, **80**, 461-466.

Kuriyama, M., Suehara, M., Marume, N., Osame, M. and Igata, A. (1984). High CSF lactate and pyruvate content in Kearns-Sayre syndrome. *Neurology (NY)*, **34**, (2) 253-5.

Kuroda, H., Ogawa, N., Yamawaki, Y., Nukina, I., Oluji, T., Yamamoto, M. and Otsuki, S. (1982). CSF GABA levels in various neurological and psychiatric diseases. *Journal of Neurology, Neurosurgery and Psychiatry*, **45**, 257-260.

Kutt H., Hurwitz, L.J., Ginsburg, S.M. and McDowell, F. (1961). CSF protein in diabetes mellitus. *Archives of Neurology*, **4**, 43.

Labadie, E.L. (1980). CSF alterations associated with CNS infections. *In* "Neurobiology of CSF". Vol. 1. (Ed. J.H. Wood). pp.433-448. Plenum Press, New York.

Labadie, E.L., Antwerp, J.V. and Bamford, C.R. (1976). Abnormal lumbar isotope cisternography in an unusual case of spontaneous hypoliquorrheic headache. *Neurology*, **26**, 135-139.

Lake, C.R., Wood, J. H., Ziegler, M.G., Ebert, M.H. and Kopin, I.J. (1978). Probenecid-induced norepinephrine elevations in plasma and CSF. *Archives of General Psychiatry*, **35**, 237-240.

Lake, C.R., Polinsky, R.J., Gullner, H.G., Ebert, M.H., Ziegler, M.G. Bartter, F.C. and Kopin, I.J. (1980*a*). Dissociation between central and peripheral noradrenergic activity in essential hypertension. *Clinical Science*, **59**, (Suppl. 6) 229S-233S.

Lake, C.R., Sternberg, D.E., van Kammen, D.P., Ballenger, J.C., Ziegler, M., Post, R., Kopin, I. and Bunney, W. (1980*b*). Schizophrenia: elevated CSF norepinephrine. *Science*, **207**, 331-333.

Lake, C.R., Gullner, H.G., Polinsky, R., Ebert, M., Ziegler, M. and Bartter, F.C. (1981*a*). Essential hypertension: central and peripheral norepinephrine. *Science*, **211**, 955-957.

Lake, C.R., Major, F.L., Ziegler, M.G. *et al.* (1981*b*). The effects of disulfiram on peripheral and central norepinephrine metabolism and blood pressure. *In* "Phenomenology and Treatment of Alcoholism". (Eds W. Fann, I. Karacan and A. Pokorny). Spectrum Publishers, New York. (1979, cited in Hawley *et al.*).

Lake, C.R., Kleinman, J.E., Kafka, M.S. *et al.* (1987). Norepinephrine metabolism in schizophrenia. *In* "Neurochemistry and Neuropharmacology of Schizophrenia. Handbook of Schizophrenia". Vol. 2. (Eds F. Henn and L. De Lisi). pp. 227-256. Elsevier Publishers, Amsterdam.

Langfitt, T.W. (1972). Pathophysiology of increased ICP. *In* "Intracranial Pressure". (Eds M. Brock and H. Dietz). pp. 361-364. Springer-Verlag, Berlin.

Langman, J. (1978). "Medical Embryology". Williams and Wilkins, Co., Baltimore.

Larsson, M., Hagberg, L., Norkrans, G. and Forsman, A. (1989). Indoleamine deficiency in blood and cerebrospinal fluid from patients with human immunodeficiency virus infection. *Journal of Neuroscience Research*, **23**, 441-44.

Larsson, M., Hagberg, L., Forsman, A. and Norkrans, G. (1991). Cerebrospinal fluid catecholamine metabolites in HIV-infected patients. *Journal of Neuroscience Research*, **28**, 406-409.

Lasater, G.M. (1970). Primary intracranial hypotension. The low spinal fluid pressure syndrome. *Headache*, **10**, 63-66.

Laterre, C. and Sindic, C. (1987). Oligoclonal bands in CSF: usefulness and limits. *In* "Advances in CSF Protein, Research and Diagnosis". (Ed. E.J. Thompson). pp. 109-122. MTP Press Ltd, Lancaster.

Laurell, C-B. (1987). On the origin of major proteins. *In* "Advances in CSF Protein, Research and Diagnosis". (Ed. E.J. Thompson). pp. 123-128. MTP Press Ltd, Lancaster.

Le Quesne D.M. (1984). Neuropathy due to drugs. *In* "Peripheral Neuropathy". 2nd Edn. (Eds. P.J. Dyck *et al.*). pp. 2162-2179. W.B. Saunders, Philadelphia.

Le Witt, P., Levine, R., Lovenberg, W. *et al.* (1986). Monoamine neuro-transmitter metabolites and hydroxylase co-factor in Alzheimer-type dementia and normals. *In* "Alzheimer's and Parkinson's Disease". (Eds A. Fisher, I. Hanin and C. Lachman). pp. 323-327. Plenum Press, New York.

Le Witt, P.A. Galloway, M.P., Matson, W. *et al.* (1992). Markers of dopamine metabolism in Parkinson's disease. *Neurology*, **42**, 2111-2117.

Le Wontin, R. (1984). "Not in our Genes. Biology Ideology and Human Nature". Penguin Books, Harmondsworth.

Leckman, J.F. and Chittenden, E.H. (1990). Gilles de la Tourette's syndrome and some forms of obsessive-compulsive disorder may share a common genetic diathesis. *Encephale*, **16**, 321-3.

Leckman, J., Walker, J.M. *et al.* (1987). Tic disorders. *In* "Psychopharmacology and The Third Generation of Progress". (Ed. H. Meltzer). pp. 1239-1246. Raven Press, New York.

Leckman, J.F., Riddle, M.A., Berrettini, W.H. *et al.* (1988). Elevated CSF dynorphin A (1-8) in Tourette's syndrome. *Life Sciences*, **43**, 2015-2023.

Lee, M.C., Heaney, L.M., Jacobson, R.L. and Klassen, A.C. (1975). Cerebrospinal fluid in cerebral hemorrhage and infarction. *Stroke*, **6**, 638-41.

Lee, J.A., Atkinson, R.S. and Watt, M.J. (1985). "Sir Robert MacIntosh's Lumbar Puncture and Spinal Analgesia". Churchill Livingstone, Edinburgh.

Leech, R.W. (1989). Abnormalities of cerebrospinal fluid production and flow and hydrocephalus. *In* "The Cerebrospinal Fluid". (Eds R.M. Herndon and R.A. Brumback). Kluwer Academic Publishers, Norwell, MA.

Leenders, K.L., Palmer, A.J., Quinn, N., Clark, J.C., Firnau, G. *et al.* (1986). Brain dopamine metabolism in patients with Parkinson's disease measured with positron emission tomography. *Journal of Neurology, Neurosurgery and Psychiatry*, **49**, 853-860.

Leibowitz, S. (1989). Hypothalamus, neuropeptide Y, co-existence and amines: concepts of co-existence in relation to feeding behaviour. *Annals of the New York Academy of Science*, **575**, 221-35.

Leibowitz, S.F. (1990). The role of serotonin in eating disorders. *Drugs*, **39**, (Suppl. 3) 33-48.

Leland, A., Marton, L.J., Lubich, W.P. and Reigel, D.H. (1983). CSF polyamines in childhood. *Archives of Neurology*, **40**, 237-240.

Lemus C.Z., Lieberman, J.A *et al.* (1990). CSF 5-hydroxyindoleacetic acid levels and suicide attempts in schizophrenia. *Biological Psychiatry,* **27**, 923-926.

Lentner, C. (Ed.) (1981). "Geigy Scientific Tables". Vol. 1. Ciba Geigy Ltd, West Caldwell, New Jersey.

Leoport, C., Chaunu, M.P., Sicre, J., Brun-Vezinet, F., Hauw, J.J. and Vilde, J.L. (1987). Peripheral neuropathy in relation to LAV/HTLV III retrovirus infection. A clinical, anaomical and immunological study. 5 Cases. *Presse Médicale,* **16**, 55-58.

Lepola U., Jolkkonen, J., Rimon, R. and Riekkinen, P. (1989). Long term effects of alprazolam and imipramine on cerebrospinal fluid monoamine metabolites and neuropeptides in panic disorder. *Neuropsychobiology*, **21**, 182-186.

Lepola, U., Jolkkonen, J., Pitkanen, A., Riekkinen, P. and Rimon, R. (1990). Cerebrospinal fluid monoamine metabolites and neuropeptides in patients with panic disorder. *Annals of Medicine,* **22**, 237-239.

Lerer, B. (1987). Neurochemical and other neurobiological consequences of ECT: implications for the pathogenesis and treatment of affective disorders. *In* "Psychopharmacology: The Third Generation of Progress". (Ed. Herbert Y Meltzer). pp. 577-586. Raven Press, New York.

Lerner, P., Goodwin, F.K., Van Kammen, D.P., Post, R.M., Majov, L.F., Ballenger, J. and Lovenberg, W. (1978). DBH in the CSF of psychiatric patients. *Biological Psychiatry,* **13**, 685-694.

Leusen, I.R., Weyne, J.J. and Demeester, G.M. (1983). Regulation of acid-base equilibrium of CSF. *In* "Neurobiology of CSF". Vol. 2. (Ed. J.H. Wood). pp. 25-42. Plenum Press, New York.

Levant, B, Bissette, G., Nemeroff, C.B. (1991). Neurotensin. *In* "Neuropeptides and Psychiatric Disorders". (Ed. C.B. Nemeroff). pp. 149-168. American Psychiatric Press, Washington D.C.

Levin, E. (1977). Are the terms blood brain barrier and brain capillary permeability synonomous. *Experimental Eye Research,* **25**, (Suppl) 191-199.

Levin, E. and Tradatti, C. (1976). Penetration of proteins in the central nervous system. *Advances in Experimental Medicine and Biology*, **69**, 111-129.

Levin, E., Sepulveda, F.V. and Yudilevich, D.L. (1974). Pial vessels transport of substances from cerebrospinal fluid to blood. *Nature*, **249**, 266-268.

Levin, E., Sheline, G. and Gutin, P. (1989). Neoplasm of the central nervous system. *In* "Cancer: Principles and Practice of Oncology". (Eds De Vita Jr, S. Hellman and S. Rosenberg). pp. 1557-1611. Lippincott, Philadelphia.

Levinson, A. (1923). "Cerebrospinal Fluid in Health and in Disease". C.V. Mosby Co., St. Louis.

Levy, J.A., Hollander, H., Shimabukuro, J., Mills, J. and Kaminsky, L. (1985). Isolation of AID-associated retroviruses from cerebrospinal fluid and brain of patients with neurological symptoms. *Lancet,* **ii**, (September 14), 586.

Lichtschtein, D., Dobkin, J., Ebstein, R.R., Biederman, J., Rimon, R. and Belmaker, R.H. (1978). GABA in the CSF of schizophenic patients before and after neuroleptic treatment. *British Journal of Psychiatry,* **132**, 145-148.

Liggett, S.B., Berger, J.R. and Hush, J. (1982). CSF xanthochromia with rifampin. *American Journal of Neurology,* **12**, (2) 228-229.

Limson, R., Goldman, D., Roy, A., Lamparski, D., Ravitz, B., Adinoff, B. and Linnoila, M. (1991). Personality and cerebrospinal fluid monoamine metabolites in alcoholics and controls. *Archives of General Psychiatry,* **48**, 437-441.

Lindqvist, T. and Moberg, E. (1949). Spontaneous hypoliquorrhea: report of a case. *Acta Medica Scandinavica,* **132**, 556.

Lindstrom L.H. (1985). Low HVA and normal 5-HIAA CSF levels in drug-free schizophrenic patients compared to healthy volunteers: correlations to symptomatology and family history. *Psychiatric Research*, **14**, 265-273.

Lindstrom, L., Widerlov, E., Gunne, L.M.. Wahlstrom, A. and Terenius, L. (1978). Endorphins in human CSF: clinical correlation to some psychotic states. *Acta Psychiatrica Scandinavica,* **57**, 153-164.

Lindstrom, L., Besev, G., Gunne, L., Sjostrom, R., Terenius, L., Wahlstrom, A. and Wistedt, B. (1982). CSF content of endorphins in schizophrenia. *In* "Endorphins and Opiate Antagonists in Psychiatric Research". (Eds N. Shah and A. Donald). pp. 245-256. Plenum Press, New York.

Lindstrom, L.H., Ekman, R., Walleus, H. and Widerlov, E. (1985). Delta-sleep inducing peptide in cerebrospinal fluid from schizophrenics, depressives and healthy volunteers. *Progress in Neuropsychopharmacology and Biological Psychiatry,* **9**, 83-90.

Lindstrom L.H., Besev, G., Gunne, L.M. and Terenius, L. (1986). CSF levels of receptor-active endorphins in schizophrenic patients: correlations with symptomatology and monoamine metabolites. *Psychiatry Research*, **19**, 93-100.

Lindstrom, L.H., Wieselgren, I-M. *et al.* (1990). Relationship between abnormal brainstem auditory-evoked potentials and subnormal CSF levels of HVA and 5-HIAA in first-episode schizophrenic patients. *Biological Psychiatry,* **28**, 435-442.

Lindvall, B. and Olsson, J. E. (1990). Monoamine metabolites and neuropeptides in patients with Parkinsons disease, Huntington's chorea, Shy-Drager syndrome and torsion dystonia. *Advances in Neurology,* **53**, 117-122.

Lindvall, M., Edvinsson, L. and Owman, C. (1978). Sympathetic nervous control of cerebrospinal fluid production from the choroid plexus. *Science*, **201**, 176-178.

Link, H. (1973). Immunoglobulin abnormalities in the Guillain-Barré syndrome. *Journal of Neurological Science,* **18**, 23.

Link, H. (1987). Cerebrospinal fluid in immunological CNS diseases. *In* "Clinical Neuroimmunology". (Eds J. Aarli, W. Behan and P. Behan). pp. 444-466. Blackwell Science Publ., Oxford.

Link, H. and Tibbling, G. (1977). Principles of albumin and IgG analysis in neurological disorders. III evaluation of IgG synthesis within the CNS in multiple sclerosis. *Scandinavian Journal of Clinical Laboratory Investigations*, **37**, 385-401.

Linnoila, M., Whorton, R., Rubinow, D.R., Cowdry, R., Ninan, P., and Waters, R.N. (1982). CSF prostaglandin levels in depressed and schizophrenic patients. *Archives of General Psychiatry*, **40**, 405-406.

Linnoila, M., Cowdry, R., Lamberg, B.A., Makinen, T., and Rubinow, D. (1983*a*). CSF triiodothyronine (rT3) levels in patients with affective disorders. *Biological Psychiatry*, **18**, (12) 1489-92.

Linnoila, M., Ninan, P.T., Scheimin, M., Waters, R.N., Chang, W.H., Bartko, J. and van Kammen, D.P. (1983*b*). Reliability of norepinephrine and major monoamine metabolite measurements in CSF of schizophrenic patients. *Archives of General Psychiatry*, **40**, (12) 1290-4.

Linnoila, M., Virkkunen, M., Scheinin, M., Nuutila, A., Rimon, R. and Goodwin, F.K. (1983*c*). Low cerebrospinal fluid 5-hydroxyindoleacetic acid concentration differentiates impulsive from nonimpulsive violent behaviour. *Life Sciences*, **33**, 2609-2614.

Linnoila M., De Jong, J. and Virkkunen, M. (1989). Family history of alcoholism, violent offenders and impulsive fire setters. *Archives of General Psychiatry*, **46**, 613-616.

Lipman, I.J. (1977). Primary intracranial hypotension. The syndrome of spontaneous low cerebrospinal fluid pressure with traction headache. *Diseases of the Nervous System*, **38**, 212-213.

Lloyd, K.G., Morselli, P.L. and Bartholini, G. (1987). GABA and affective disorders. *Medical Biology*, **65**, 159-165.

Lobenthal, S.W., Hajdu, S.I., Urmacher, C. (1983). Cytologic findings in homosexual males with acquired immunodeficiency. *Acta Cytologica*, **27**, (6) 597-604.

Lolli, F., Siracusa, G., Amato, M.P., Fratiglioni, L., Dal Pozzo, G. *et al* (1991). Intrathecal synthesis of free immunoglobulin light chains and IgM in initial multiple sclerosis. *Acta Neurologica Scandinavica*, **83**, 239-243.

Lorenberg, W., Levine, R.A. and Robinson, D.S. (1979). Hydroxylase cofactor activity in CSF of normal subjects and patients with Parkinson's disease. *Science*, **204**, 624-626.

Lorenzo, A.V. (1974). Amino acid transport mechanisms of the cerebrospinal fluid. *Federation Proceedings*, **33**, 2079-2085.

Lorenzo, A.V. (1977). Factors governing the composition of the cerebrospinal fluid. *Experimental Eye Research*, **25**, (Suppl) 205-228.

Lorenzo, A.V. and Spector, R. (1976). The distribution of drugs in the central nervous system. *Advances in Experimental Medicine and Biochemistry*, **69**, 447-461.

Loscher, W. (1982). Relationship between GABA concentrations in CSF and seizure excitability. *Journal of Neurochemistry*, **38**, 293-295.

Losonczy, M.F., Mohs, R.C. and Davis, K.L. (1984). Seasonal variations of human lumbar CSF neurotransmitter metabolite concentrations. *Psychiatric Research*, **12**, 79-87.

Losy, J., Mehta, P.D. and Wisniewski, H.M. (1990). Identification of IgG subclasses' oligoclonal bands in multiple sclerosis CSF. *Acta Neurologica Scandinavica*, **82**, 4-8.

Lotstra F., Verbanck, P.M.P. *et al.* (1985). Reduced cholecystokinin levels in cerebrospinal fluid of Parkinsonian and schizophrenic patients. *Annals New York Academy of Sciences*, 507-516.

Lowenthal, A. (1972). Chemical physiopathology of the cerebrospinal fluid. *In* "Handbook of Neurochemistry". (Ed. A. Lajtha). pp. 429-464. Plenum Press, New York.

Lowenthal, A. (1977). The problem of CSF. *In* "MS: A Critical Conspectus". (E.J. Field). pp. 207-224. MTP Press, England.

Lowenthal, A. and Karcher, D. (1980). Cerebrospinal fluid in clinical neurology. *Progress in Clinical and Biological Research*, **39**, 265-274.

Lowenthal, A., Crols, R., DeSchulter, E., Ghevens, J., Karcher, D., Noppe, M. and Tasner, A. (1984). Cerebrospinal fluid proteins in neurology. *International Reviews of Neurobiology*, **25**, 95-138.

Luerssen, T.G. and Robertson, G.L. (1980). CSF Vasopressin and vasotocin in health and disease. *In* "Neurobiology of CSF". (Ed. J.H. Wood). pp. 613-624. Plenum Press, New York.

Luger, A., Schmidt, B.L., Steyrer, K. and Schonwald, E. (1981). Diagnosis of neurosyphilis by examination of the cerebrospinal fluid. *British Journal of Venereal Diseases*, **57**, 232-7.

Lukehart, S.A., Hook III, E.W., Baker-Zander, S.A. *et al.* (1988). Invasion of the central nervous system by Treponema pallidum: implications for diagnosis and treatment. *Annals of Internal Medicine*, **109**, 855-862.

Lumsden, C.E. (1972). The clinical pathology in MS. *In* "MS: A Reappraisal". (Eds D. McAlpine, C. Lumsden and E. Acheson). pp. 311-621. Williams and Wilkins, Balitmore.

Maas, J., Kocsis, J., Bowden, C. *et al.* (1982). Pre-treatment neurotransmitter metabolites and responses to imipramine or amitriptyline treatment. *Psychological Medicine*, **12**, 37-43.

Mackay, A.V.P., Yates, C.M., Wright, P., Hamilton, P. and Davies, P. (1978). Regional distribution of monoamines and their metabolites in the human brain. *Journal of Neurochemistry*, **30**, 841-848.

Magnaes, B. (1982). Cerebrospinal fluid hydromechanics in adult patients with benign noncommunicating hydrocephalus: one-way test shunting and balanced cerebrospinal fluid infusion test to select patients for intracranial bypass operation. *Neurosurgery*, **11**, 765-775.

Magnaes, B. (1983). Body position and CSF pressure. *In* "Neurobiology of CSF". Vol. 2. (Ed. J.H. Wood). pp. 629-642. Plenum Press, New York.

Maida, E. and Kristoferitsch, W. (1981). Cyclic AMP in CSF of MS patients. *Journal of Neurology*, **225**, (Abstr.) in E.M. *Neural Neurosurgery*, **53**, 484.

Major, L.F., Ballenger, J.C., Goodwin F.K. and Brown, G.L. (1977). Cerebrospinal fluid homovanillic acid in male alcoholics: effects of disulfiram. *Biological Psychiatry*, **12**, (5) 635-642.

Major, L.F., Lerner, P., Goodwin, F.K., Ballenger, J., Brown, G. and Lovenberg,

W. (1980). Dopamine β-hydroxylase in CSF: relationship to personality measures. *Archives of General Psychiatry*, **37**, 308-310.

Major, L.F., Lerner, P., Dendel, P.S. and Post, R.M. (1983). Dopamine-β-hydroxylase in CSF: putative indicator of central adrenergic activity. *In* "Neurobiology of CSF". Vol 2. (Ed. J.H. Wood). pp. 179 -196. Plenum Press, New York.

Major, L.F., Lerner, P. and Ziegler, M.G. (1984). Norepinephrine and Dopamine-beta-hydroxylase in CSF: indicators of central noradrenergic acitivity. *In* "Noreppinephrine" (Eds M.G. Ziegler and C.R. Lake). Williams and Wilkins, Baltimore.

Malison, R.T. and Price, L.H. (1991). Panic disorder: neurobiological advances. *Current Opinion in Psychiatry*, **4**, 255-261.

Manberg, P.J., Nemeroff, C., Bissette, G. *et al.* (1985). Neuropeptides in CSF and post-mortem brain tissue of normal controls, schizophrenics and Huntington's Choreics. *Progress in Neuropsychopharmacology and Biological Psychiatry*, **9**, 97-108.

Mann, J.D., Johnson, R.N., Butler, A.B. and Bass, N.H. (1983a). CSF circulatory dynamics in pseudotumor cerebri and response to steroid therapy. *In* "Neurobiology of CSF". Vol. 2. (Ed. J.H.Wood). pp. 739-752. Plenum Press, New York.

Mann, J.J., Stanley, M., Kaplan, R.D., Sweeney, J. and Neophytides, A. (1983b). Central catecholamine metabolism *in vivo* and the cognitive and motor deficits in Parkinson's disease. *Journal of Neurology, Neurosurgery and Psychiatry*, **46**, (10) 905-1010.

Manno, N.J., Uihlein, A. and Kernohan, J.W. (1962). Intraspinal epidermoids. *Journal of Neurosurgery*, **19**, 754-65.

Mansour, M.M., Guindi, S. and Girgis, N.I. (1981). Levels of individual serum and CSF proteins in purulent and tuberculous meningitis. *European Neurology*, **20**, 40-45.

Manyam, N.V. (1982). Low CSF GABA levels in Parkinson's disease. *Archives of Neurology*, **39**, 391-392.

Manyam, N.V., Hare, R.A. and Katz, L. (1979). CSF GABA levels in Huntington's disease, "At Risk" for Huntington's disease, and normal controls. *Advances in Neurology*, **23**, 547-556.

Manyam, B., Ferraro, T. and Hare, T. (1988). CSF amino compounds in Parkinson's disease. *Archives of Neurology*, **45**, 48-50.

Mao, C., Guidotti, A. and Costa, E. (1974). The regulation of cGMP in rat cerebellum. *British Research*, **79**, 510-514.

Mardh, P.A., Larsson, L., Hoby, N., Engbaek, H.C. and Odham, G. (1983). Tuberculostearic acid as a diagnostic marker in tuberculous meningitis. *Lancet* i, pp. 367 (letter).

Maren, T.H. (1977). Ion secretion into cerebrospinal fluid. *Experimental Eye Research*, **25**, 157-159.

Markovitz, D.C. and J.Fernstrom, D. (1977). Diet and uptake of aldomet by the brain: competition with natural large neutral amino acids. *Science*, **197**, 1014-1015.

Marmarou, A, Shulman, K. and La Morgese, J. (1975). Compartmental analysis of compliance and outflow resistance of the cerebrospinal fluid system. *Journal* of Neurosurgery, **43**, 523-534.

Marmarou, A, Shulman, K. and Rosende, R. (1978). A nonlinear analysis of the cerebrospinal fluid system and intracranial pressure dynamics. *Journal of Neurosurgery*, **48**, 332-344.

Marrazzi, M. and Luby, E. (1989). Anorexia nervosa as an auto-addiction: clinical and basic studies. *Annals of the New York Academy of Science*, **575**, 545-7.

Marshall, D.W., Brey, R.L. and Butzin, C.A. (1989). Lack of cerebrospinal fluid myelin basic protein in HIV-infected asymptomatic individuals with intrathecal synthesis of IgG. *Neurology*, **39**, 1127-29.

Martensson, B., Nyberg, S., Toresson, G., Brodin, E. and Bertilsson, L. (1989). Fluoxetine treatment of depression. *Acta Psychiatrica Scandinavica*, **79**, 586-596.

Martin, W.J. (1983). Rapid and reliable techniques for the laboratory detection of bacterial meningitis. *American Journal of Medicine*, **75**, (lB), 119-23.

Martin, P.R., Adinoff, B., Eckardt, J.J., Stapleton, J.M. et al. (1989). Effective pharmacotherapy of alcoholic amnestic disorder with fluvoxamine. *Archives of General Psychiatry*, **46**, 617-621.

Martinot, J.L., Paillere-Martinot, M.L., Loc'h, C. et al. (1991.). The estimated density of D_2 striatal receptors in schizophrenia. A study with positron emission tomography and [76]Br-bromolisuride. *British Journal of Psychiatry*, **158**, 346-350.

Marton, L.J. (1981). CSF polyamines: potential as brain tumor markers. *Archives of Neurology*, **38**, 73-74.

Marton, K.I. and Gean, A.D. (1986). The spinal tap: a new look at an old test. *Annals of Internal Medicine*, **104**, 840-848.

Marton, L.J., Edwards, M.S., Levin, V.A., Lubich, W.P. and Wilson, C.B. (1981). CSF polyamines: a new and important means of monitoring patients with medulloblastoma. *Cancer*, **47**, 757-760.

Marynick, S.P., Wood, J.H. and Loriaux, D.L. (1980). CSF steroid hormones. *In* "Neurobiology of CSF". (Ed. J.H. Wood). pp. 605-612. Plenum Press, New York.

Mathé, A.F., Wiesel, A., Sedvall, G. and Nyback, H. (1980). Increased content of immunoreactive PGE in CSF of patients with schizophrenia. *Lancet*, i, 16-.19.

Matthews, W.B. (1984). Sarcoid neuropathy. *In* "Peripheral Neuropathy". 2nd Edn. (Eds. P.J. Dyck, P.K. Thomas, E.H. Lambert and R. Burge). pp. 2018-26. W. B. Saunders, Philadelphia.

Matthysse, S. (1978). Central catecholamine metabolism in psychosis. *In* "Neurotransmission and Disturbed Behavior". (Eds H.M. van Praag and J. Bruinvels). S.P. Medical Books, New York.

Mattias-Guiu, J., Martinez-Vazquez, J., Ruibal, A., Colomer, R., Boada, M. and Codina, A. (1986). Myelin basic protein and creatine kinase BB isoenzyme as CSF markers of intracranial tumours and stroke. *Acta Neurologica Scandinavica*, **73**, 461-465.

Mattson, D.H., Roos, R. and Arnason, B. (1982). Oligoclonal IgG in multiple sclerosis and SSPE brains. *Journal of Neuroimmunology*, **2**, 261-76.

Maurer, J. and Rieder, H.P. (1978). Total protein und elektrophophortische Proteinfraktionen des Liquors im Kindesalter. *Schweizerische Medizinische Wochenschrift*, **108**, 1854-1860.

May, C., Kaye, J.A., Atack, J.R., Schapiro, M.B., Friedland, R.P. and Rapoport, S.I. (1990). Cerebrospinal fluid production is reduced in healthy aging. *Neurol-*

ogy, **40**, 500-503

Mayer, D.J. and Frenk, H. (1988). The role of neuropeptides in pain. *In* "Neuropeptides in Psychiatric and Neurological Disorders". (Ed. C.B. Nemeroff). Chapter 9. Johns Hopkins University Press, Baltimore.

McArthur, J.C. (1987). Neurologic manifestations of AIDS. *Medicine*, **66**, (6) 407-37.

McArthur, J.C., Cohen, B.A., Farzedegan, H., Cornblath, D.R. *et al*. (1988). Cerebrospinal fluid abnormalities in homosexual men with and without neuropsychiatric findings. *Annals of Neurology*, **23**, S34-S37.

McArthur, J.C., Sipos, E., Cornblath, D.R., Welch, D. Chupp, M. Griffin, D.E. and Johnson, R.T. (1989). Identification of mononuclear cells in CSF of patients with HIV infection. *Neurology*, **39**, 66-70.

McAuthur, J.C., Nance-Sproson, T.E., Griffin, D.E. *et al*. (1992). The diagnostic utility of elevation in CSF β2-microglobulin in HIV-1 dementia. *Neurology*, **42**, 1707-1712.

McCarthy, B.W., Gomes, U.R., Neethling, A.C., Shanley, B.C., Taljaard, J., Potgieter, L. and Roux, J.T. (1981). GABA concentration in CSF in schizophrenia. *Journal of Neurochemistry*, **36**, 1406-1408.

McComb, J.G. (1983). Recent research into the nature of cerebrospinal fluid – formation and absorption. *Journal of Neurosurgery*, **59**, (3) 369-83.

McDonald W.I. and Kocen, R.S. (1984). Diptheritic neuropathy. *In* "Peripheral Neuropathy". 2nd Edn. (Eds P.J. Dyck, P.K. Thomas, E.H. Lambert and R. Burge). pp. 2010-17. W. B. Saunders, Philadelphia.

McDonald, W.M. and Krishnan, K.R.R. (1991). Vasopressin. *In* "Neuropeptides and Psychiatric Disorders". (Ed.C.B. Nemeroff). pp. 109-128. American Psychiatric Press, Washington D.C.

McGale, E.H.F., Pye, I., Stonier, L., Hutchinson, E. and Aber, G. (1977). Studies of the inter-relationship between CSF and plasma amino acid concentrations in normal individuals. *Journal of Neurochemistry*, **29**, 291-297.

McGinnis, M.R. (1983). Detection of fungi in cerebrospinal fluid. *American Journal of Medicine*, July, 129-138.

McLeod, I.G. (1982). Multiple sclerosis – a review. *Australian and New Zealand Journal of Medicine*, **12**, 302-308.

McLeod, J.G. (1984). Carcinomatous neuropathy. *In* "Peripheral Neuropathy". 2nd Edn. (Eds P.J. Dyck, P.K. Thomas, E.H. Lambert and R. Burge). pp. 2180-91. W. B. Saunders, Philadelphia.

McLeod, J.G. and Walsh, J.C. (1984) Peripheral neuropathy associated with lymphomas and other reticuloses. *In* "Peripheral Neuropathy". 2nd Edn. (Eds. P.J. Dyck, P.K. Thomas, E.H. Lambert and R. Burge). pp. 2192-2203. W. B. Saunders, Philadelphia.

McLeod, J.G., Walsh, J.C., Prineas, J.W. and Pollard, J.D. (1976). Acute idiopathic polyneuritis: A clinical and electrophysiological follow up study. *Journal of Neurological Science*, **27**, 145.

McLeod, J.G., Walsh, J.C. and Pollard, J.D. (1984). Neuropathies associated with paraproteinemias and dysproteinemia. *In* "Peripheral Neuropathy". 2nd Edn. (Eds. P.J. Dyck, P.K. Thomas, E.H. Lambert and R. Burge). pp. 1847-65. W. B. Saunders, Philadelphia.

McRae-Degueurce, A., Klawans, H., Penn, R. *et al*. (1988). An antibody in the

CSF of Parkinson's disease patients disappears following adrenal medulla transplantation. *Neuroscience Letters*, **94**, 192-197.

Meeks, G.R., Morrison, J. C., Fish, S.A. and Wiser, W.L. (1983). CSF alterations in pregnancy and eclampsia. *In* "Neurobiology of CSF". Vol. 2. (Ed. J.H. Wood). pp. 603-614. Plenum Press, New York.

Meena, C.E., Olson, W.H. and Yam, L.T. (1989). Light microscopic cytology of cerebrospinal fluid. *In* "The Cerebrospinal Fluid". Chapter 9. (Eds R.M. Herndon and R.A. Brumback), Kluwer Academic Publishers, Norwell, MA.

Mehl, A.L. (1986). Interpretation of traumatic lumbar puncture. *Clinical Pediatrics*, **25**, (10) 575-577.

Mehl, E., Ruther, E. and Redemann, J. (1977). Endogenous ligands of a putative LSD-serotonin receptor in the CSF: higher level of LDF in unmedicated psychotic patients. *Psychopharmology*, **54**, 9-16.

Mehta, L.J. and Wisniewski, H.M. (1990). Identification of IgG subclasses. Oligoclonal bands in multiple sclerosis CSF. *Acta Neurologica Scandinavica*, **82**, 4-8.

Mehta, P.D., Patrick, B.A. and Miller, J.A. (1984). Absence of oligoclonal Ig A in CSF and serum of multiple sclerosis patients. *Journal of Neuroimmunology*, **6**, (1) 67-9.

Meldrum, B. (1978). Neurotransmitters and epilepsy. *In* "Neurotransmitter Systems and Their Clinical Disorders". (Ed. N.J. Legg). pp. 167-182. Academic Press, New York.

Meltzer, H.Y. (1987). Biological studies in schizophrenia. *Schizophrenia Bulletin*, **13**, (1) 77-110.

Meltzer, H.Y. (1990). Role of serotonin in depression. *Annals of the New York Academy of Sciences,* **600**, 486-499.

Mens, W.B., Andringa-Bakker, E., Van Wimer, J.M. and Grerdanus, T.B. (1982). Changes in CSF levels of vasopressin and oxytocin of the rat during various light and dark regimes. *Neuroscience Letters,* **34**, (1) 51-56.

Merritt, H. and Fremont-Smith, H. (1938). "The Cerebrospinal Fluid". W.B. Saunders, Philadelphia.

Merritt, H.H., Adams, R.D. and Solomon, H.C. (1946). "Neurosyphilis". Oxford University Press, New York.

Mikheyeva, Y. (1963). Study of CSF in schizophrenics – a review of the literature. *Zhurnal Nevropatologic i Psikhiatrii.* **63**, 920-930, Translated by Pearson, E. in (1973). *Psychopharmacology Bulletin*, **9**, 59-72.

Milhorat, T.H. (1975). The third circulation revisited. *Journal of Neurosurgery*, **42**, 628-45.

Milhorat, T.H. (1976). Structure and function of the choroid plexus and other sites of cerebrospinal fluid formation. *International Review of Cytology*, **47**, 225-288.

Milhorat, T.H. (1985). Hydrocephalus: pathophysiology and clinical features. *In* "Neurosurgery". (Eds R.Wilkins and S. Rengachary). McGraw-Hill, New York.

Milhorat, T.H. and Hammock, M.K. (1983). CSF as reflection of internal milieu. *In* "Neurobiology of CSF". (Ed. J.H. Wood). pp. 1-24. Plenum Press, New York.

Millen, J. and Woollam, D. (1962). "The Anatomy of the Cerebrospinal Fluid". Oxford University Press, London.

Miller, R. (1989). Schizophrenia as a progressive disorder: relation to EEG, CT, neuropathological and other evidence. *Progress in Neurobiology*, **33**, 17-44.

Miller, T.B. and Ross, C.R. (1976). Transport of organic cations and anions by choroid plexus. *Journal of Pharmacology and Experimental Therapy*, **196**, 771-777.

Miller, J.R., Burke, A. M. and Bever, C.T. (1983). Occurrence of oligoclonal bands in MS and other CNS diseases. *Annals of Neurology*, **13**, 53-58.

Miyamato, H., Walker, J., Ginsberg, A., Burks, J., McIntosh, K. and Kempe, L.H. (1976). Antibodies to vaccines and measles viruses in MS patients. *Archives of Neurology*, **33**, 414-17.

Moar, J.J. (1982). Determining the so-called moment of death in homicide victims. *South African Medical Journal*, **62**, 64-66.

Modigh, K. (1975). The relationship between the concentrations of tryptophan and 5-HIAA – in rat brain and CSF. *Journal of Neurochemistry*, **25**, 351-352.

Mohan, A., Nag, O., Misra, R.N., Gujrati, V.R., Shanker, K., Doval, D.C., Saxena, R.C. and Bhargava, K.P. (1982). Serotonergic and dopaminergic metabolites in cerebrospinal fluid of epileptics. *Die Pharmazie*, **37**, 803.

Moir, A.T. (1974). Tryptophan concentration in the brain. *In* "Aromatic Amino Acids in the Brain". CIBA Symposium 22, pp. 197-206. Elsevier, Amsterdam.

Moir, A.T.B., Ashcroft, G.W., Crawford, T.B.B., Eccleston, D. and Guldberg, H.C. (1970). Cerebral metabolites in cerebrospinal fluid as a biochemical approach to the brain. *Brain*, **93**, 357-368.

Molavi, A. and Le Frock, J.L. (1985). Tuberculous meningitis. *Medical Clinics of North America*, **69**, 315-331

Montgomery, S. and Montgomery, D. (1982). Drug treatment of suicidal behavior. *In* "Typical and Atypical Antidepressants". (Eds E. Costa and Racagni), Raven Press, New York.

Moore, C.M. and Ross, M. (1973). Acute bacterial meningitis with absent or minimal cerebrospinal fluid abnormalities – a report of three cases. *Clinical Paediatrics*, **12**, (2) 117-118.

Mori, K. (1990). Hydrocephalus – revision of its definition and classification with special reference to "intractable infantile hydrocephalus". *Child's Nervous System*, **6**, 198-204.

Morimoto C., Hafler, D.A. and Weiner, H.L. (1987). Selective loss of the suppressor-inducer T-Cell subset in progressive multiple sclerosis. *New England Journal of Medicine*, **316**, 67-72.

Moroni, G., Rombardi, G., Carla, N., Lal, S., Etienne, P. and Nair, N.P. (1986). Increase in the content of quinolinic acid in cerebrospinal fluid and frontal cortex of patients with hepatic failure. *Journal of Neurochemistry*, 1667.

Moss, R.L., Dudley, C.A. and Riskind, P.N. (1991). Gonadotropin-releasing hormone and human sexual behaviour. *In* "Neuropeptides and Psychiatric Disorders". (Ed. C.B. Nemeroff). American Psychiatric Press, Washington D.C.

Mouret, J., Debilly, G., Renaud, B. and Blois, R. (1976). Narcolepsy and hypersomnia diseases or symptoms? Polygraphic and pharmacologic studies. *In* "Narcolepsy". (Eds C. Guillemnnault *et al.*). pp. 571-584. S.P. Books, New York.

Mullen, K., Szuater, K., Kaminsky-Russ, K. (1990). 'Endogenous" benzodiazepine activity in body fluids of patients with hepatic encephalopathy. *Lancet*, **336**,

81-83.

Mumenthaler, M. (1990). "Neurologie", p. 475. George Thieme Nesley, Stuttgart-New York.

Murata, R. and Vemura, T. (1981). The diagnostic value of CSF lactic acid levels in meningitis. *Folia Psychiatrica et Neurologica Japonica*, **35**, 175-179.

Murros, K. and Fogelholm, R. (1983). Spontaneous intracranial hypotension with slit ventricles. *Journal of Neurology, Neurosurgery and Psychiatry*, **46**, 1149-1151.

Myers, R.D. (1985). Multiple metabolite theory, alcohol drinking and the alcogene. *In* "Aldehyde Adducts in Alcoholism". pp. 201-220.

Myllyla, V.V., Hokkanen, E., Nousiainen, H., Heikkinen, E.R. and Vapaatalo, H. (1977). CSF cyclic AMP and epilepsy. *In* "Epilepsy: The Eighth International Symposium". (Ed. J.K. Penry). pp. 313-316. Raven Press, New York.

Naber, D. and Pickar, D. (1983). The measurement of endorphins in body fluids. *Psychiatric Clinics of North America*, **6**, (3), 443-456.

Nadis, S.M. and Klawans, H.L. (1989). Cerebrospinal fluid in stroke. *Handbook of Clinical Neurology*, **10**, (54) 195.

Nair, N., Lal, S. and Bloom, D. (1986). CCK and schizophrenia. *Progress in Brain Research*, **65**, 237-258.

Navaratnam, D.S., Priddle, J.D., McDonald, B., Esiri, M.M., Robinson, J.R. and Smith, A.D. (1991). Anomalous molecular form of acetylcholinesterase in cerebrospinal fluid in histologically diagnosed Alzheimer's disease. *The Lancet*, **23**, 337, 447-449.

Navia, B.A., Jordan, B.D. and Price, R.W. (1986). The AIDS dementia complex: I clinical features. *Annals of Neurology*, **19**, 517-524 .

Nemeroff, C.B. (1991a). "Neuropeptides and Psychiatric Disorders". American Psychiatric Press, Washington D.C.

Nemeroff, C.B. (1991b). Corticotropin-releasing factor. *In* "Neuropeptides and Psychiatric Disorders". (Ed. C.B. Nemeroff). pp. 75-92. American Psychiatric Press, Washington D.C.

Nemeroff, C. and Bissette, G. (1987). The role of neuropeptides in schizophrenia. *In* "Handbook of Schizophrenia". Vol. 2. (Eds F. Hem and L. De Lisi). Elsevier Publishers, Amsterdam.

Nemeroff, C. and Bissette, G. (1988). Neuropeptides, dopamine and schizophrenia. *Annals of the New York Academy of Science*, **537**, 273-91.

Nemeroff C.B., Manberg, P.J. *et al.* (1983). Neuropeptides in cerebrospinal fluid and postmortem brain tissue of schizophrenics, Huntington's choreics, and normal controls. *Psychopharmacology Bulletin*, **19**, (3) 369-374.

Nemeroff, C.B., Bissette, G., Widerlov, E. *et al.* (1989). Neurotensin-like immunoreactivity in CSF of patients with schizophrenia, depression, anorexia nervosa-bulimia and premenstrual syndrome. *Journal of Neuropsychiatry and Clinical Neuroscience*, **1**, (1) 16-20.

Netsky, M.G. and Shuangshoti, S. (1975). "The Choroid Plexus in Health and Disease". University Press of Virginia, Charlottesville, VA.

Neu, I. (1981a). Essentielle fettsauren in serum and liquor cerebrospinalis bei patienten mit multipler sklerose. *Nervanarzt*, **52**, 100-107.

Neu, I. (1981b). EFA's in serum and CSF of patients during MS. *Nervanartzt*, **52**, 100-107, (Abst.) in E.M. *Neurology and Neurosurgery*, **53**, 345.

Neu, I.S. (1984). Essential fatty acids in the serum and CSF of multiple sclerosis patients. *In* "Gansette and Delmotte". pp. 184, 194.

Neuwelt E.A. and Rapoport, S.I. (1984). Modification of the blood-brain barrier in the chemotherapy of malignant brain tumors. *Federation Proceedings*, **43**, 214-219.

Neuwelt, E.A. (1989). "Implications of the Blood-Brain Barrier and its Manipulation". Vols 1 and 2. Plenum Press, New York.

Neville, B.G.R. (1988). When not to do a lumbar puncture. *Archives of Disease in Childhood*, **63**, 569-575.

Nijst, T.Q., Wevers, R.A., Schoonderwaldt, H.K., Hommes, O.R. and de Haan, A.F. (1990). Vitamin B12 and folate concentrations in serum and CSF of neurological patients with special reference to multiple sclerosis and dementia. *Journal of Neurology, Neurosurgery and Psychiatry*, **53**(ii), 951-954.

Niklasson, F., Agren, H. and Hallgren, R. (1983). Purine and monoamine metabolites in CSF: parallel purinergic and monoaminergic activation in depressive illness. *Journal of Neurology, Neurosurgery and Psychiatry*, **46**, 255-260.

Ninan, P.T., van Kammen, D.P. *et al.* (1984). CSF 5-hydroxyindoleacetic acid levels in suicidal schizophrenic patients. *American Journal of Psychiatry*, **141**, (4) 566-569.

Nishi, K., Kondo, T. Narabayashi, H. *et al* (1989). Unresponsiveness to L-DOPA in Parkinsonian patients: a study of HVA concentration in the CSF. *Journal of Neurological Sciences*, **92**, 65-70.

Nisijima K, and Ishiguro, T. (1989). Neuroleptic malignant syndrome: a study of CSF monoamine metabolism. *Biological Psychiatry*, **27**, 280-288.

Noble, E.P. and Tewari, S. (1977). Metabolic aspects of alcoholism in the brain. *In* "Metabolic Aspects of Alcoholism". (Ed. C.S. Lieber). pp. 149-185. MTP Press, Lancaster, England.

Nordin, C. (1988). Relationships between clinical symptoms and monoamine metabolite concentrations in biochemically defined subgroups of depressed patients. *Acta Psychiatrica Scandinavica*, **78**, 720-729.

Nordin, C., Siwers, B. and Bertilsson, L. (1982). Site of lumbar puncture influences levels of monoamine metabolites. *Archives of General Psychiatry*, **39**, (12) 1445.

Nornes, H., Magnaes, B. and R. Aaslid (1975). Observations in intracranial pressure plateau waves. *In* "Intracranial Pressure II". (Ed. N. Lunderg). pp. 421-6. Springer-Verlag, Berlin.

Norrby, E., Link, H., Olsson, J., Panelius, M., Salmi, A. and Vandvik, B. (1974). Comparison of antibodies against different viruses in CSF and serum samples from patients with multiple sclerosis. *Infection and Immunology*, **10**, 688-94.

Norris, M.C., Leighton, B.L. and DeSimone, C.A. (1989). Needle bevel direction and headache after inadvertent dural puncture. *Anaesthesiology*, **70**, 729-731.

Nosik, W.A. (1955). Intracranial hypotension secondary to lumber nerve sleeve tear. *Journal of the American Medical Association*, **157**, 1110.

Nowak, T.S. and Munro, H.W. (1977). Effects of protein, calorie malnutrition on biochemical aspects of brain development. *In* "Nutrition and the Brain". (Ed. J. Wurtman). pp. 194-247. Raven Press, New York.

Nutt, D.J. (1986). Increased central α-2 adrenoceptor sensitivity in panic disorder. *Psychopharmacology*, **90**, 268-269.

Nutt, J.G. (1983). Substance P in human CSF. *In* "Neurobiology of CSF". Vol. 2. (Ed. J.H. Wood). pp. 67-76.

Nyback, H., Berggren, B.M., Hindmarsh, T., Sedvall, G. and Wiesel, F.A. (1983). Cerebroventricular size and cerebrospinal fluid monoamine metabolites in schizophrenic patients and healthy volunteers. *Psychiatry Research*, **9**, (4) 301-8.

Nyberg, F. and Terenius, L. (1982). Endorphins in human cerebrospinal fluid. *Life Science*, **31**, 1737.

Nyberg, F., Wahlstrom, A., Sjolund, B. and Terenius, L. (1983). Characterization of electrophoretically separable endorphins in human CSF. *Brain Research*, **259**, 267-274.

Nyman, H., Nyback, H., Wiesel, F-A. *et al.* (1986). Neurophyschological test performance, brain morphological measures and CSF monoamine metabolites in schizophrenic patients. *Acta Psychiatrica Scandinavica*, **74**, (3) 292-301.

Oehmichen, M. (1976). "CSF Cytology: An Introduction and Atlas". W.B. Saunders, Co., Philadelphia.

Ogawa, S.K., Smith, M.A., Brennessel, D.J. and Lowry, F.D. (1987). Tuberculosis meningitis in an urban medical center. *Medicine*, **66**, 317-326.

Oksanen, V., Fyhrquish, F., Somer, H. and Gronhagen-Riska, C. (1985*a*). Angiotensin converting enzyme in cerebrospinal fluid: a new assay. *Neurology*, **35**, 1220-1223.

Oksanen, V., Fyhrquist, F., Gronhagen-Riska, C. and Somer, H. (1985*b*). CSF angiotensin-converting enzyme in neurosarcoidosis. *Lancet*, i, (8436), 1050-1.

Olanow, C.W., Gauger, I.L. and Cedarbaum, J.M. (1991). Temporal relationships between plasma and cerebrospinal fluid pharmacokinetics of levodopa and clinical effect in Parkinson's disease. *Annals of Neurology*, **29**, 556-539.

Oldendorf, W.H. (1977). The blood-brain barrier. *Experimental Eye Research*, 177-190.

Oliver, C., Ben-Jonathan, N., Mical, R.S. and Porter, J.C. (1975). Transport of TRH from CSF to hypophysial portal blood and the release of thyrotropin. *Endocrinology*, **97**, 1138-1143.

Ollat, H. and Sebban, C. (1983). Lesions histologiques et modifications des systèmes neurotransmetteurs du cerveau agé. *Presse Médicale*, **12**, 809-814.

Olney, J.W. (1989). Excitatory amino acids and neuropsychiatric disorders. *Biological Psychiatry*, **26**, 505-525.

Olsen, K.S. (1987). Epidural blood patch in the treatment of post-lumbar puncture headache. *Pain*, **30**, 293-301.

Olson, L.C. and Arnoldi, S.H. (1982). The CSF anion gap. *Journal of Pediatrics*, **100**, 91-93.

Olson, M.E., Chernik, N.L. and Posner, J. (1974). Infiltration of the leptomeninges by systemic cancer: A chemical and pathological study. *Archives of Neurology*, **30**, 122-137.

Orenberg, E.K., Zarcone, V., Renson, J. and Barchas, J.D. (1976). The effects of ethanol ingestion on cyclic AMP, HVA, and 5-HIAA in human CSF. *Life Science*, **19**, 1669-1672.

Ouvrier, R.A. (1978). Progressive dystonia with marked diurnal fluctuation. *Annals of Neurology*, **4**, 412-417.

Palfreyman, M.G., Huot, S. and Greve, J. (1983). Total GABA and homocarnasine in CSF as indices of brain GABA concentrations. *Neuroscience Letters*, **35**,

161-166.

Pall, H.S., Williams, A., Blake, D. *et al.* (1987). Raised CSF copper concentrations in Parkinson's disease. *Lancet*, ii, 238-241.

Pall, H.S., Brailsford, S., Williams, A., Lunic, J. and Blake, D. (1990). Ferritin in the CSF of patients with Parkinson's disease. *Journal of Neurology, Neurosurgery and Psychiatry*, **53**, 803.

Palm, R. and Hallmans, G. (1982). Zinc concentrations in the CSF of normal adults and patients with neurological diseases. *Journal of Neurology, Neurosurgery and Psychiatry*, **45**, (8) 685-90.

Palm, G., Hallmans, G. and Sjostrom, R. (1982). Zinc concentrations in normal and pathological CSF. *Acta Neurologcia Scandinavica*, **65**, 184-185.

Panitch, H., Hafler, D. and Johnson, K. (1980a). Antibodies to MBP in CSF of patients with M.S. *In* "Progress in MS Research". (Eds H. Bauer, *et al.*). pp. 98-105. Springer-Verlag, New York.

Panitch, H.S., Hooper, C.J. and Johnson, K.P. (1980b). CSF antibody to myelin basic protein. *Archives of Neurology*, **37**, 206-209.

Papageorgious, C., Gyftaki, H., Mavrikakis, M., Kesse-Elias, M. and Alevizou-Terzaki, V. (1983). Cerebrospinal fluid cyclic adenosine 3. 5. - monophosphate in cases of severe cerebral ischemia and meningitis. *European Journal of Neurology*, **22**, 12-16.

Pappu, L.D., Purohit, D.M., Levkoff, A.H. and Kaplan, B. (1982). CSF cytology in the neonate. *American Journal of Diseases of Children*, **136**, 297-298.

Parkes, J.D. (1985). "Sleep and its Disorders". W.B. Saunders, London.

Parkes, J., Fenton, G., Struthers, G., Curzan, G., Kantamaneni, B.D., Buxton, B. and Record, C. (1974). Narcolepsy and cataplexy: clinical features, treatment and CSF findings. *Quarterly Journal of Medicine*, **43**, 525-536.

Parry, G.J. (1988). Peripheral neuropathies associated with human immunodeficiency virus infection. *Annals of Neurology*, **23**, S49-553.

Parsons, M. (1988). Diagnosis in tuberculous meningitis. *In* "Tuberculous Meningitis. A Handbook for Clinicians". 2nd Edn, (Ed. M. Parsons). pp. 14-26. Oxford Medical Publications, Oxford.

Parsons, M.A., Royds, J.A., Taylor, C.B. and Timperley, W. (1981). Enolase isoenzymes as markers of cellular differentiation in the normal human fetus and adult. *Journal of Pathology*, **134**, 314-31.

Paty, D.W., McFarlin, D.E. and McDonald, W.I. (1991). MRI and laboratory aids in the diagnosis of Multiple Sclerosis. *Annals of Neurology*, **29**, (1) 3-6.

Paulson, G.W. and Stickney, D. (1971). Cerebrospinal fluid after death. *Conf. Neurology*, **33**, 149-162.

Peake, G.T., Buckman, M.T., Davis, L.E. and Standefer, J. (1983). Pituitary and placentally derived hormones in CSF during normal human pregnancy. *Journal of Clinical Endocrinology and Metabolism*, **56**, (1) 46-52.

Pedersen, C.A. (1991). The psychiatric significance of oxytocin. *In* "Neuropeptides and Psychiatric Disorders". (Ed. C.B. Nemeroff). pp. 129-148. American Psychiatric Press, Washington D.C.

Pedersen, H.E. (1974). CSF cholesterol and phospholipids in MS. *Acta Neurologica Scandinavica*, **50**, 171-182.

Peltier, L. (1988). The classic – The first description of the spinal fluid – Domenico Cotugno (1964). *In* "The Orthopedics and Related Research". pp. 6-9.

Penn, R.D. and Kroin, J.S. (1987). Long-term intrathecal baclofen infusion for treatment of spasticity. *Journal of Neurosurgery,* **66,** 181-185.

Perkin, G.D., Sethi, K. and Muller, B.R. (1983). IgG ratios and oligoclonal IgG in multiple sclerosis and other neurological disorders. *Journal of Neurological Science,* **60,** (3) 325-36.

Perlow, M.J. and Lake, C.R. (1980). Daily fluctuations in catecholamines, monoamine metabolites, cAMP and GABA. *In* "Neurobiology of CSF". (Ed. J.H. Wood). pp. 63-70. Plenum Press, New York.

Perry, S.W. (1990). Organic mental disorders caused by HIV: update on early diagnosis and treatment. *American Journal of Psychiatry,* **147,** (6), 696-710.

Perry, T.L. (1982). Normal CSF and brain glutamate levels in schizophrenic do not support the hypothesis of glutamatergic neuronal dysfunction. *Neuroscience Letters,* **28,** 81-85.

Perry, T.L., Hansen, S., Wall, R.A. and Gauthier, S.G. (1982a). Human CSF GABA concentrations: revised downward for controls, but not decreased in Huntington's chorea. *Journal of Neurochemistry,* **38,** 766-773.

Perry, T.L., Hansen, S., Quinn, N. and Marsden, C.D. (1982b). Concentrations of GABA and other amino acids in CSF from torison dystonia patients. *Journal of Neurochemistry,* **39,** 1188.

Perry T.L., Hansen, S. and Jones, K. (1989). Schizophrenia, tardive dyskinesia, and brain GABA. *Biological Psychiatry,* **25,** 200-206.

Persson L., Hardemark, H-G., Gustafsson, J. *et al.* (1987). S-100 protein and neuron-specific enolase in cerebrospinal fluid and serum: markers of cell damage in human central nervous system. *Stroke,* **18,** 911-18.

Peter, J. (1993). "Use and Interpretation of Laboratory Tests in Neurology". Specialty Laboratories, Inc., Santa Monica, CA.

Pezzoli, G., Panerai, A., Di Giulio, A. *et al.* (1984). Methionine-enkephalin, substance P, and HVA in the CSF of Parkinsonian patients. *Neurology,* **34,** 516-19.

Pfister, H-W., Preac-Mursic, V., Wilske, B., Einhaupl, K-M. and Weinberger, K. (1989). Latent lyme neuroborreliosis: presence of borrelia burgdorferi in the cerebrospinal fluid without concurrent inflammatory signs. *Neurology,* **39,** 1118-1120.

Pickar, D., Cohen, M.R. Naber, D. and Cohen, R.M. (1982a). Clinical studies of the endogenous opioid system. *Biological Psychiatry,* **17,** (11) 1243-1269.

Pickar, D., Naber, D., Post, R.M., van Kammen, D.P., Ballenger, J., Rubinow, D., Waters, R., Kaye, W.H. Ebert, M.H. and Bunney, W.E. (1982b). Endogenous opioids and psychiatric illness: CSF studies. *In* "Brain Peptides and Hormones". (Eds R. Collu, *et al.*). pp. 207-219. Raven Press, New York.

Pickar D., Labarca, R., Linnoila, M. *et al.* (1984). Neuroleptic-induced decrease in plasma homovanillic acid and antipsychotic activity in schizophrenic patients. *Science,* **225,** 954-956.

Pickar, D., Roy, A., Breier, A. *et al.* (1986a). Suicide and aggression in schizophrenia. Neurobiologic correlates. *Annals of the New York Academy of Science,* **487,** 189-96.

Pickar, D., Labarca, R., Doran, A.R. *et al.* (1986b). Longitudinal measurement of plasma homovanillic acid levels in schizophrenic patients. *Archives of General Psychiatry,* **43,** 669-676.

Pickar, D., Reier, A.B. and Kelsoe, J. (1988). Plasma HVA as an index of central dopaminergic activity: studies in schizophrenic patients. *Annals of New York Academy of Science,* **537**, 339-375.
dopaminergic activity: studies in schizophrenic patients. *Annals of New York Academy of Science,* **537**, 339-375.

Pickar, D., Breier, A., Hsiao, J.K. *et al.* (1990). Cerebrospinal fluid and plasma monoamine metabolites and their relation to psychosis. *Archives of General Psychiatry,* **47**, (7) 641-648.

Pitkanen, A., Jolkkonen, J. and Riekkinen, P. (1987). Beta-endorphin, somatostatin, and prolactin levels in cerebrospinal fluid of epileptic patients after a generalised convulsion. *Journal of Neurology, Neurosurgery and Psychiatry,* **50**, 1294-1297.

Pitkanen, A., Jolkkonen, J. Sirvio, M.A.J., Sivenius, J. and Riekkinen, P.J. (1988*a*). Somatostatin-like immunoreactivity in cerebrospinal fluid of patients with complex partial epilepsy. *European Neurology,* **28**, 1-5.

Pitkanen, A., Matilainen, R. Halonen, T., Kutvonen, R. Hartikainen, P. and Riekkinen, P. (1988*b*). Inhibitory and excitatory amino acids in cerebrospinal fluid of chronic epileptic patients. *Journal of Neural Transmission,* **76**, 221-230.

Pitkanen, A., Lepola, U., Ylinen, A. and Riekkinen, P.J. (1989). Somatostatin and beta-endorphin levels in cerebrospinal fluid of nonmedicated and medicated patients with epileptic seizures. *Neuropeptides,* **13**, 9-15.

Pitts, A.F., Carroll, B.T., Gehris, T.L., Kathol, R.G. and Samuelson, S.D. (1990). Elevated CSF. Protein in male patients with depression. *Biological Psychiatry,* **28**, 629-637.

Plum, F. and Posner, J.B. (1968). Inhomogeneity of cisternal and lumbar CSF acid-base balance during acute metabolic alterations. *Scandinavian Journal of Laboratory and Clinical Medicine,* (Suppl.) **102**, 1B.

Pohl, P., Schmutzhard, E. and Stanek, G. (1986). Cerebrospinal fluid findings in neurological manifestations of Lyme disease. *Zentralblatt für Bakteriologie, Mikrobiologie und Hygiene,* A**263**, 314-320.

Polini, A. (1954). EEG changes induced by injection of CSF of schizophrenic and epileptic patients. *Electroencephalography and Clinical Neurophysiology,* **6**, 535.

Pollay, M. (1974). Transport mechanisms in the choroid plexus. *Federation Proceedings,* **33**, 2064-2069.

Pollay, M. (1975). Formation of cerebrospinal fluid. *In* "Intracranial Pressure II". (Eds N. Lundberg, U. Ponten and M. Brock). pp. 20-23. Springer-Verlag, New York.

Pomara, N., Singh, R.R., Deptula, D., LeWitt, P.A., Bissette, G., Stanley, M. and Nemeroff, C.B. (1989). CSF corticotropin-releasing factor (CRF) in Alzheimer's disease: its relationship to severity of dementia and monoamine metabolites. *Biological Psychiatry,* **26**, 500-504.

Portegies, P., Epstein, L.G., Tjong, S., Hung, A., de Gans, J., (1989). Human immunodeficiency virus type 1 antigen in cerebrospinal fluid. Correlation with clinical neurologic status. *Archives of Neurology,* **46**, 261-264.

Portnoy, J.M. and Olson, L.C. (1985). Normal cerebrospinal fluid values in children: another look. *Pediatrics,* **75**, (3) 484-487.

Poso, A.M., Hillbom and Eriksson, L. (1981). Acetaldehyde penetrates the blood-liquor barrier of goats. *Toxicology Letters,* **8**, 57-62.

Post, R. and Goodwin, F. (1974a). Effects of amitriptyline and imipramine on amine metabolites in the CSF of depressed patients. *Archives of General Psychiatry*, **30**, 234-239.

Post, R.M. and Goodwin, F.K. (1974b). Estimation of brain amine metabolism in affective illness: CSF studies utilizing probenicid. *Psychotherapy, Psychosomatics*, **23**, 142-158.

Post, R.M. and Goodwin, F.K. (1978). Approaches to brain amines in psychiatric patients. *Handbook of Psychopharmacology*, **13**, 147-85.

Post, R., Fink, E., Carpenter, W. and Goodwin, F. (1975). CSF amine metabolites in acute schizophrenia. *Archives of General Psychiatry*, **32**, 1063-9.

Post, R.M., Lake, C.R., Jimerson, D.C., Bunney, W.E., Wood, J.H., Ziegler, M.G. and Goodwin, F.K. (1978a). Cerebrospinal Fluid Norepinephrine in Affective Illness. *American Journal of Psychiatry*, **135**, (8) 907-911.

Post, R., Gerner, R., Carman, J., Gillin, J., Jimerson, D., Goodwin, F.K. and Bunney, W. (1978b). Effects of a dopamine agonist piribedil in depressed patients. *Archives of General Psychiatry*, **35**, 609-615.

Post, K.D., Biller, B.J. and Jackson, I.M.D. (1980a). CSF pituitary hormone concentrations in patients with pituitary tumors. *In* "Neurobiology of CSF". (Ed. J. H. Wood). pp. 685-718. Plenum Press, New York.

Post, R.M., Ballenger, J.C. and Goodwin, F.K. (1980b). Cerebrospinal fluid studies of neurotransmitter function in manic and depressive illness. *In* "Neurobiology of CSF". Vol I. (Ed. J.H. Wood). pp. 685-717. Plenen Press, New York.

Post, R.M., Gold, P., Rubinow, D.R., Ballenger, J. C., Bunney, W.E. and Goodwin, F.K. (1982). Peptides in the CSF of neuropsychiatric patients: An approach to central nervous system peptide function. *Life Science*, **31**, 1-15.

Post, R.M., Gold, P.W., Rubinow, D.R., Bunney, W.E., Ballenger, J.L. and Goodwin, F.K. (1983). CSF as a neuroregulatory pathway. *In* "Neurobiology of Cerebrospinal Fluid". Vol. 2. (Ed. J.H. Wood). Plenum Press, New York.

Post, R.M., Jimerson, D.C., Ballenger, J.C., Lake, C.R. Uhde, T.W. and Goodwin, F.K. (1984a). Cerebrospinal fluid norepinephrine and its metabolites in manic-depressive illness. *In* "Neurobiology of Mood Disorders". Chapter 34. (Eds R.M. Post and J.C. Ballenger), Williams and Wilkins, Baltimore.

Post, R.M., Pickar, D., Ballenger, J.C., Naber, D. and Rubinow, D.R. (1984b). Endogenous opiates in cerebrospinal fluid: relationship to mood and anxiety. *In* "Neurobiology of Mood Disorders". Chapter 23. (Eds R.M. Post and J.C. Ballenger). Williams and Wilkins, Baltimore.

Post, R.M., Rubinow, D.R. and Gold, P.W. (1988). Neuropeptides in manic-depressive illness. *In* "Neuropeptides in Psychiatric and Neurological Disorders". Chapter 4. (Ed. C.B. Nemeroff). Johns Hopkins University Press, Baltimore.

Potkin, S.G., Shore, D., Torrey, E.F., Weinberger, D.R., Gillin, J.C., Henkin, R.I., Agarwal, R.P. and Wyatt, R.J. (1982). CSF zinc concentrations in ex-heroin adults and patients with schizophrenia: some preliminary observations. *Biological Psychiatry*, **17**, (11) 1315-1322.

Potkin S.G., Weinberger, D.R. *et al.* (1983). Low CSF 5-hydroxyindoleacetic acid in schizophrenic patients with enlarged cerebral ventricles. *American Journal of Psychiatry*, **140**, (1) 21-25.

Powers, W. (1985). Cerebrospinal fluid lymphocytes in acute bacterial meningitis.

American Journal of Medicine, **79**, 216-20.

Powers, W.J. (1986). Should lumbar puncture be part of the routine evaluation of patients with cerebral ischemia? *Stroke*, **17**, 332-333.

Praus, D.J., Brown, G.R., Rundell, J.R. and Paolucci, S.L. (1990). Associations between cerebrospinal fluid parameters and high degrees of anxiety or depression in United States Air Force personnel infected with human immunodeficiency virus. *Journal of Nervous and Mental Disease*, **178**, (6) 392-395.

Prockop L.D. and C.P. Shah (1989). Disorders of cerebrospinal and brain fluids – hydrocephalus. *In* "Meritt's Textbook of Neurology". Chapter 4 (Ed L.P. Rowlands). Lea and Febiger, Philadelphia.

Procter, A.W., Palmer, A.M., Francis, P.T., Lowe, S.L., Neary, D., Murphy, E., Doshi, R. and Bowen, D.M. (1988). Evidence of glutamatergic denervation and possible abnormal metabolism in Alzheimer's Disease. *In* "Journal of Neurochemistry". pp. 790. Raven Press Ltd, New York.

Pruitt, A., Rubin, R., Karchmer A. and Duncan, G. (1978). Neurologic complications of bacterial endocarditis. *Medicine*, **57**, 329-343.

Pycock, C. (1978). Other neurotransmitters in Parkinson's disease. *In* "Neurotransmitter Systems and their Clinical Disorders". (Ed. N.J. Legg). pp. 99-114. Academic Press, New York.

Quality Standards Subcommittee of the American Academy of Neurology (1993). Practice parameters: lumbar puncture. *Neurology*, **43**, 625-627.

Rainero, I., Kaye, J., May, C. *et al.* (1988a). Alpha-MSH-like immuno-reactivity is increased in CSF of patients with Parkinson's disease. *Archives of Neurology*, **45**, 1224-1227.

Rainero I., May, C., Kaye, J.A., Friedland, R.P. and Rapoport, S.I. (1988b). CSF Alpha-MSH in dementia of the Alzheimer type. *Neurology*, **38**, 1281-1284.

Rapoport J.L. (1986). Childhood obsessive compulsive disorder. *Journal of Child Psychology and Psychiatry*, **27**, 289-295.

Rapoport, S.I. (1976). "Blood-Brain Barrier in Physiology and Medicine". Raven Press, New York.

Rapoport, S.I., Hori, M. and Klatzo, I. (1972). Testing of a hypothesis for osmotic opening of the blood-brain barrier. *American Journal of Physiology*, **223**, (2) 323-330.

Raskin, N.H. (1990). Lumbar puncture headache: a review. *Headache*, **30**, 197-200.

Raskind, M.A., Peskind, E.R., Lampe, T.H., Risse, S.C., Taborsky, G.J. and Dorsa, D. (1986). Cerebrospinal fluid vasopressin, oxytocin, somatostatin, and beta endorphin in Alzheimer's disease. *Archives of General Psychiatry*, **43**, 382-388.

Rasmussen A.G., Adolfsson, R. and Karlsson, T. (1988). New method specific for acetylcholinesterase in cerebrospinal fluid: application to Alzheimer's disease. *The Lancet*, Sept 3, pp. 571-572.

Rastogi, S., Clausen, J., Tourtellotte, W. and Potvin, A. (1983). Multiple-sclerosis-specific CNS antigens (MSG2): a blind study. *European Neurology*, **22**, 17-21.

Read, D. and Warlow, C. (1978). Peripheral neuropathy and solitary plasmacytoma. *Journal of Neurology, Neurosurgery and Psychiatry*, **41**, 177-184.

Redmond, D.E. Jnr., Katz, M.M., Maas, J.W. , Swann, A., Casper, R. and Davis, J.M. (1986). Cerebrospinal fluid amine metabolites. Relationships with behavioural measurements in depressed, manic, and healthy control subjects. *Archives of General Psychiatry*, **43**, 938-947.

Refsum, S. (1946). Heredopathia atactica polyneuritiformis: a familial syndrome not hitherto described. *Acta Psychiatrica Scandinavica*, Suppl. 38.

Refsum, S. (1984). Heredopathia atactica polyneuritiformis (Refsum disease). *In* "Peripheral Neuropathy". 2nd edn. (Eds P.J. Dyck, P.K. Thomas, E.H. Lambet and R. Burge). pp. 1680-1703. W.B. Saunders, Philadelphia.

Regland, B., Abrahamsson, L., Blennow, K., Gottfries, C.G. and Wallin, A. (1992). Vitamin B12 in CSF: reduced CSF/serum B12 ratio in demented men. *Acta Neurologica Scandinavica*, **85**, 276-281.

Reimherr, F.W., Wender, P. H., Ebert, M.H. and Wood, D.R. (1984). Cerebrospinal fluid homovanillic acid and 5-hydroxy-indoleacetic acid in adults with attention deficit disorder, residual type. *Psychiatry Research*, **11**, (1) 71-8.

Reinhard, J, Liebmann, J. and Schlosberg, A. (1979). Serotonin neurons project to small blood vessels in the brain. *Science*, **206**, 85-86.

Randu, T. and Fishman, R.A. (1992). Spontaneous intracranial hypotension: report of two cases and review of the literature. *Neurology*, **42**, 481-487.

Reske, A., Haferkamp, G. and Hopl, H.C. (1981). Influence of artificial blood contamination of the analysis of CSF. *Journal of Neurology*, **226**, 187-193.

Resnick, L., DiMarzo-Veronese, F., Schupback, J. *et al*, (1985). Intra-blood-brain barrier synthesis of HTLV-III-Specific IgG in patients with neurologic symptoms associated with AIDS or AIDS-related complex. *New England Journal of Medicine*, **313**, 1498-504.

Reunanen, M. and Ilonen, J. (1982). DNA synthesizing mononuclear cells in the CSF of MS patients. *Acta Neurologica Scandinavica*, **65**, (Suppl. 90) 262-3.

Reveley, M.A., De Belleroche, J., Recordati, A. *et al*. (1987). Increased CSF amino acids and ventricular enlargement in schizophrenia: a preliminary study. *Biological Psychiatry*, **22**, 413-420.

Reynolds, E.H. (1981). A pilot study of monoamine precursors in epilepsy. *In* "Neurotransmitters, Seizures and Epilepsy". (Ed. P.L. Morselli). pp. 301-304. Raven Press, New York.

Reynolds, G.P. (1989). Beyond the dopamine hypothesis. The neurochemical pathology of schizophrenia. *British Journal of Psychiatry*, **155**, 305-316.

Ricci, L.C. and Wellman, M. (1990). Monamines: biochemical markers of suicide. *Journal of Clinical Psychology*, **46**, (1) 106-16.

Rich, A.R. and McCordock, H.A. (1933). The pathogenesis of tuberculous meningitis. *Bulletin Johns Hopkins Hospital*, **62**, 5-37.

Richards, P.T. and Cuzner, M.L. (1977). Proteolytic activity in CSF. *Advances in Experimental and Medical Biology*, **100**, 521-8.

Ridley, A. (1984). Porphyric neuropathy. *In* "Peripheral Neuropathy". 2nd Edn. (Eds P.J. Dyck, P.K. Thomas, E.H. Lambert and R. Burge). pp. 1704-1716. W.B. Saunders, Philadelphia.

Rimon R., Roos, B-E., Rakkolainen, V. and Alanen, Y. (1971). The content of 5-hydroxyindoleacetic acid and homovanillic acid in the cerebrospinal fluid of patients with acute schizophrenia. *Journal of Psychosomatic Research*, **15**, 375-378.

Rimon R., Terenius, L., Averbuch, I., Belmaker, R.H. (1983). High-dose haloperidol increases CSF opioid activity in patients with chronic schizophrenia.

Pharmacopsychiatry **16**, 9-12.

Rimon, R., Le Greves, P., Nyberg, F., Heikkila, L., Salmela, L. and Terenius, L. (1984). Elevation of substance P-like peptides in the CSF of psychiatric patients. *Biological Psychiatry,* **19**, (4) 509-516.

Rimon R., Kampman, R., Laru-Sompa, R. and Heikkila, L. (1985). Serum and cerebrospinal fluid prolactin patterns during neuropeptide treatment in schizophrenic patients. *Pharmacopsychiatry,* **18**, 252-254.

Rindler, M.J., Bashor, M.M., Spitzer, N. and Saier, M.H. (1978). Regulation of cAMP reflux from animal cells. *Journal of Biological Chemistry,* **253**, 5431-5436.

Rinne, U.K. and Riekkinen, P. (1968). Esterase, peptidase and proteinase activity of human CSF in MS. *Acta Neurologica Scandinavica,* **44**, 156-67.

Risby, E.D., Hsiao, J.K., Sunderland, T., Agren, H., Rudorfer, M.V. and Potter, W.Z. (1987). The effects of antidepressants on the cerebrospinal fluid homovanillic acid/5-hydroxyindoleacetic acid ratio. *Clinical Pharmacological Therapy,* **42**, (5), 547-554.

Risch, S.C. (1991). Growth hormone-releasing factor and growth hormone. *In* "Neuropeptides and Psychiatric Disorders". (Ed. C.B. Nemeroff). pp. 93-108. American Psychiatric Press, Washington D.C.

Roberts, G.D. (1988). Bacteriology and bacteriological diagnosis of tuberculosis. *In* "Tuberculosis". 2nd Edn. (Ed. D. Schlossberg). pp. 23-31. Springer, New York, Heidelberg, Tokyo.

Robinson, I. (1983). Neurohypophysial peptides in CSF. *Progress in Brain Research,* **60**, 129-145.

Robertson, M.M. (1989). The Gilles de la Tourette syndrome: the current status. *British Journal of Psychiatry,* **154**, 147-169.

Rocchelli, B., Poloni, M., Mazzarello, P. and Delodovice, M. (1983). Clinical and CSF findings in MS patients with or without oligoclonal bands at isoelectric focusing examination of CSF and serum proteins. *European Neurology,* **22**, 35-42.

Rodriguez, A.F., Kaplan, S.L. and Mason, E.O. (1990). CSF values in the very low birthweight infant. *Journal of Pediatrics,* **116**, 971-974.

Roos, B-E. (1989). Schizophrenia and viral and autoimmune issues. *Psychopharmacology Bulletin,* **20**, pp. 514-518.

Rosenberg, G.A. (1990). "Brain Fluids and Metabolism". Oxford University Press, New York.

Rosenblum, W.I. (1975). Effects of PG's on cerebral blood vessels: interaction with vasoactive amines. *Neurology,* **25**, 1169-1171

Rosman, N.P. and K.N. Shands, (1978). Hydrocephalus caused by increased intracranial venous pressure: a clinicopathological study. *Annals of Neurology,* **3**, 445-450.

Ross, D., Klykylo, W. and Hitzemann, R. (1987). Reduction of elevated CSF beta-endorphin by fenfluramine in infantile autism. *Pediatric Neurology,* **3**, 83-86.

Rossier, J., Bloom, F.E. and Guillemin, R. (1979). Stimulation of human periacqueductal gray for pain relief increases immunoreactive β-endorphin in ventricular fluid. *Science,* **203**, 279-281.

Rossor, M.N. (1988). Peptides and dementia. *In* "Neuropeptides in Psychiatric and Neurological Disorders". Chapter 5. (Ed. C.B. Nemeroff). Johns Hopkins

University Press, Baltimore.

Rothstein, J.D., McKhann, G., Guarneri, P., Barbaccia, M.H.,Guidotti, A. and Costa, C. (1989a). Cerebrospinal fluid content of diazepam binding inhibotors in chronic hepatic encephalopathy. *Annals of Neurology*, **26**, 57-62.

Rothstein, J.D., McKhann, G., Guarneri, P., Barbaccia, M.H.,Guidotti, A. and Costa, C. (1989b). Increased endogenous neuropeptide ligand for benzodiazepine receptors in hepatic encephalopathy. *Annals of Neurology*, **26**, 708-709.

Rothstein, J.D., Tsai, G., Kuncl, R.W., Clawson, L. Cornblath, D.R., Drachman, cerebrospinal fluid. *Acta Psychiatrica Scandinavica*, **80**, 287-291.

Roy, A., Berrettini, W., Adinoff, B. and Linnoila, M. (1990a). CSF galanin in alcoholics, pathological gamblers and normal controls: a negative report. *Biological Psychiatry*, **27**, 923-926.

Roy, A., DeJong, J., Gold, P., Rubinow, D., Adinoff, B., Ravitz, B., Waxman, R. and Linnoila, M. (1990b). Cerebrospinal fluid levels of somatostatin corticotropin-releasing hormone and corticotropin in alcoholism. *Acta Psychiatrica Scandinavica*, **82**, 44-48.

Roy, A., Lamparski, D., De Jong, J., Adinoff, B., Ravitz, B., George, D.T., Nutt, D. and Linnoila, M. (1990c). Cerebrospinal fluid monoamine metabolites in alcoholic patients who attempt suicide. *Acta Psychiatrica Scandinavica*, **81**, 58-61.

Roy, A., DeJong, J., Lamparski, D., George, T. and Linnoila, M. (1991). Depression among alcoholics. *Archives of General Psychiatry*, **48**, 428-432.

Royds, J.A., Parsons, M.A. Taylor, C.B. and Timperley, W.R. (1981a). The correlation between CSF enolase activity and localization of enolase isoenzymes in human brain tumors. *Journal of Pathology*, **134**, 315.

Royds, J.A., Timperley, W.R. and Taylor, C.B. (1981b). Levels of enolase and other enzymes in the CSF as indices of pathological change. *Journal of Neurology, Neurosurgery and Psychiatry*, **44**, 1129-1135.

Ruberg, M., Villageois, A., Bonnet, A.M. *et al.* (1988). ACHE and butylcholinesterase in CSF from patients with dystonia. *Advances in Neurology*, **50**, 211-3.

Rubin, S.J. (1983). Detection of viruses in spinal fluid. *American Journal of Medicine*, July, 124-128.

Rubinow, D.R. (1986). CSF somatostatin and psychiatric illness. *Biological Psychiatry*, **21**, 341-365.

Rubinow, D., Post, R., Pickar, D. *et al.* (1981). Relationship between urinary free cortisol and CSF opioid binding activity in depressed patients and normal volunteers. *Psychiatry Research*, **5**, 87-93.

Rubinow, D.R., Gold, P.W., Post, R.M., Ballenger, J.C., Cowdry, R., Bollinger, J. and Reichlin, S. (1983a). CSF somatostatin in affective illness. *Archives of General Psychiatry*, **40**, 409-412.

Rubinow, D.R., Gold, P.W., Post, R.M., Ballenger, J.C. and Reichlin, S. (1983b). Cerebrospinal fluid somatostatin in primary affective disorder. *Psychopharmacology Bulletin*, **19**, (3) 422-425.

Rubinow, D.R., Post, R.M., Gold, P.W., Ballenger, J.C. and Reichlin, S. (1985). Effects of carbamazepine on cerebrospinal fluid somatostatin. *Psychopharmacology*, **85**, 210-213.

Rubinow, D.R., Post, R.M. and Davis, C.L. (1991). Somatostatin. *In* "Neuropeptides and Psychiatric Disorders". (Ed. C.B. Nemeroff). pp. 29-50.

American Psychiatric Press, Washington D.C.

Ruckebusch, M. and Sutra, J.F. (1984). On the significance of monoamines and their metabolites in the cerebrospinal fluid of sheep. *Journal of Physiology, (Lond)* **348**, 457-69.

Rudman, D., Fleischer, A. and M. Kutner, (1976). Concentration of cAMP in VCSF of patients with prolonged coma after head trauma or intracranial hemorrhage. *New England Journal of Medicine*, **295**, 635-638.

Rudman, D., Hollins, B. Lewis, N.C. and Scott, J.W. (1977). Effects of hormones of cAMP in choroid plexus. *American Journal of Physiology*, **232**, 353-357.

Ruff, R.L. and Dougherty, J.H. (1981). Evaluation of acute cerebral ischemia for anticoagulant therapy: computed tomography or lumbar puncture. *Neurology* **31**, 736-740.

Rundles, R.W. (1945). Diabetic neuropathy: general review with report of 125 cases. *Medicine, (Balt)* **24**, 111.

Rust, R.S., Dodson, W.E. and Trotter, J.L. (1986). Cerebrospinal fluid immunoglobulins in childhood: normal values. *Annals of Neurology*, **20**, 63-69.

Ryberg, B., Hindfelt, B., Nilsson, B. and Olsson, J.E. (1984). Antineural antibodies in Guillain-Barre syndrome and lymphocytic meningoradiculitis (Bannworth's syndrome) *Archives of Neurology*, **41**, (12) 1277-1281.

Rytel, M.W. (1975). Rapid diagnostic methods in infectious diseases. *Advances in Internal Medicine*, **20**, 37-60.

Sabetta, J.R. and Andriole, V.T. (1985). Cryptococcal infection of the CNS. *Medical Clinics of North America*, **69**, 333-344.

Sahs, A.L. and Joynt, R.J. (1956). Brain swelling of unknown cause. *Neurology* (Minneap). **6**, 791-802.

Sakula, A. (1991). A hundred years of lumbar puncture: 1891-1991. *Journal of Royal College of Physicians of London*, **25**, (2) 171-175.

Salmi, A.A. (1989). Current diagnostic methodology. *In* "Handbook of Clinical Neurology". Vol. 12. (56) Viral Disease, Chapter 6. (Ed. R.R. McKendall). Elsevier Scientific Publishers, B.V.

Salmi, A.A, Ziola, B., Reunanen, M., Julkunen, I. and Wager, O. (1982). Immune complexes in serum and CSF of MS. patients and patients with other neurological diseases. *Acta Neurologica Scandinavica*, **66**, 1-15.

Samanin, R. and Garrattini, S. (1989.). Serotonin and the pharmacology of eating disorders. *Annals of the New York Academy of Science*, **575**, 194-208.

Samuel, A.M., Kadival, G.V., Irani, S., Pandya, S.K. and Ganatra, R.D. (1983). A sensitive and specific method for diagnosis of tubercular meningitis. *Indian Journal of Medical Research*, **77**, 752-7.

San Joaquin, V.H., Khai, N. Seale, T.W. and Rennert, O.M. (1982). Increased CSF free amino acid concentrations in children with bacterial meningitis. *Scandinavian Journal of Infectious Disease*, **14**, 23-26.

Sand, T. and Sulg, I. (1990). Evoked potentials and CSF-immunoglobulins in MS: relationship to disease duration, disability, and functional status. *Acta Neurologica Scandinavica*, **82**, 217-221.

Sandberg-Wollheim, M. (1987). Immunoglobulin synthesis within the central nervous system in multiple sclerosis. *In* "Advances in CSF Protein, Research and Diagnosis". (Ed. E.J. Thompson). pp. 99-108. MTP Press Ltd, Lancaster.

Sandyk, R. (1988). Enkephalinergic mechanisms in the "compensated" phase of

Parkinson's disease. *International Journal of Neuroscience,* 42, 301-303.

Sandyk, R. (1989a). The protective function of beta-endorphin in movement disorders. *International Journal of Neuroscience,* 46, 61-63.

Sandyk, R. (1989b). Dynorphin deficiency in Tourette's syndrome. *International Journal of Neuroscience,* 46, 65.

Sandyk, R. and Bamford, C.R. (1988a). Heightened cortisol response to administration of naloxone in Tourette's syndrome. *International Journal of Neuroscience,* 39, 225-26.

Sandyk, R. and Bamford, C.R. (1988b). Opioid modulation of gonadotrophin release in Tourette's syndrome. *International Journal of Neuroscience,* 39, 233.

Saran, R., Sahuja, R., Gupta, N., Hasan, M., Bhargava, K., Shanker, K. and Kishor, K. (1978). MHPG in CSF and VMA in urine of humans with hypertension. *Science,* 200, 317-318.

Sarff, L.D., Platt, L.H. and McCracken, Jr. G.H. (1976a). Cerebrospinal fluid evaluation in neonates: comparison of high-risk infants with and without meningitis. *Journal of Pediatrics,* 88, (3) 473-477.

Savoldi, F., Mazzella, G.L., Facchinetti, F., Nappi, G., Petraglia, F., Sinforiani, E., Parrini, D. and Genazzani, A. R. (1983). Beta-endorphin, beta-lipotropin and adrenocorticotropic hormone levels in cerebrospinal fluid, and brain damage in chronic alcoholics. *European Neurology,* 22, (4) 265-71.

Sayk, J. (1974). The cerebrospinal fluid in brain tumours. *In* "Handbook of Clinical Neurology". (Eds. P. Vinken and G. Bruyn). pp. 360-417. North Holland Publishing Co., Amsterdam.

Sayk, J., Olischer, R. and Lehmitz, R. (1980). Cytological findings in CSF as criteria of process activity in MS. *In* "Progress in MS Research". (Eds H. Bauer *et al.*). pp. 331-335. Springer-Verlag, New York.

Schacker, W.T., Nadi, N.S., Wyer, A.R. and Porter, R.J. (1987). Neuropeptides in the human epileptic focus: a neurochemical comparison with nonfocal tissue. *Neurology,* 37, (Suppl. 1) 105.

Schadlich, H.J. Mohrmann, G., Nekic, M. and Felgenhauer, K. (1990). Intrathecal synthesis of virus antibodies: a diagnostic test for multiple sclerosis. *European Neurology,* 30, 302-304.

Schain, R.J. (1960). Neurotumors and other pharmacologically active substances in CSF: a review of the literature. *Yale Journal of Biological Medicine,* 33, 15-36.

Schaltenbrand, V.G. (1938). Neure Anschauungen zur Pathophysiologie der Liquorzirkulation. *Zentralblatt für Neurochirurgie,* 3, 290-299.

Schapira, F. (1962). L'activite aldolasique normale du LCR. *Clinica Chemica Acta,* 7, 566-571.

Schatzberg, A., Rothschild, A., Langlais, P. *et al.* (1985.). A corticosteroid/dopamine hypothesis for psychotic depression and related states. *Journal of Psychiatric Research,* 19, 57-64.

Schaumburg H.H., and P.S. Spencer (1984). Human toxic neuropathy due to industrial agents. *In* "Peripheral Neuropathy". 2nd edn. (Eds P.J. Dyck, P.C. Thomas, E.H. Lambert and Burge). pp. 2115-32. W.B. Saunders, Philadelphia.

Schenberg, L.C., Giessen, B.S. and Schaumberg, H.H. (1983). "The Neurology Handbook of Medical Examinations". Publ. Co., New Hyde Park, New York.

Schipper, H., Posa, S., Wuzel, S. and Behrens-Baumann, W. (1984). Prognostic Value of CSF IgG in monosymptomatic optic neuritis. *In* "Immunological and

Clinical Aspects of Multiple Sclerosis". (Eds R. Gansette and P. Delmotte). pp. 278-281. MTP Press, Hingham, MA.

Schmidli, J. and Meyer, J. (1990). Lyme borreliosis: report from the IVth International Conference on Lyme borreliosis (Stockholm, (1990). submitted for publication.

Schmidt, R. and Neumann, V. (1980). CSF oligoclonal bands in MS. *In* "Progress in MS Research". (H. Bauer, *et al.*). pp. 123-128. Springer-Verlag, New York.

Schmidt, R.M. (1983). Classification of cells in the cerebrospinal fluid. *Schweizer Archiv für Neurologie Neurochirurgie und Psychiatrie,* **132**, (2), 309-14.

Schmidt, D. and Loscher, W. (1982). Plasma and CSF GABA in neurological disorders. *Journal of Neurology, Neurosurgery and Psychiatry,* **45**, 931-935.

Schoen, E.J. (1984). Spinal fluid chloride: a test 40 years past its time. (letter). *Journal of the American Medical Association,* **251**, (1) 70-2.

Schold, S.C. and Bullard, D.E. (1980). CSF analysis in CNS cancer. *In* "Neurology of CSF". Vol. 1. (Ed. J.H. Wood). pp. 549-560. Plenum Press, New York.

Schold, S.C., Wasserstrom, W.R., Fleischer, M. Schwartz, M.K. and Posner, J.B. (1980). CSF biochemical markers of CNS metastases. *Annals of Neurology,* **8**, 597-604.

Schoning, P. and Strafuss, A.C. (1980). Postmortem biochemical changes in canine CSF. *Journal of Forensic Science,* **25**, 60-66.

Schuckit, M.A. (1987). Biology of risk for alcoholism. *In* "Psychopharmacology: The Third Generation of Progress". (Ed Herbert Y. Meltzer). pp. 1527. Raven Press, New York.

Schwartz, W., Coleman, R. and Reppert, S. (1983). A daily vasopressin rhythm in rat CSF. *Brain Research,* **263**, (1) 105-112.

Schwersenski, J., McIntyre, L. and Bauer, C.R. (1991). Lumbar puncture frequency and CSF analysis in the neonate. *American Journal of Disorders of Children,* **145**, 54-58.

Scott, T.F. (1988). New cause of cerebrospinal fluid Eosinophilia: neurosarcoidosis. *American Journal of Medicine,* **84**, 973-974.

Scott, T.F., Seay, A.R. and Goust, J.M. (1989). Pattern and concentration of IgG in cerebrospinal fluid in neurosarcoidosis. *Neurology,* **39**, 1637-39.

Scriabine, A., Clineschmidt, B.V. and Sweet, C.S. (1976). Central noradrenergic control of blood pressure. *Annual Review in Pharmacology and Toxicology,* **16**, 113-123.

Sechzer, P and Abel, L. (1978). Post-spinal anaesthesia headache treated with caffeine. *Current Therapeutic Research,* **24**, 307-312.

Sedvall, G. (1990). Monamines and schizophrenia. *Acta Psychiatrica Scandinavica,* **82**, (Suppl. 358) 7-13.

Sedvall, G and Wode-Helgodt, B. (1980). Aberrant monoamine metabolite levels in CSF and family history of schizophrenia; their relationships in schizophrenic patients. *Archives of General Psychiatry,* **37**, 1113.

Sedvall, G., Fyro, B., Nyback, H. and Wiesel, F.A. (1975). Actions of dopaminergic antagonists in the striatum. *In* "Advances in Neurology". (Eds D. Calne, T. Chase and A. Barbeau). pp. 131-140. Raven Press, New York.

Sedvall, G., Alfredsson, G., Bjerkenstedtr, L., Eneroth, P., Fyro, B. Harnryd, L. and Wade-Helgodt, B. (1977). Central biochemical correlates to antispychotic drug action in man. *In* "The Impact of Biology on Modern Psychiatry". (Eds L.

Gershan, R. Belmaker, S. Kety, and M. Rosenbaum). pp. 41-55, Plenum Press, New York.

Sedvall, G. Fyro, B., Gullberg, B. and Nyback, H. (1980). Relationships in healthy volunteers between concentrations of monoamine metabolites in cerebrospinal fluid and family history of psychiatric morbidity. *British Journal of Psychiatry*, **136**, 366-374.

Sedvall, G., Iselius, L., Nyback H. *et al.* (1984). Genetic studies of CSF monoamine metabolites. *Advances in Biochemical Psychopharmacology*, **39**, 79-98.

Seebacher, J., Ribeiro, V., Le Guillou, J-L., Lacomblez, L., Henry, M., Thorman, F. *et al.* (1989). Epidural blood patch as treatment for post lumbar puncture headache – a double blind controlled trial. Paper presented at the Headache Congress, Sydney, Australia, October 185-186.

Seeman P. (1987). Dopamine receptors and the dopamine hypothesis of schizophrenia. *Synapse,* **1**, 133-152.

Seeman, M.V. and Seeman, P. (1988). Psychosis and positron tomography. *Canadian Journal of Psychiatry,* **33**, (5) 299-304.

Segal, M.B. and Pollay, M. (1977). The secretion of cerebrospinal fluid. Experimental Eye Research, **25**, (Suppl.) 127-148.

Segura, R.M., Pascual, C., Ocana, I., Martinez-Vazquez, J.M., Ribera, E. and Ruiz, I. (1989). Adenosine deaminase in body fluids: a useful diagnostic tool in tuberculosis. *Clinical Biochemistry,* **22**, 141-148.

Segurado, O.G., Kruger, H. and Mertens, H.G. (1986). Clinical significance of serum and CSF findings in the Guillain-Barré syndrome and related disorders. *Journal of Neurology*, **233**, 202-208.

Seidel, D. (1982). Polyunsaturated fatty acids and their importance in pathogenesis diagnosis, and therapy of Multiple Sclerosis. *Fortschrift für Neurologie und Psychiatrie,* **50**, 173-189.

Seidel, D., Heipertz, R. and Buck, R. (1980). CSF lipids in demyelinating disease. *In* "Progress in MS Research". (Eds H. Bauer, *et al.*). pp. 157-160. Springer-Verlag, New York.

Seller, M.J. and Adinolfi, M. (1975). Blood-brain barrier in the human fetus. *Lancet*, i, 1030-1031.

Serratric G. and Roux, H. (1979). "Peronial Atrophies and Related Disorders". Masson, New York.

Servo, C., Bergstrom, L. and Fogelholm, R. (1977). Cerebrospinal fluid sorbitol and myoinosital in diabetic polyneuropathy. *Acta Medica Scandinavica,* **202**, 301-304.

Shah, N.T. (1982). Cytology and CSF. *American Journal of Medical Technology*, **48**, (10) 829-831.

Shah, N. and Donald, A. (1982). Endorphins and opiate antagonists. *In* "Psychiatric Research". Plenum Press, New York.

Shankar, P., Manjunath, N., Mohan, K.K., Prasad, K., Behari, M. and Ahuja, G.K. (1991). Rapid diagnosis of tuberculosis meningitis by polymerase chain reaction. *Lancet*, **337**, 5-7.

Shapiro, W. (1988). CSF circulation and the blood-brain barrier. *Annals of the New York Academy of Science,* **531**, 9-14.

Shapiro, A., Shapiro, E., Bruun, R. and Sweet, R. (1978). "Gilles de la Tourette Syndrome". Raven Press, New York.

Sharief, M.K. and Thompson, E.J. (1991). The predictive value of intrathecal immunoglobulin synthesis and magnetic resonance imaging in acute isolated syndromes for subsequent development of multiple sclerosis. *Annals of Neurology*, **29**, 147-150.

Sharma, R., Javaid, J.I. *et al.* (1988). Effect of trifluoperazine on CSF and plasma HVA levels in schizophrenic subjects. *American Journal of Psychiatry*, **145**, (11) 1480-1481.

Shaywitz, B.A. (1972). Brief clinical and laboratory observations: Epidermoid spinal cord tumors and previous lumbar punctures. *Journal of Pediatrics*, **80**, (4) 638-640.

Shaywitz, B.A., Cohen, D.J. and Bowers, M.P. (1977). CSF monoamine metabolites in children with MBD: evidence for alteration of brain dopamine. *Journal of Pediatrics*, **90**, 67-71.

Shaywitz, B.A., Cohen, D.J. and Bowers, B.M. (1980). CSF monoamine metabolites in neurological disorders of children. *In* "Neurobiology of CSF". (Ed. J.H. Wood). pp. 219-36. Plenum Press, New York.

Shealy, C.N. (1969). "Spinal Acuology". Charles C. Thomas, Springfield, Illinois.

Shen, L. and Rutter, W. (1984). Sequence of the human somatostatin I gene. *Science*, **224**, 168-70.

Shetty, T. and Chase, T. (1976). Central monoamines and hyperkinesis of childhood. *Neurology*, **26**, 1000-1002.

Shimode, K., Fujihara, S., Nakamura, M. *et al.* (1991). Diagnosis of cerebral amyloid angiopathy by ELISA of cystatin C in CSF. *Stroke*, **22**, 860-866.

Shrikhande, S., Hirsch, S.R., Coleman, J.C. Reveley, M.A. and Dayton, R. (1985). Cytomegalovirus and schizophrenia. A test of a viral hypothesis. *British Journal of Psychiatry*, **146**, 503-506.

Siever, L., Guttmacher, L. and Murphy, D. (1984.). Serotonergic receptors: evaluation of their possible role in the affective disorders. *In* "Neurobiology of Mood Disorders". (Eds R. Post and J. Ballenger). William and Wilkins, Baltimore.

Silverstone, T. (1985). Dopamine in manic depressive illness. *Journal of Affective Disorders*, **8**, 225-231.

Simon, R.P. and Abele, J.S. (1978). Spinal fluid pleocytosis estimated by the tyndal effect. *Annals of Internal Medicine*, **89**, 75-6.

Simon, R.P. and Fishman, R.A. (1986). Lumbar puncture in the treatment of neurosyphilis. *Archives of Internal Medicine*, **146**, 409-412.

Sindic, C, Cambiaso, C. Masson, P. and Laterre, E. (1980). Clinical relevance of the determination of Ig M in the CSF with special reference to MS patients. *In* "Progress in MS Research". (Eds H. Bauer *et al.*). pp. 176-179. Springer-Verlag, New York.

Sindic, C., Collet-Cassart, D., Cambiaso, C., Masson, P. and Laterre, E. (1981). The clinical relevance of ferritin concentration in the CSF. *Journal of Neurology, Neurosurgery and Psychiatry*, **44**, 329-333.

Sindic, C., Chalon, M., Cambiaso, C., Laterre, E. and Masson, P.L. (1982). Assessment of damage to the CNS by determination of S-100 protein in the CSF. *Journal of Neurology, Neurosurgery and Psychiatry*, **45**, 1130-1135.

Singer, H., Butler, I., Tune, L. *et al.* (1982a). Dopaminergic dysfunction in Tourette syndrome. *Annals of Neurology*, **12**, 361-366.

Singer, H., Tune, L., Butler, I. *et al.* (1982*b*). Clinical symptomatology, CSF neurotransmitter metabolites and serum haloperidol levels in Tourette syndrome. *In* "Gilles de la Tourette Syndrome". (Eds A. Friedhoff and T. Chase). pp. 177-184. Raven Press, New York.

Singer, H. S., Oshida, L. and Coyle, J.T. (1984). CSF cholinesterase activity in Gilles de la Tourette's syndrome. *Archives of Neurology, 41*, 756.

Singhol, S.C., Lall, J.C., Singh, H., Aggarwal, V.P. and Rao, K.N. (1981). CSF lactic acid levels in meningitides in children. *Indian Pediatrics, 18*, 891-894.

Sjolund, B., Terenius, L. and Eriksson, M. (1977). Increased CSF levels of endorphins after electro-acupuncture. *Acta Physiologica Scandinavica, 100*, 382-384.

Sjoquist, B., Borg, S. and Kvande, H. (1981). Catecholamine derived compounds in urine and CSF from alcoholics during and after long-standing intoxication. *In* "Substance and Alcohol Actions". Vol. 2. "Misuse". pp. 63-72. Pergamon Press.

Sjostrom, R., Ekstedt, A. and Anggard, E. (1975). Concentration gradients of monoamine metabolites in human cerebrospinal fluid. *Journal of Neurology, Neurosurgery and Psychiatry, 38*, 666-668.

Sklar, F.H. (1980). Non-steady-state measurements of CSF dynamics. *In* "Neurobiology of CSF". Vol. 1. (Ed. J.H. Wood). pp. 365-379. Plenum Press, New York.

Smidt, D. and Loscher, W. (1981). GABA concentrations in CSF and plasma of patients with epileptic seizures. *In* "Neurotransmitters, Seizures and Epilepsy". (Ed. P.L. Morselli). pp. 315-322. Raven Press, New York.

Smith, A.D. and Thompson, R.H.S. (1977). Lipids and multiple sclerosis. *In* "MS: A Critical Conspectus". (Ed. E.J. Field). pp. 225-224. MTP Press, Great Britain.

Smith, C.C., Tallman, J.F., Post, R.M., van Kammen, D.P., Jimerson, D.C. and G.L. Brown, (1976). An examination of baseline and drug-induced levels of cyclic nucleotides in the CSF of control and psychiatric patients. *Life Science, 19*, 131-136.

Smith I.S., Kahn, S.N., Lacey, B. W. *et al.* (1983). Chronic demyelinating neuropathy associated with benign IgM paraproteinaemia. *Brain, 106*, 169-195.

Soininen, H., Halonen, T. and Tiekkinen, P.J. (1981*a*). Acetylcholinesterace activity in SCF of patients with senile dementia of Alzheimer type. *Acta Neurologica Scandinavica, 64*, 217-224.

Soininen, H.S., MacDonald, E., Rekonen, M. and Riekkinen, P.J. (1981*b*). HVA and 5-HIAA levels in CSF of patients with senile dementia of Alzheimer type. *Acta Neurologica Scandinavica, 64*, 101-107.

Soininen, H., Riekkinen, P.J., Partanen, J. *et al.* (1988). CSF somatostatin correlates with spectral EEG variables and with parietotemporal cognitive dysfunction in Alzheimer patients. *Neuroscience Letters, 85*, 131-136.

Sonninen, V., Rinne, U.K., Marttila, R., Molser, P. and Rautakorpi, I. (1982). HVA in the CSF as an index of brain dopamine turnover. *Acta Neurologica Scandinavica* (Suppl.) *90*, 64-65.

Sorensen, S.C. (1971). Factors regulating H^+ and HCO_3^- in brain ECF. *In* "Ion Homestasis of the Brain". (Eds S.C. Sorensen and B.K. Siesjo). Academic Press, New York.

Sorensen, P.S., Hammer, M. and Gjerris, F. (1982). CSF vasopressin in benign intracranial hypertension. *Neurology, 32*, 1255-1259.

Sorensen, P.S., Gjerris, A. and Hammer, M. (1985). Cerebrospinal fluid vasopressin in neurological and psychiatric disorders. *Journal of Neurology, Neurosurgery and Psychiatry*, **48**, 50-57.

Sornas, R., Ostlund, H. and Muller, R. (1972). Cerebrospinal fluid cytology after stroke. *Archives of Neurology*, **26**, 489-500.

Spector, R. and Ellis, J. (1984). Deoxynucleoside and vitamin transport into the central nervous system. *Federation Proceedings*, **43**, (2) 196-200.

Sperschneider, H., Spustova, V., Stein, G. and Dzurik, R. (1982). Middle molecular weight substances in the CSF of uremic patients. *Clinical Nephrology*, **17**, 298-301.

Stahl, S. and Wets, K. (1987). Indoleamines and schizophrenia. *In* "Handbook of Schizophrenia". Vol. 2. (Eds F.Henn and L. De Lisi). pp. 257-296. Elsevier, Amsterdam,

Stanley, M., Traskman-Bendz, L. and Dorovini-Zis, K. (1985). Correlations between aminergic metabolites simultaneously obtained from human CSF and brain. *Life Sciences*, **37**, 1279-1286.

Statz, A. and Felgenhauer, K. (1983). Development of the blood-CSF barrier. *Developmental Medicine and Child Neurology*, **25**, 152-161.

Steardo, L. and Nathanson, J.J.A. (1987). Brain barrier tissues: end organs for atriopeptins. *Science* **235**, 470-473.

Steardo, L., Barone, P. and Hunnicutt, E. (1986). Carbamazepine lowering effect on CSF somatostatin-like immunoreactivity in temporal lobe epileptics. *Acta Neurologica Scandinavica*, **74**, 140-144.

Steere, A.C., Bartenhagen, N.H., Craft, J.E., Hutchinson, G.J., Newman, J.H., Rahn, D.W., Sigal, L.H., Spieler, P.H. *et al.* (1983). The early clinical manifestations of Lyme disease. *Annals of Internal Medicine*, **99**, 76-82.

Steere, A.C., Bartenhagen, N.H., Craft, J.E., Hutchinson, G.J., Newman, J.H., Pachner, A.R., Rahn, D.W., Sigal, L.H., Taylor E. and Malawista, S.E. (1986). Clinical manifestations of Lyme disease. *Zentralblatt für Bakteriologie, Microbiologie und Hygiene*, **263**, 201-205.

Steere, A.C., Berardi, V.P., Weeks, K.E. Logigian, E.L. and Ackermann, R. (1990). Evaluation of the intrathecal antibody response to *Borrelia burgdorferi* as a diagnostic test for Lyme Neuroborreliosis. *Journal of Infectious Diseases*, **161**, 1203-1209.

Steinbrook, R.A., Carr, D.B., Datta, S., Naulty, J.S., Lee, C. and Fisher, J. (1982). Dissociation of plasma and cerebrospinal fluid-endorphin-like immunoactivity levels during pregnancy and parturition *Anesthesia and Analgesia*, **61**, 893 897.

Stendahl-Brodin, L. and Link, H. (1983). Optic neuritis: oligoclonal bands increases the risk of multiple sclerosis. *Acta Neurologica Scandinavica*, **67**, (5) 301-4.

Stendahl-Brodin, L., Link, H. and Kristensson, K. (1979). Myelintoxic activity on tadpole optic nerve of CSF from patients with optic neuritis. *Neurology*, **29**, 882-86.

Stern, B.J., Krumholz, A., Johns, C., Scott, P. and Nissim, J. (1985). Sarcoidosis and its neurological manifestations. *Archives of Neurology*, **42**, 909-917.

Stern, B.J., Griffin, D.E., Luke, R.A., Krumholz, A. and Johns, C.J. (1987). Neurosarcoidosis: cerebrospinal fluid lymphocyte subpopulations. *Neurology*, **37**, 878-881.

Sternberg, D.E., van Kammen, D.P., Ballenger, J.C., Lerner, P., Marder, S.R.

and Post, R.M. (1978). "CSF Dopamine-β-hydroxylase and Schizophrenia". Presented at the Annual Meeting of the American Psychiatric Association. New Research, Abstract pp. 32, (1978), cited in van Kammen and Sternberg, (1980).

Sternberg D.E., Bowers Jnr. M.B., Heninger, G.R. and Charney, D.S. (1983a). Lithium prevents adaptation of brain dopamine systems to haloperidol in schizophrenic patients. *Psychiatric Research*, **10**, 79-86.

Sternberg, D.E., van Kammen, D.P., Lerner, P., Ballenger, J.C., Marder, S.R., Post, R.M. and Bunney, Jr. W.E. (1983b). CSF dopamine beta-hydroxylase in schizophrenia. *Archives of General Psychiatry*, **40**, (7) 743-7.

Strand, T., Alling, C., Karlsson, B., Karlson, I. and Winblad, B. (1984). Brain and plasma proteins in spinal fluid as markers for brain damage and severity of stroke. *Stroke,* **15**, (1) 138-44.

Subrahmanyam, S. (1975). Role of biogenic amines in certain pathological conditions. *Brain Research*, **87**, 355-362.

Suckling, A, Rumsby, M. and Bradbury, M. (eds), (1986). "The Blood-Brain Barrier in Health and Disease". Ellis Horwood, Chichester.

Sullivan, H.G. and Allison, J.D. (1985). Physiology of cerebrospinal fluid. *In* "Neurosurgery". (Eds R. Wilkins and S. Rengachary). McGraw-Hill, New York.

Sullivan, P., Mornaghan, D., Callaghan, N., Kantamaneni, B. and Curzon, G. (1980). Effect of dialysis on plasma and CSF tryptophan and CSF 5-HIAA in advanced renal disease. *Journal of Neurology, Neurosurgery and Psychiatry,* **43**, 739-743.

Sunderland, T., Rubinow, D.R., Tariot, P.N., Cohen, R.M., Newhouse, P.A., Mellow, A.M., Mueller, E.A. and Murphy, D.L. (1987). CSF somatostatin in patients with Alzheimer's disease, older depressed patients, and age-matched control subjects. *American Journal of Psychiatry,* **144**, 1313-1316.

Sundquist, J., Forsling, M., Olsson, J.E. and Akerland, M. (1983). CSF arginine vasopressin in degenerative disorders and other neurological diseases. *Journal of Neurology, Neurosurgery and Psychiatry,* **46**, 14-17.

Svennerholm, L. and Vanier, M.T. (1978). Lipid and FA composition of human cerebral myelin during development. *Advances in Experimental Medicine and Biology,* **100**, 27-41.

Swahn, C-G. and Sedvall, G. (1988). CSF creatinine in schizophrenia. *Biological Psychiatry*, **23**, 586-594.

Swart, J.A.A. and Korf, J. (1987.). Commentary: *in vivo* dopamine receptor assessment for clinical studies using positron emission tomography. *Biochemical Pharmacology*, **36**, (14) 2241-2250.

Swartz, M.N. (1980). Intracranial infections. *In* "The Science and Practice of Clinical Medicine". Vol. 5. (Ed. J.M. Dietsch). pp. 1-40. Grune and Stratten, New York.

Swedo, S.E., Leonard, H.L., Kruesi, M. *et al.* (1992). CSF neurochemistry in children and adolescents with O.C.D. *Archive of General Psychiatry*, **49**, 29-36.

Szczepanska-Sadowska, E., Gray, D. and Simon-Oppermann, C. (1983). Vasopressin in blood and third ventricle CSF during dehydration, thirst, and hemorrhage. *American Journal of Physiology*, **245**, (4) 549-55.

Szilagyi, A.K. (1988). Increased CSF amino acids and ventricular enlargement. *Biological Psychiatry*, **23**, 317-323.

Szilagyi, A.K., Lavinha, F. and Mardens, Y. (1974). Studies of free amino acid pattern in human CSF along the cerebrospinal axis. *Acta Neurologica Belgica*, **74**, 329-336.

Szukiewicz, H. and Jaskolska, A. (1982). CSF as an element of biological protection of the spinal cord. *Folia Morphologica, (Warz)* **41**, (1) 17-31.

Tabaddor, K., Wolfson, L. and Sharpless, N. (1978a). Ventricular fluid HVA and 5-HIAA concentrations in patients with movement disorders. *Neurology*, **28**, 1249-1253.

Tabaddor, K., Wolfson, L. and Sharpless, N.S. (1978b). Diminished VCSF dopamine metabolites in adult-onset dystonia. *Neurology*, **28**, 1254-1258.

Tabakoff B. and Hoffman, P.L. (1987). Biochemical pharmacology of alcohol. *In* "Psychopharmacology: The Third Generation of Progress". (Ed. Herbert Y. Meltzer). pp. 1521-1526. Raven Press, New York.

Tabakoff, B., Melchior, C. , Urwyler, S. and Hoffman, P.L. (1980). Alterations in neurotransmitter function during the development of ethanol tolerance and dependence. *Acta Psychiatrica Scandinavica*, (Suppl. 286) **62**, 153-159.

Tabira, T., De, H., Webster, F. and Wray, S. (1977). *In vivo* test for myelotoxicity of CSF. *Brain Research*, **120**, 103-112.

Takahashi, S., Kondo, H. and Kato, N. (1975). Effect of L-5HTP on brain monoamine metabolism and evaluation of its clinical effect in depressed patients. *Journal of Psychiatric Research*, **12**, 177-187.

Takeoka, T., Shinohara, Y., Furumi, K. and Mori, K. (1983). Impairment of blood-cerebrospinal fluid barrier in multiple sclerosis. *Journal of Neurochemistry*, **41**, (4) 1102-8.

Tamai, I., Takei, T., Maekawa, K. and Ohta, H. (1983). Prostaglandin F2 alpha concentrations in the cerebrospinal fluid of children with febrile convulsions, epilepsy and meningitis. *Brain Development*, **5**, (4) 357-62.

Tamminga, C.A., Foster, N.L., and Chase, T.N. (1985). Reduced brain somatostatin levels in Alzheimer's disease. *New England Journal of Medicine*, **313**, (20) 1294-1295.

Tandon R. and Greden, J.F. (1989). Cholinergic hyperactivity and negative schizophrenic symptoms. *Archives of General Psychiatry*, **46**, (8) 745-753.

Tanimoto, K., Kuo, S., Crawley, J.N. and Tamminga, C.A. (1991). Cholecystokinin in the mammalian central nervous system: review and analysis. *In* "Neuropeptides and Psychiatric Disorders". (Ed. C.B. Nemeroff). pp, 193-206. American Psychiatric Press, Washington D.C.

Tapia, E.J., Polak, J., Barbosa, A., Bloom, S., Marangos, P. and Pearse, A. (1981). Neuron specific enolase as a cytochemical marker for peripheral endocrine tumors. *Journal of Pathology,* **134**, 316.

Tavolato, B., Gallo, P. and DeZanche, C. (1984). The transferrin - Tau ratio of the CSF. *In* "Gansette and Delmotte". pp. 63-69.

Taylor, G., Crow, T., Ferrier, I., Johnstone, E., Parry, R. and Tyrrell, D. (1982). Virus-like agent in CSF of schizophrenia and some neurological disorders. *Lancet*, ii, 1166-67.

Taylor, G., Carter, G. and Crow, T. (1985a). A comparison of the effects of cytotoxic CSF on cell cultures and other cytopathic agents. *Experiments in Medical Pathology,* **42**, 401-410.

Taylor, G., Roberts, G., Crow, T., Royds, J., Gamble, S., Taylor, G., Carter, G. and Timperley, H. (1985b). The cytopathic agent in CSF: evidence for a relationship with enolase levels. *Journal of Neurology, Neurosurgery and Psychiatry*, **48**, 281.

Taylor, P.L., Garrick, N.A., Burns, R.S., Tamarkin, L., Murphy, D. and Markey, S. (1982). Diurnal rhythms of serotonin in monkey CSF. *Life Science.* **31**, (18) 1993-1999.

Teoh, R., O'Mahony, S.G. and Yeung, V.T.F. (1986). Polymorphonuclear pleocytosis in the cerebrospinal fluid during chemotherapy for tuberculous meningitis. *Journal of Neurology*, **233**, 237-241.

Terenius L. and Nyberg, F. (1986). Opioid peptides in the cerebrospinal fluid of psychiatric patients. *Progress in Brain Research*, **65**, 207-219.

Terenius, L. and Wahlstrom, A. (1979). Endorphins in human CSF as indicators of central endorphin activity. *In* "Radioimmunology". (Ed C.A. Bizollon). Elsevier/North Holland Press, Amsterdam.

Terent, A and Ronquist, G. (1980). CSF markers of disturbed brain cell metabolism in patients with stroke and global cerebral ischemia. *Acta Neurologica Scandinavica,* **62**, 327-35.

Teychenne, P., Lake, C. and Zeigler, M. (1980). CSF studies in Parkinson's disease: norepinephrine and GABA concentrations. *In* "Neurobiology of CSF". (Ed. J.H. Wood). pp. 197-206. Plenum Press, New York.

Thadepalli, H., Gangopadhyay, P.K., Ansari, A., Overturf, G.D., Dhawan, U.K. and Mandol, A.K. (1982). Rapid differentiation of bacterial meningitides by direct gas-liquid chromatography. *Journal of Clinical Investigation*, **69**, 979-984.

Thaker G.K., Tamminga, C.A. *et al.* (1987). Brain γ-aminobutyric acid abnormality in tardive dyskinesia. *Archives of General Psychiatry,* **44**, (6) 522-529.

Thomas P.K, and Eliasson, S.G. (1984). Diabetic Neuropathy. *In* "Peripheral Neuropathy". 2nd edn. (Eds P.J. Dyck, P.K. Thomas, E.H. Lambert, R. Burge). pp. 1773-1810. W.B. Saunders, Philadelphia.

Thomas P.K., Lascelles, R.G., Hallpike, J.F., Hewer, R.L. (1969). Recurrent and chronic relapsing Guillain-Barré polyneuritis. *Brain*, **92**, 589.

Thompson, E.J. (1977). Laboratory diagnosis of multiple sclerosis: immunological and biochemical aspects. *British Medical Bulletin,* **33**, 28-33.

Thompson, E.J. (1988). "The CSF Proteins". Elsevier Publishers, Amsterdam.

Thompson, J. and Salinsky, M. (1988). The utility of cerebrospinal fluid examination in patients with partial epilepsy. *Epilepsia*, **29**, (2) (195-7.

Thompson, E.J., Kaufmann, P. and Rudge, P. (1983). Sequential changes in oligoclonal patterns during the course of Multiple Sclerosis. *Journal of Neurology, Neurosurgery and Psychiatry*, **46**, 115-118.

Thompson, A.J., Hutchinson, M., Martin, E.A., Mansfield, M., Whelan, A. and Feighery, C. (1985). Suspected and clinically definite multiple sclerosis: the relationship between CSF immunoglobulins and clinical course. *Journal of Neurology, Neurosurgery and Psychiatry*, **48**, 989-994.

Thoren, P., Asberg, M. Bertilsson, L., Mellstrom, B., Sjoqvist, F. and Traskman, L. (1980). Clomipramine treatment of obsessive-compulsive disorder. *Archives of General Psychiatry*, **37**, 1289-1294.

Thornberry, E. and Thomas T. (1988). Posture and post-spinal headache. A controlled trial in 80 obstetric patients. *British Journal of Anaesthesia.* **60**, (195-7.

Tibbling, G., Link, H. and Ohman, S. (1977). Principles of albumin and IgG analyses in neurological disorders I. Establishment of reference values. *Scandinavian Journal of Clinical Laboratory Investment*, **37**, 385-390.

Timperley, W.R., Royds, J.A., Taylor C.B. and Parsons, M.A. (1982). Enolase studies in the CSF and in tumors of the human nervous system. *Journal of Neurology, Neurosurgery and Psychiatry*, **45**, 281.

Torack, R.M. (1982). Historical aspects of normal and abnormal brain fluids I. cerebrospinal fluid. *Archives of Neurology*, **39**, 197-201.

Torrey, E., Yolken, R. and Winfieg, C. (1982). CMV antibody in CSF of schizophrenic patients detected by enzyme immunoassay. *Science*, **216**, 892-894.

Tourtellotte, W.W. (1970). Cerebrospinal fluid in multiple sclerosis. *In* "Handbook of Clinical Neurology". (Ed. P.J. Vinken and G.W. Bruyn). pp. 324-382. North-Holland, Amsterdam.

Tourtellotte, W.W. (1984). CSF studies in EAE and MS. *Progress in Clinical and Biological Research*, **146**, 329-33.

Tourtellotte, W.W. (1985). The cerebrospinal fluid in multiple sclerosis. *In* "Handbook of Clinical Neurology". Vol. 3. (Ed. J.C. Koetsier), pp. 79-130. Elsevier Science Publishers.

Tourtellotte, W.W. (1987). Cerebrospinal fluid profile indicative of clinical definite multiple sclerosis: a proposal, facts, issues, opportunities and perspective. *In* "Advances in CSF Protein, Research and Diagnosis". (Ed. E.J. Thompson). pp. 17-34. MTP Press Ltd, Lancaster.

Tourtellotte, W.W. and Ma, B.I. (1978). Multiple sclerosis: the blood-brain barrier and the measurement of the novo central nervous system IgG synthesis. *Neurology*, **28**, 76-83.

Tourtellotte, W.W. and Shorr, R.J. (1982). Cerebrospinal fluid. *In* "Neurological Surgery". Chapter 1, (Ed. J.R. Yovmans). W.B. Saunders, Philadelphia, PA.

Trabucci, M., Cerri, C., Spano, P. and Kumakura, K. (1977). cGMP in the CSF of neurological patients. *Archives of Neurology*, **34**, 12-13.

Tramont, E. (1991). Syphilis of the central nervous system. *In* "Infections of the Central Nervous System). (Ed. H. Lambert), B.C. Decker, Philadelphia.

Traskman-Bendz, L., Asberg, M., Bertilsson, L. *et al.* (1979). Plasma levels of chlorimipramine and its dimethyl metabolite during treatment of depression. *Clinical Pharmacology and Therapeutics*, **26**, 600-610.

Traskman-Bendz, L., Asberg, M., Bertilsson, L. and Thoren, P. (1984). CSF monoamine metabolites of depressed patients during illness and after recovery. *Acta Psychiatrica Scandinavica*, **69**, (4) 333-42

Traskman-Bendz, L., Stanley, M., Stanley, B., Matthews, B. and Brown, L. (1988). N-acetylation and serotonergic measures in a group of psychiatric patients. *Acta Psychiatrica Scandinavica*, **77**, 736-740.

Trimble, M., Chadwick, D., Reynolds, E. and Marsden, C. (1975). L-5-HTP and mood. *The Lancet*, **1**, 583.

Tripathi, B. and Tripathi R. (1974). Vacuolar transcellular channels on a drainage pathway for CSF. *Journal of Physiology (London)*, **239**, 195-206.

Trotter, J.L. and Brooks, B.R. (1980). Pathophysiology of CSF immunoglobulins. *In* "Neurobiology of CSF". (Ed. J.H. Wood). pp. 465-486. Plenum Press, New York.

Trotter J.L. and Rust, R.S. (1989). Human cerebrospinal fluid immunology. *In*

"The Cerebrospinal Fluid". Chapter 8. (Eds R.M. Herndon and R.A. Brumback). Kluwer Academic Publishers, Norwell, M.A.

Trupp, M. (1977). Stylet Injury syndrome. *Journal of the American Medical Association*, **237**, (23) 2524.

Turner, S.M., Beidel, D.C. and Nathan, R.S. (1985). Biological factors in obsessive-compulsive disorders. *Psychiatry Bulletin*, **97**, (3) 430-450.

Tyce, G., Ahlskog, J., Carmichael, S. *et al*. (1989). Catecholamines in CSF, plasma and tissue of autologous transplantation of adrenal medulla to the brain in patients with Parkinson's Disease. *Journal of Laboratory Clinical Medicine*, **114**, 185-192.

Tyrrell, D., Crow, T., Parry, R., Johnstone, E. and Ferrier, I. (1979). Possible virus in schizophrenia and some neurological disorders. *Lancet*, **i**, 839-43.

Tyrrell, D.A.J., Parry, R., Davies, H. *et al*. (1983). Further studies of the cytopathic effect in tissue cultures innoculated with CSF from patients with schizophrenia and other nervous system diseases. *British Journal of Experimental Pathology*, **64**, 445-450.

Udayakumar, M.A., Dinaker, I., Ramanamurthy, P.S., Devasankaraiah, G. and Haranath, P. (1982). Biogenic amine changes in human VCSF during sleep and wakeful states. *Indian Journal of Medical Research*, **75**, 428-434.

Uhl, G.R. (1988). Neuropeptide systems in Parkinson's disease. *In* "Neuropeptides in Psychiatric and Neurological Disorders". Chapter 7. (Ed. C.B. Nemeroff), Johns Hopkins University Press, Baltimore.

Unger, W., Toifl, K., Bohm, M.P. and Bayer, P.M. (1983). Adenylate kinase activity of CSF in CNS disorders. *European Neurology*, **22**, 65-69.

Van den Doel, E.M.H. (1987). Balzac's serous apoplexies. The hesitant acceptance of the discovery of the cerebrospinal fluid by Magendie. *Archives of Neurology*, **44**, (12) 1303-1305.

Van Kammen, D.P. and D.F. Sternberg (1980). Cerebrospinal fluid studies in schizophrenia. *In* "Neurobiology of CSF". (Ed. J.H. Wood). pp. 719-42. Plenum Press, New York.

Van Kammen D.P. and De Lisi, L.E. (1984). The viral hypothesis of schizophrenia: Smoke – But is there fire? – summary. *Psychopharmacology Bulletin*, **20**, (3) 523-24.

Van Kammen, D., Waters, R., Gold, P. *et al*. (1981). Spinal fluid vasopressin, angiotensin I and II, beta endorphin and opioid activity. *In* "Schizophrenia: a Preliminary Evaluation in Biological Psychiatry". (Eds C. Perris, G. Struwe and B. Jansson). pp. 339-344. Elselvier Publishers, North Holland, Amsterdam.

Van Kammen, D.P., Sternberg, D.E., Hare, T.A., Waters, R.N. and Bunney, W.E. (1982). CSF levels of GABA in schizophrenia. *Archives of General Psychiatry*, **39**, 91-97.

Van Kammen D.P., Mann, L.S. *et al*. (1983). Dopamine β-hydroxylase activity and homovanillic acid in spinal fluid of schizophrenics with brain atrophy. *Science*, **220**, 974-977.

Van Kammen, D.P., Mann, L. *et al*. (1984*a*). Spinal fluid monamine metabolites and anti-cytomegalovirus antibodies and brain scan evaluation in schizophrenia. *Psychopharmacology Bulletin*, **20**, (3) 519-521.

Van Kammen, D.P., Mann, L.S., Sternberg, D.E. *et al*. (1984*b*). Cortical atrophy and enlarged ventricles associated with low levels of cerebrospinal fluid monoamine metabolites and dopamine-β-hydroxylase activity in schizophrenia. *In* "Catecholamines: Neuropharmacology and Central Nervous System – Therapeutic Aspects". pp. 167-172.

Van Kammen D.P., Rosen, J., Peters, J. *et al.* (1985a). Are there state-dependent markers in schizophrenia? *Psychopharmacology Bulletin*, **21**, (3) 497-502.

Van Kammen, D.P., Wood, J.H. and Nemeroff, C. B. (1985b). Neuroendocrinology of various hormones in CSF. *Progress in Neuropsychopharmacology and Biological Psychiatry*, **9**, 53-54.

Van Kammen, D.P., Peters, J. *et al.* (1986a). Cerebrospinal fluid studies of monoamine metabolism in schizophrenia. *Psychiatric Clinics of North America*, **9**, (1) 81-97.

Van Kammen, D.P., van Kammen, W.B., Mann, L.S. *et al.* (1986b). Dopamine metabolism in the cerebrospinal fluid of drug-free schizophrenic patients with and without cortical atrophy. *Archives of General Psychiatry*, **43**, (10) 978-983.

Van Kammen, D., Yao, J. and Goetz, K. (1988). Polyunsaturated fatty acids, prostaglardins, and schizophrenia. *Annals of the New York Academy of Science*, **559**, 411-423.

Van Kammen, D.P., Peters, J. *et al.* (1989a). CSF norepinephrine in schizophrenia is elevated prior to relapse after haloperidol withdrawal. *Biological Psychiatry*, **26**, 176-188.

Van Kammen, D.P., Peters, J.L. *et al.* (1989b). Clonidine treatment of schizophrenia: can we predict treatment response? *Psychiatry Research*, **27**, 297-311.

Van Kammen, D.P. and Peters, J. *et al.* (1990). Norepinephrine in acute exacerbations of chronic schizophrenia. Negative symptoms revisited. *Archives of General Psychiatry*, **47**, (2) 161.

Van Nostrand, W.E., Wagner, S.L., Bakker, E. and Roos, R.A.C. (1992a). Alzheimer's disease and heriditary cerebral hemorrhage – dutch type share a decrease in CSF levels of amyloid β-protein precursor. *Annals of Neurology*, **32**, 215-218.

Van Nostrand, W.E. Wagner, S.L., Rodman Shankle, W. *et al.* (1992b). Decreased levels of soluble amyloid β-protein precursor in CSF of live Alzheimer disease patients. *Proceedings of the National Academy of Science*, **89**, 2551-2555.

Van Praag, H. (1979). Central serotonin: its relation to depression vulnerability and depression prophylaxis. *In* "Biological Psychiatry Today". (Eds J. Otiolo, C. Ballus, E. Gonzalez Mondus and J. Pujol). pp. 485-498. Elsevier/North Holland Press, Amsterdam.

Van Praag, H.M. (1980a). Central monoamine metabolism in depression. 1. Serotonin and related compounds. *Comprehensive Psychiatry*, **21**, 30-43.

Van Praag, H.M. (1980b). Central monoamine metabolism in depression. II catecholamines and related compounds. *Comprehensive Psychiatry*, **21**, 44-53.

Van Praag, H.M. (1982). Biochemical and psychopathological predictors of suicidality. *Bibliotheca Psychiatrica*, **162**, 42-60.

Van Praag, H. (1986). Affective disorders and aggression disorders: evidence for a common biological mechanism. *Suicide and Life Threatening Behaviour*, **16**, 21-50.

Van Praag, H.M. and Korf, J. (1975). Neuroleptics, catecholamines and psychoses: a study of their interrelations. *American Journal of Psychiatry*, **132**, (6) 595-597.

Van Praag, H.M., Kahn, R, Asnis, G.M., Lemus, C.Z. and Brown, S.L. (1987). Therapeutic indications for serotonin-potentiating compounds: a hypothesis. *Biological Psychiatry*, **22**, 205-212.

Van Praag, H.M. Asnis, G.M., Kahn, R.S., Brown, S.L., Korn, M., Harkavy, J.M. Friedman, and Wetzler, S. (1990). Nosological tunnel vision in biological psychiatry. A plea for a functional psychopathology. *Annals of the New York Academy of Science,* **600**, 501-509.

Van Tiggelen, C.J., J. P. Peperkamp, and H.J. Tertoolen, (1984). Assessment of vitamin B12 status in CSF. (letter) *American Journal of Psychiatry,* **141**, (1) 136-7.

Van Woert, M.H. and Sethy, V.H. (1975). Therapy of intention myoclonus with L-5-HTP and a peripheral decarboxylase inhibitor, MK 486. *Neurology,* **25**, 135-140.

Van Woert, M., Jutkowitz, R., Rosenbaum, D. and Bowers, M. (1976). Gilles de la Tourette syndrome: biochemical approaches. *In* "The Basal Ganglia". (Ed. M. Yahr). pp. 359-465. Raven Press, New York.

Vandam, L.D. and Dripps, R.D. (1956). Long-term follow-up of patients who received 10,098 spinal anaesthetics. *Journal of the American Medical Association,* **161**, (7) 57-591.

Vandenbark, A., Van Rompaey, F., Nijst, D., Heyligen, H. and Raus, J. (1984). CSF antibodies detect brain antophy. *In* "Gansette and Delmotte". pp. 16-19.

Vanderheyden, J.E., Noel, G. and Mendlewicz, J. (1982). Apport du test probenecid dans le diagnostic et le traitement de la maladie de Parkinson. *Acta Neurologica Belgica,* **82**, 339-352.

Vecsei, L., and Widerlov, E. (1988). Brain and CSF somatostatin concentrations in patients with psychiatric or neurological illness. An overview. *Acta Psychiatrica Scandinavica,* **78**, 657-667.

Vedeler C.A., Matre, R. Nyland, H. (1986). Immunoglobulins in serum and cerebrospinal fluid from patients with acute Guillain-Barré syndrome. *Acta Neurologica Scandinavica,* **73**, 388-393.

Verbanck, P.M.P., Lotstra, F., Gilles, C., Linkowski, P., Mendlewicz, J. and Vanderhaeghen, J.J. (1984). Reduced cholecystokinin immunoreactivity in the cerebrospinal fluid of patients with psychiatric disorders. *Life Sciences,* **34**, 67-72.

Verhoeven,W. and Van Praag, H.M. (1982). Endorphins in psychiatric research and treatment. *In* "Endorphins and Opiate Antagonists in Psychiatric Research". (Eds N. Shah and A. Donald). pp. 213-229. Plenum Press, New York.

Vermuyten, K., Lowenthal, A. and Karcher, D. (1990). Detection of neuron specific enolase concentrations in cerebrospinal fluid from patients with neurological disorders by means of a sensitive enzyme immunoassay. *Clinica Chimica Acta,* **187**, 69-78.

Vestergaard, P., Sorensen, T., Hoppe, E., Rafaelson, O., Yates, C.M. and Nicolaou, N. (1978). Biogenic amine metabolites in CSF of patients with affective disorders. *Acta Psychiatrica Scandinavica,* **58**, 88-96.

Vilkov, G.A. *et al.* (1986). Biochemical and ultrastructural changes in animal brain after intracisternal administration of the CSF from patients with schizophrenia. *Voprosy Meditsinskoi Khimii,* **32**, (4) 91-93.

Vilkov, G.A. *et al.* (1987). Biochemical and ultrastructural changes in the brain of the rat exposed to the cerebrospinal fluid of schizophrenics. *Zhurnal*

Neuropatologii Psikhiatrii Imeni. S.S. Korsakova, **87**, (5) 735-738.

Vincent, D., Dubas, F., Hauw, J.J., Godeau, P., Lhermitte, F., Buge, A. and Castaigne, P. (1986). Nerve and muscle microvasculitis in peripheral neuropathy: a remote effect of cancer? *Journal of Neurology, Neurosurgery and Psychiatry,* **49**, 1007-1010.

Virji, M.A., Diven, W.F. and Kelly, R. H. (1985). CSF α-2-macroglobulin and C-reactive protein as aids to rapid diagnosis of acute bacterial meningitis. *Clinica Chimica Acta,* **148**, 31-37.

Virkkunen, M. (1988). CSF: Monoamine metabolites among habitually violent and impulsive offenders. *In* "Biological Contributions to Crime Causation". (Eds T. Moffitt, and S. Medwick). pp. 147-157. Martinus Nijhoff Publishers, Dardrecht.

Virkkunen, M., Nuutila, A., Goodwin, F.K. and Linnoila, M. (1987). CSF monoamine metabolites in male monoamine arsonists. *Archives of General Psychiatry,* **44**, 241-7.

Vivekanandan, S., Kamalakara-Rao, A. Selvam, R. and Kanaka, T.S. (1982). Sequential determinations of CSF lactate dehydroglenase in human brain tumors on treatment. *Acta Neruologica Scandinavica,* **66**, 347-354.

Vogt, M. (1975). Metabolites of cerebral transmitters entering the cerebrospinal fluid; their value as indicators of brain function. *In* "Fluid Environment of the Brain". (Eds H.F. Cserr, J.D. Fenstermacher and V. Fencl). Academic Press, New York.

Volavka, J., Mallya, A., Baig, S. and Perex-Cruet, J. (1977). Naloxone in chronic schizophrenia. *Science,* **196**, 1227-1228.

Von Knorring, L., Almory, B., Johansson, F., Terenuis, L. and Wahlstrom, A. (1982). Circannual variation in concentrations of endorphins in CSF. *Pain,* **12**, (3) 265-272

Von Knorring, L., Terenius, L. and Wahlstrom, A. (1983). Fraction I endorphin in CSF: clinical studies. *In* "Neurobiology of CSF". Vol. 2. (Ed. J.H. Wood). pp. 83-96. Plenum Press, New York.

Waal-Manning, H.J. (1974). Serum dopamine-hydroxylase activity in relatives of a man with autosomal dominant torsion dystonia. *New Zealand Medical Journal,* **79**, 583.

Waddington, J.L. (1989.). Sight and insight: brain dopamine receptor occupancy by neuroleptics visualised in living schizophrenic patients by positron emission tomography. *British Journal of Psychiatry,* **154**, 433-436.

Wagner, J., Vitali, P., Palfreyman, M., Zraiker, M. and Hout, S. (1982). Simultaneous determinations of 3-4-dihydroxyphenylalamine, DA, 3-hydroxy-3-methoxyphylalamine, NE, 3-4, dihydroxyphenylacetic acid, HVA, serotonin, 5-hydroxytryptophan and 5-HIAA, in rat CSF and brain by HPLC with electrochemical detection. *Journal of Neurochemistry,* **38**, 1241-1254.

Wagner, S. (1992). Personal communication (November). The Salk Institute of Biotechnology (SIBIA), La Jolla, CA.

Walker, A.E. (1971). The cerebrospinal fluid from ancient times to the atomic age. *In* "Cerebrospinal Fluid in Health and Disease". (Eds A. Walker and Arana-Inigvez). pp. 1-10. .

Walker, M.D. (1982). Brain and peripheral nervous system tumors. *In* "Cancer Medicine". (Eds J.F. Holland and E. Frei), pp. 1603-1633. Lea and Febiger, Philadelphia.

Walker, R.W. and Thompson, E.J. (1983). The cerebrospinal fluid in subacute sclerosing panencephalitis and multiple sclerosis. *Progress in Brain Research*, **59**, 375-90.

Wall, M. and George, D. (1987). Visual loss in pseudotumour cerebri – Incidence and defects related to visual field strategy. *Archives of Neurology*. **44**, 170-175.

Wallach, J. (1980). Diseases of the central and peripheral nervous system. *In* "Interpretation of Diagnostic Tests". (Ed. J. Wallach). pp. 238-59. Little, Brown and Co., Boston.

Wallen, W.C., Biggar, R.J. Levine., P.H. and Iivanainen, M.U. (1983). Oligoclonal bands in CSF of patients with african Burkett's lymphoma. *Archives of Neurology*, **40**, 13.

Warren, K.G. and Catz, K. (1985). The relationship between levels of cerebrospinal fluid myelin basic protein and IgG measurements in patients with multiple sclerosis. *Annals of Neurology*, **17**, 475-480.

Warren, K.G. and Catz, I. (1986). Diagnostic value of cerebrospinal fluid anti-myelin basic protein in patients with multiple sclerosis. *Annals of Neurology*, **20**, 20-25.

Warren, K.G. and Catz, K. (1987). A correlation between cerebrospinal fluid myelin basic protein and anti-myelin basic protein in multiple sclerosis patients. *Annals of Neurology*, **21**, 183-189.

Warren, K.G. and Catz, I. (1988). Neutralisation of anti-myelin basic protein by cerebrospinal fluid of multiple sclerosis patients in clinical remission. *Journal of of Neurological Science*, **88**, 185-194.

Wasserstrom, W.R., Schwartz, M.K., Fleischer, M. and Posner, J.R. (1981). CSF biochemical markers on CNS tumors: a review. *Annals of Clinical Laboratory Science*, **11**, 239-251.

Watson, S.J., Berger, P.A., Akil, H., Mills, M.J. and Barchas, J.D. (1978). Effects of naloxone on schizophrenia: reduction in hallucinations in a subpopulation of subjects. *Science*, **201**, 73-76.

Waziri, R. (1988). Glycine therapy in schizophrenia. *Biological Psychiatry*, **23**, 209-214.

Weenink H.R. and Bruyn, G.W. (1988). Cryptococcosis. *In* "Handbook of Clinical Neurology". Vol. 8. (Ed A.A. Harris). Elsevier Sci Publishers, B.V.

Wehrenberg, W., McNicol, D., Frantz, A. and Ferin, M. (1980). The effects of serotonin on prolactin and growth hormone concentrations in normal and pituitary stalk-sectioned monkeys. *Endocrinology*, **107**, 1747-1750.

Weinberger, D.R., Berman, K.F. and Illowsky, B.P. (1988). Physiological dysfunction of dorsolateral prefrontal cortex in schizophrenia. III. A new cohort and evidence for a monoaminergic mechanism. *Archives of General Psychiatry*, **45**, (7) 609-615.

Weinstein, M.A., Lederman, R.J., Rothner, A.D., Duchesneau, P.M. and Norman, D. (1978). Internal computed tomography in MS. *Radiology*, **129**, 689-94.

Weir, R.L., Chase, T.N., Ng, L. and Kopin, I.J. (1973). 5-hydroxyindoleacetic acid in spinal fluid: relative contribution from brain and spinal cord. *Brain Research*, **52**, 409-412.

Weisner, B. and Bernhardt, W. (1978). Protein fractions of lumbar, cisternal, and ventricular CSF. *Journal of Neurological Science*, **37**, 205-214.

Weisner, B. and Roethig, H. (1983). The concentration of prealbumin in CSF, indicator of CSF circulation disorders. *European Neurology*, **22**, (2) 96-105.

Weitbrecht, W. and Cramer, H. (1980). Depression of cyclic AMP and cyclic GMP in the CSF of rats after acute administration of ethanol. *Brain Research in Anesthesia*, **200**, 478-480.

Welch, K., (1975a). The principles of physiology of the cerebrospinal fluid in relation to hydrocephalus including normal pressure hydrocephalus. *Advances in Neurology*, **13**, 247-332.

Welch, K., (1975b). The dynamics of the cerebrospinal fluid. *In* "Intracranial Pressure II". (Eds N. Lundberg, U. Ponton and M. Brock). pp. 13-16. Springer-Verlag, New York.

Welch, K.M.A. and Meyer, J.S. (1980). Neurochemical alterations in CSF in cerebral ischemia and stroke. *In* "Neurobiology of CSF". (Ed. J.H. Wood). pp. 325-36. Plenum Press, New York.

Welch, K.M.A., Meyer, J.S. and Chee, A.N.C. (1975). Evidence for disordered cAMP metabolism in patients with cerebral infarction. *European Neurology*, **13**, 144-154.

Welch, K., Chabi, E., Nell, J., Bartosh, K., Chee, A., Mathew, N. and Achar, U. (1976a). Biochemical comparison of migraine and stroke. *Headache*, **16**, 160-167.

Welch, K., Nell, J., Chabi, E., Mathew, N., Neblett, C. and Meyer, J. (1976b). Cyclic nucleotide studies in migraine. (Abst). *Neurology*, **26**, 380-381.

Welch, M.J., Markham, C.H. and Jenden, D.J. (1976c). ACh and Ch in CSF of patients with Parkinson's disease and Huntington's chorea. *Journal of Neurology, Neurosurgery and Psychiatry*, **39**, 367-374.

Wen H.L., Lo, C.W. and Ho, W.K.K. (1983). Met-enkephalin level in the cerebrospinal fluid of schizophrenic patients. *Clinica Chimica Acta*, **128**, 367-371.

Wenzel, D, and Felgenhauer, K. (1976). The development of the blood-CSF barrier after birth. *Neuropediatrics*, **7**, 175-181.

Wester, P., Eriksson, S., Forsell, A., Puu, G. and Adolfsson, R. (1988). Monoamine metabolite concentrations and cholinesterase activities in cerebrospinal fluid of progressive dementia patients: relation to clinical parameters. *Acta Neurologica Scandinavica*, **77**, 12-21.

Weyne, J. and Leusen, I. (1975). Lactate in CSF in relation to brain and blood. *In* "Fluid Environment of the Brain". (Eds H.F. Cserr, J.D. Fenstermacher and V. Fencl). pp. 255-276. Academic Press, New York.

Wheat, L.J., Kohler, R.B. and Tewari, R.P. (1986). Diagnosis of disseminated histoplasmosis by detection of histoplasma capsulation antigenin serum and urine. *New England Journal of Medicine*, **314**, 83-88.

White, R.P., Hagen, A. and Robertson, J. (1983). Prostaglandins in CSF: possible role in cerebrovascular and neurological disease. *In* "Neurobiology of CSF". Vol. 2. (Ed. J.H.Wood). pp. 579-590. Plenum Press, New York.

Widerlov, E. (1988a). The future of neuropeptides in psychiatry and neurology. *In* "Neuropeptides in Psychiatric and Neurological Disorders". Chapter 10. (Ed. C.B. Nemeroff). Johns Hopkins University Press, Baltimore.

Widerlov, E. (1988b). A critical appraisal of CSF monoamine metabolite studies in Schizophrenia. *Annals of the New York Academy of Science*, **537**, 273-91.

Widerlov, E., Lindstrom, L.H., Wahlestedt, C. and Ekman, R. (1988a).

Neuropeptide Y and peptide YY as possible cerebrospinal fluid markers for major depression and schizophrenia, respectively. *Journal of Psychiatric Research,* **22**, (1) 69-79.

Widerlov, E., Bissette, G. and Nemeroff, C.B. (1988*b*). Monoamine metabolites, corticotropin releasing factor and somatostatin as CSF markers in depressed patients. *Journal of Affective Disorders,* **14**, 99-107.

Widerlov, E., Heilig, M. Bjartell, A. and R. Edman, (1991). Involvement of Neuropeptide Y and delta-sleep-inducing peptide in neuropsychiatric illnesses. *In* "Neuropeptides and Psychiatric Disorders". (Ed. C.B. Nemeroff). pp. 225-260. American Psychiatric Press, Washington D.C.

Wiederholt W.C. and Mulder, D.W. (1965). Cerebrospinal fluid findings in the Landry-Guillain-Barré-Strohl syndrome. *Neurology (Minneapolis),* **15**, 184.

Wiesel, J., Rose, D.N., Silver, A.L., Sacks, H.S. and Bernstein, R.H. (1985). Lumbar puncture in asymptomatic late syphilis. An analysis of the benefits and risks. *Archives of Internal Medicine,* **145**, 465-468.

Wilkinson, P. and P. Carlen, (1982). Reversibility of brain and CSF abnormalities in abstient chronic alcoholics. *In* "Brain Neurotransmitters and Hormone". (Eds R. Collu, A. Barbeau, J. Ducharme and G. Tolis). pp. 391-397. Raven Press, New York.

Williams, A., Houff, S., Lees, A. and Calne, D.B. (1979). Oligoclonal banding in the CSF of patients with postencephalitic Parkinsonism. *Journal of Neurology, Neurosurgery and Psychiatry,* 42, 790-792

Williams, H.C., Levine, R.A., Chase, T.N., Lovenberg, W. and Calne, D.B. (1980). CSF hydroxylase cofactor levels in some neurological diseases. *Journal of Neurology, Neurosurgery and Psychiatry,* **43**, 735-738.

Wilske B., Schierz, G., Preac-Mursic, V., von Busch, K., Kuhbeck, R., Pfister, H.W. *et al.* (1986). Intrathecal production of specific antibodies against Borrelia Burgdorfer in patients with lymphocytic meningoradiculitis. (Bannwarth's syndrome) *Journal of Infectious Diseases,* **153**, 304-314.

Windebank A.J., McCall, J.J., Dyck, P.J. (1984). Metal neuropathy. *In* "Peripheral Neuropathy". 2nd Edn. (Eds P.J. Dyck, P.K. Thomas, E.H. Lambert and R. Burge). pp. 2133-61. W. B. Saunders, Philadelphia.

Winfield, J.B., Shaw, M., Silverman, L.M., Eisenberg, R.A., Wilson, H.A. and Koffler, D. (1983). Intrathecal IgG synthesis and blood-brain barrier impairment in patients with systemic lupus erythematosus and central nervous system dysfunction. *American Journal of Medicine,* **74**, 837-844.

Winn, H., Rubio, G. and Berne, R. (1983). Metabolic fate of adenosine in CSF. *In* "Neurobiology of CSF". Vol. 2. (Ed. J.H. Wood). pp. 591-602. Plenum Press, New York.

Winokur, A.(1991). The relevance of thyrotropin-releasing hormone to psychiatric disorders. *In* "Neuropeptides and Psychiatric Disorders". (Ed. C.B. Nemeroff). pp. 13-28. American Psychiatric Press, Washington D.C.

Winsberg, B.G., Sverd, J., Castells, S. *et al.* (1980.). Estimation of monoamine and cAMP turnover and amino acid concentrations of spinal fluid in autistic children. *Neuropediatrics,* **11**, 250-255.

Wisniewski, H.M. and Kozlowski, P.B. (1982). Evidence for blood-brain barrier changes in senile dementia of the Alzheimer type (SDAT). *Annals of the New York Academy of Science,* **396**, 119.

Wolfe, L.S., Marion, J. *et al.* (1975). The biosynthesis of PG's and thromboxanes by nervous tissue. *Advances in Experimental Medicine and Biology*, **83**, 465-467.

Wolfe, N., Katz, D.I., Albert, M.L., Almozlino, A., Durso, R., Smith, M.C. and Volicer, L. (1990). Neuropsychological profile linked to low dopamine in Alzheimer's disease, major depression, and Parkinson's disease. *Journal of Neurology, Neurosurgery and Psychiatry*, **53**, 915-917.

Wolfson, L.I. and Escriva, A. (1976). Clearance of 3-methoxy-4-hydroxyphenyl-glycol for the cerebrospinal fluid. *Neurology*, **26**, 781-784.

Wolfson, L.I., Sharpless, N.S., Thal, L.J., Waltz, J.M. and Shapiro, K. (1983). Decreased ventricular fluid norepinephrine metabolite in childhood-onset dystonia. *Neurology*, **33**, 369-372.

Wolfson, L. Sharples, N. and Thal, L. (1988). Diminished levels of ventricular fluid NE metabolite and somatostatin in childhood-onset dystonia. *Advances in Neurology*, **50**, 177-81.

Wolintz A.H., Jacobs, L.D., Christoff, N., Solomon, M. and Chernik, N. (1969). Serum and cerebrospinal fluid enzymes in cerebrovascular disease. *Archives of Neurology*, **20**, 54-61.

Wolkowitz, O.M., Rubinow, D.R., Breier, A., A.R., Doran, Davis, C. and Pickar, D. (1987). Prednisone decreases CSF somatostatin in healthy humans: implications for neuropsychiatric illness. *Life Sciences*, **41**, 1929-1933.

Wolpow, E.R. (1978). Neurologic Emergencies. *In* "MGH Textbook of Emergency Medicine", (Ed. E.W. Wilkins). pp. 270-300. Williams and Wilkins Co., Baltimore.

Wolstenholme, G. and O'Connor, C. (eds). (1958). "CIBA Symposium on the Cerebrospinal Fluid". Little, Brown, and Co., Boston.

Wolters, E.C. (1986). Lumbar puncture in late syphilis. *Archives of Internal Medicine*, **146**, 408.

Wolters, E.C. Hische, E.A.H., Tutuarima, J.A., van Trotsenburg, L., van Eijk, V.V.W. *et al.* (1988). Central nervous system involvement in early and late syphilis: the problem of asymptomatic neurosyphilis. *Journal of Neurosciences*, **88**, 229-239.

Wong, D.F., Wagner, Jr. H.N., Tune, L.E. *et al.* (1986). Positron emission tomography reveals elevated D_2 dopamine receptors in drug-naive schizophrenics. *Science*, **234**, 1558-9.

Wood, M. and Anderson, M. (1988). "Neurological Infections". Saunders, London.

Wood, J.H. (1980*a*). "Neurobiology of Cerebrospinal Fluid". Vol. 1. Plenum Press, New York.

Wood, J.H. (1980*b*). Neurochemical analysis of cerebrospinal fluid. *Neurology*, **30**, 645-651.

Wood, J.H. (1980*c*). Sites of origin and CSF concentration gradients. *In* "Neurobiology of CSF". Vol. 1. (Ed. J.H. Wood). pp. 53-62. Plenum Press, New York.

Wood, J.H. (1982*a*). Physiological neurochemistry of CSF. *In* "Handbook of Neurochemistry". Vol. 1. (Ed. A. Lajtha). pp. 415-87. Plenum Press, New York.

Wood, J.H. (1982*b*). Neuroendocrinology of cerebrospinal fluid: peptides, steroids and other hormones. *Neurosurgery*, **11**, 293-305.

Wood, J.H (ed.). (1983). "Neurobiology of CSF". Vol. 2. Plenum Press, New York.

Wood, J.H. (1985). Cerebrospinal fluid: techniques of access and analytical interpretation. *In* "Neurosurgery". (Eds. R. Wilkins and S. Rengacharg). McGraw-Hill, New York.

Wood, J.H. and Brooks, B.R. (1980). Neurotransmitter metabolite, and cyclic nucleotide alterations in CSF of seizure patients. *In* "Neurobiology of CSF". (Ed. J.H. Wood). pp. 259-278. Plenum Press, New York.

Wood, J.H., Glaeser, B.S., Enna, S.J. and Hare, T.A. (1978). Verification and quantification of GABA in human CSF. *Journal of Neurological Chemistry,* **30,** 291-293.

Wood, J.H., Hare, T.A., Glaeser, B., Ballenger, J. and Post, R. (1979). Low CSF GABA content in seizure patients. *Neurology,* **29,** 1203-1208.

Wood, P.L., Etienne, P., Lal, S., Gauthier, S., Cajal, S. and Nair, N.P.U. (1982). Reduced lumbar CSF somatostatin levels in Alzheimer's disease. *Life Science,* **31,** 2073-2079.

Woods, C. and Gibbs, J. (1989). The regulation of food intake by peptides. *Annals of the New York Academy of Science,* **575,** 236-243.

Woollam, D.H. (1957). The historical significance of the cerebrospinal fluid. *Medical History,* **1,** 91-113.

Wright, E.M. (1977). Regulation of weak acids and bases in the cerebrospinal fluid. *Journal of Physiology,* **272,** 30-31.

Wright, P.M., Nogueira, G.J. and Levin, E. (1971). Role of the pia matter in the transfer of substances in and out of the cerebrospinal fluid. *Experimental Brain Research,* **13,** 294-305.

Wurster, V., Patzold, U. and Haas, J. (1984). CSF findings in isolated optic neuritis compared to multiple sclerosis. *In* "Gansette and Delmotte". pp. 282-291.

Wurtman, R.J., Larin, F., Mostafapour S. and Fernstrom, J. (1974). Brain catechol synthesis: control by brain tyrosine concentration. *Science,* **3,** 183-184.

Yaksh, T., Carmichael, S. Stoddard, S. *et al,* (1990). Measurement of LCSF of met-enkephalin, encripted met-enkephalin and neuropeptide Y in normal patients and in patients with Parkinson's Disease before, and after autologous transplantation of adrenal medulla into the Caudate nucleus. *Journal of Laboratory and Clinical Medicine,* 115, 346-351.

Yatsu, F.M. (1975). Lipid disorders of the nervous system. *In* "Biochemistry of Neural Disease". (Ed. M. Cohen). pp. 79-140, Harper and Row, Hagerstown, Maryland.

Yergey, J.A., Karanian, J.W., Salem, N., Heyes, M.P., Ravitz, B. and Linnoila, M. (1989). Prostaglandins in cerebrospinal fluid of healthy human volunteers, abstinent alcoholics and rhesus monkeys. *Prostaglandins,* **37,** (4), 505-513.

Yesavage, J.A., Holmon, C.A. and Berger, P.A. (1982). CSF lactate levels and aging: findings in normals and patients with major depressive disorders. *Gerontology,* **28,** (6), 377-380.

Young, J., Cohen, D., Kavanagh, M. *et al.* (1981). CSF, plasma and urinary MHPG in children. *Life Sciences,* **28,** 2837-45.

Young, J.G., Leven, L.I., Newcorn, J.H. and Knott, P.J. (1987). Genetic and neurobiological approaches to the pathophysiology of autism and the pervasive developmental disorders. *In* "Psychopharmacology: The Third Generation of Progress". (Ed. Herbert Y. Meltzer). pp. 825-836 . Raven Press, New York.

Young, S., Garelis, E., Lal, S., Martin, J., Molina-Negro, P., Ethier, R. and Sourkes, T. (1974). Tryptophan and 5-HIAA in human CSF. *Journal of*

Neurochemistry, **22,** 777-779.

Young, D.A. and Burney, R.E. (1971). Complications of myelography-transsection and withdrawal of a nerve filament by the needle. *New England Journal of Medicine,* **285,** (3) 156-7.

Zacarias, J., Harum, A. and Brinck, P. (1971). Glutamine values in cerebrospinal fluid of children: some observations on clinical application. *Journal of Pediatrics,* **78,** 318-321.

Zarcone, V., Schreier, L., Barchas, J., Orenberg E. and Benson, K. (1977). Alcohol, sleep and CSF changes in alcoholics: cyclic AMP and biogenic amine metabolites in CSF. *Advances in Experimental Medicine and Biology,* **85A,** 593-599.

Zeeberg, B.R., Gibson, R.E. and Reba, R.C. (1988). Elevated D2 dopamine receptors in drug-naive schizophrenics. *Reports,* Feb. 789.

Ziegler, M.G. and Lake, C.R. (eds.). (1984). "Norepinephrine". Williams and Wilkins, Baltimore.

Ziegler, M.G., Lake, C.R., Foppen, F.H., Shoulson, I. and Kopin, I.J. (1976). Norepinephrine in CSF. *Brain Research,* **108,** 436-440.

Ziegler, M., Lake, C., Wood, J., Brooks, B. and Ebert, M. (1977a). Relationship between norepinephrine in blood and CSF in the presence of a blood-CSF barrier for norepinephrine. *Journal of Neurochemistry,* **28,** 677-679.

Ziegler, M.G., Wood, J.H., Lake, C.R. and Kopin, I.J. (1977b). Norepinephrine and MHPG gradients in human CSF. *American Journal of Psychiatry,* **134,** 565-568.

Ziegler, M.G., Lake, C., Wood, J. and Ebert, M.H. (1980). Norepinephrine in CSF: basic studies, effects of drugs and disease. *In* "Neurobiology of CSF". (Ed. J.H. Wood). pp. 141-152. Plenum Press, New York.

Zimmer, J.R., Cramer, H., Athen, D. and Bechmann, H. (1982). Changes in CSF cyclic nucleotides in alcohol-dependant patients suffering from delirium tremens. *Biological Psychiatry,* **17,** 837-843.

Zimmer, R., Teelken, A.W., Trieling, W.B., Weber, W., Weihmayr, T. and Lauter, H. (1984). Gamma-aminobutyric acid and homovanillic acid concentration in the CSF of patients with senile dementia of Alzheimer's type. *Archives of Neurology,* **41,** (6) 602-4.

Zohar, J., Biederman, J., Rimon, R., Ebstein, R. and Belmaker, R.H. (1978). Clinical correlates of CSF cyclic nucleotides in schizophrenia. *American Journal of Psychiatry,* **35,** 253-255.

Zwibel, II.L. and Schwartzman, R.J. (1974). Evaluation of the nitroblue tetrazoline test as applied to PMN leukocytes in the CSF, *Neurology,* 995-998.

Zvaifler, N.J. and Bluestein, H.G. (1982). The pathogenesis of central nervous system manifestations of systemic lupus erythematosus, *Arthritis Rheumatology,* **25,** 862-866.

Index